# GERIATRIC
# NUTRITION

# GERIATRIC
# NUTRITION

Daphne A. Roe

Division of Nutritional Sciences
Cornell University

PRENTICE-HALL, INC.
Englewood Cliffs, New Jersey 07632

*Library of Congress Cataloging in Publication Data*

Roe, Daphne A.
   Geriatric nutrition.
   Includes bibliographies and index.
    1. Aged—Nutrition. 2. Geriatrics.
I. Title. [DNLM: 1. Nutrition—In old age.
WT 100 R698G]
TX361.A3R63   1983   613.2'0880565   82-13298
ISBN 0-13-354035-9

©1983 by Prentice-Hall, Inc., Englewood Cliffs, N.J. 07632

Printed in the United States of America

10 9 8 7 6 5 4 3 2 1

Editorial/production supervision and design by Virginia Rubens
Cover design by Wanda Lubelska
Manufacturing buyer: Harry P. Baisley

0-13-354035-9

PRENTICE-HALL INTERNATIONAL,INC., *London*
PRENTICE-HALL OF AUSTRALIA PTY. LIMITED, *Sidney*
EDITORA PRENTICE-HALL DO BRASIL, LTDA., *Rio de Janeiro*
PRENTICE-HALL CANADA INC., *Toronto*
PRENTICE-HALL OF INDIA PRIVATE LIMITED, *New Delhi*
PRENTICE-HALL OF JAPAN, INC., *Tokyo*
PRENTICE-HALL OF SOUTHEAST ASIA PTE. LTD., *Singapore*
WHITEHALL BOOKS LIMITED, WELLINGTON, *New Zealand*

# Contents

## CHAPTER THREE
### The Nutritional Status of the Elderly

**56**

## CHAPTER FOUR
### Nutritional Requirements

**64**

## CHAPTER FIVE
### Factors Determining Food Intake

**75**

## CHAPTER SIX
### Assessment of Nutritional Status

**87**

## CHAPTER SEVEN
## Nutritional Deficiencies                                                                    **119**

## CHAPTER EIGHT
## Diseases Which Respond to Diet Modification                                    **141**

## CHAPTER NINE
## Drugs and Nutrition in the Elderly                                                  **155**

## CHAPTER TEN
Nutrition Services    **174**

cussed, including federal guidelines and evaluation to determine whether the programs meet the economic, social, and medical needs of recipients. Federal and state standards for dietary services in nursing homes and domiciliary care facilities are explained. The role of the nutritionist or dietitian in developing, implementing, and evaluating the nutrition component of patient care plans in geriatric institutions is discussed.

Readers are encouraged to test their knowledge of geriatric nutrition by answering the test questions at the end of each chapter. Chapter references are supplemented by additional reading suggestions in the Resource Materials section at the end of the book.

It is my hope that this book will encourage young nutritionists to specialize in geriatric nutrition, where their expertise is so much needed.

# Preface

This book is a basic text on geriatric nutrition. Intended primarily for a course on this subject in a senior undergraduate or graduate nutrition curriculum, it will also serve as a reference book for health professionals working with elderly people.

The need for a textbook on geriatric nutrition accompanies the broader current commitment to geriatrics that has resulted from the steadily increasing percentage of our population over 65 years of age. Health care for the elderly is no longer limited to the treatment of disease, but includes community nutrition programs aimed at enhancing the quality of life of older people and reducing the burden of their care which otherwise would reside with families and institutions.

In this book, the student of nutrition will be familiarized with the effects aging, particularly as they change food habits, alter digestive processes, decrease nutrient utilization. Causes of nutrient overload and nutritional deficiency are described. Nutritional assessment of elderly people is explained together with precautions that must be taken in interpreting findings.

Geriatric nutrition is a major responsibility of nutritionists working in community as well as in hospitals and extended care facilities. Prevention goals which are addressed in the book include avoidance of obesity, sodium overload, and deficiency states, whether these are caused by diet, disease drugs. Goals and strategies of nutrition counselling for the elderly are considered. Specific diet therapy is described for chronic disease patients Title VII and Title III community feeding programs for the elderly a

# Acknowledgments

First I want to acknowledge my graduate students, past and present, with whom I have learned about the nutrition of the elderly. My special thanks go to Bonnie Liebman, who studied the factors determining the nutritional status of nursing home patients; Susan Weinberg, who is presently investigating the food habits of very independent, active elderly women; Olha Shevchuk and Ellen Levine, who want to know whether age affects vitamin requirements; Karen Kinsell, who is interested in the specificity of clinical signs suggesting malnutrition in geriatric patients; and Jennifer Carl, who examined shopping lists to find out about the eating habits of housebound elderly people.

I would like to thank Susan Bogusz, who has helped me to select and analyze sample diets which are discussed and recommended in this book.

Among my colleagues I am particularly grateful to Professor Ruth Klippstein for information on the Title III program, and to Joan Koch for an update on dietetic services in skilled nursing homes.

I am most pleased to thank Mr. Mark Zwerger, administrator of Ithacare, a domiciliary care facility, who has enabled me and my students to see a center of excellence in geriatric care.

I have greatly enjoyed working with Marion Van Soest, who has illustrated this book. She assisted me in selecting photographs to show how elderly people, with and without disabilities, live, feed themselves, or are assisted in getting nourishment.

My secretary, Beverly Hastings, has given me inestimable help and encouragement by reading my writing, by transcribing my tapes, by typing and correcting the manuscript, by assisting me in checking references, and by reading proof.

Finally and most of all, I want to thank my husband, Shad (Albert Roe). His support and encouragement have enabled me to write this book while sitting at my own dining table where the light is good enough for me to see the pages.

# CHAPTER ONE
# The Elderly
# In Our Society

In the United States about 11 percent of the population is over 65 years of age. It is estimated that by the year 2030, 20 percent of the population will be over the age of 65 (Kane, 1980).

This change in the age structure of the population can be attributed to a recent decline in the fertility rate and a long-term decline in the mortality rate. The decline in the mortality rate is due to improved means of combating disease in middle-aged and older people. Because of the growing number of older people in our society, more and more scholarly papers, health programs, and popular books discuss what to do with the elderly, where they should be housed, and what they should be fed.

"Getting old" is a derogatory term suggesting that a person can no longer function efficiently, that thought processes are slowed down, or that senility is imminent. The expressed or implied goals of programs for the elderly are to create unequal opportunities in the workplace, to segregate them in living situations, to offer them an inferior social position, to deny them decision-making roles in community policy-making, and to provide them with health and nutrition programs which deny them freedom to choose their own facility, physician, or food. The elderly in our society are you, I, and the next person grown older. Demographically, the elderly are heterogeneous. They vary in age, sex, marital status, education, job skills, work experience, social background, living situation, and health (Shanas, 1974). Variability in the health status of the elderly has been attributed to the presence or absence of health-seeking behavior earlier in life. We assume (without very good evidence) that the healthy elderly have had "healthy" eating patterns throughout

1

life and have maintained the nutritional quality of their diets. Likewise, we assume that the unhealthy elderly have indulged in self-abusive behaviors like smoking, alcohol abuse, overeating, consuming an excessive amount of sodium, cholesterol, fat or sugar, and leading a sedentary life. We have not, however, identified many of the factors which contribute to good physical and mental health in later years. In the present state of knowledge, it appears that "biological intactness," the ability to function well to an advanced age, is the outcome of life advantages, including:

1. *Genetic potential for extended longevity.* Stated differently, this means that the individual has inherited characteristics which confer protection from, or lack of susceptibility to, degenerative diseases.

2. *Intelligence.* Highly intelligent people tend to retain their capacity for productive intellectual pursuits longer.

3. *Motivation.* Individuals who believe they can shape their own destiny and plan their own lives can resist societal pressures to play a passive role in later life.

4. *Curiosity.* The continued desire for new knowledge and new experience means that as a person grows older, he or she can find new and challenging occupations and activities.

5. *Socialization.* Older people who maintain an active role in local affairs find they are still indispensable. Senior citizens' groups foster this idea.

6. *Religious belief.* Religious conviction, with or without external observation, allows celebration of life and reduces fear of death.

7. *Responsibility.* Elderly people function well when they have responsibility for the care of others, including other elderly and young children.

8. *Family integrity.* Older people thrive in situations where family bonds are strong. The traditional responsibility of the family is to take care of their own membership. Older people function best in a family atmosphere in which love, understanding, respect, and sharing of household duties are combined to give meaning to life.

9. *Intimacy.* Marriage or sustained intimate friendships based on love and mutual understanding not only bring joy. The partners also accept responsibility for each other's welfare. When two older people live together, keeping up personal appearance, organization of the daily routine, cooking of nutritious meals, and sharing of experiences are common benefits which have positive impact on health and social functioning.

10. *Prudent diet.* Adherence to a prudent diet with avoidance of dietary excesses of food-energy, fat, cholesterol, and sodium diminishes the risk of killer diseases such as atherosclerotic vascular disease, essential hypertension, and maturity-onset diabetes. Complications of these diseases such as angina, late effects of stroke, and diabetic gangrene with amputation restrict the mobility of the elderly inside and outside the home. For the prudent diet to have a protective effect against these diseases and their complications, it is assumed that the elderly individual has followed such a dietary pattern throughout adult life or, better still, since childhood.

11. *Slimness.* In addition to increasing the agility of the elderly, slimness is associated with dietary moderation, which lowers the risk of hypertension, maturity-onset diabetes, and the disabling symptoms of osteoarthritis.

12. *Avoidance of substance abuse.* Nonsmokers who have never smoked heavily or who stopped smoking in early middle life have a substantially reduced risk of chronic disease including bronchitis and emphysema, lung cancer and heart attacks. Lifelong nonsmokers and ex-smokers tend to be more health conscious than smokers and follow general guidelines for health maintenance. Moderate drinkers and abstainers avoid alcohol-related disease.

    Avoidance of over-the-counter self-medication and prescription drugs other than with specific indication reduces the risk of adverse drug reactions including drug-induced nutritional deficiencies.

13. *Community health care.* Elderly people who are willing and able to make optimal use of community health services are better able to lead independent lives and avoid institutionalization. The type of people who make use of these services tend to have more support available within the community setting from their family members or friends and are less impaired in the areas of mental health and social resources (Smyer, 1980).

    Community health personnel necessary to the elderly include: a family physician who knows and cares about his or her older patients; a health clinic which provides a broad range of medical, dental, and ancillary services without financial barriers on the elderly; an efficiently organized public health nursing service which can provide health care to the elderly in their own homes; a podiatrist to supply care for the feet of the elderly; a dentist who has special knowledge of the dental needs of the elderly, including servicing of dentures; a physical therapist who can instruct elderly persons in exercise to promote mobility and offer advice on the purchase and use of special cooking appliances for the elderly disabled; a pharmacist who can interpret prescriptions; and a community nutritionist who can give guidance on the selection and preparation of foods to meet nutritional needs and comply with special diets.

14. *Living arrangements.* Housing for the elderly in an urban setting is most successful in low-level apartment complexes providing units for one or two persons. Each apartment unit should be designed to allow tenants to prepare their own food, and a ground floor congregate meal center would provide tenants with a main meal on weekdays. The facility should be within walking distance of food markets, or bus service could be provided for elderly people of limited mobility. Provision of low income housing for the elderly is the responsibility of all urban communities. In rural areas, housing for the elderly may be arranged as grouped cottage homes. Housing units for the elderly in urban and rural areas should be served both by a public health nurse and by community nutritionists who can define and address the health and nutritional needs of residents. It should be emphasized that better housing for the elderly is often with younger people, preferably family, and that the best housing for vigorous elderly people is in their own established homes, with or without a spouse or companion.

15. *Financial independence.* Elderly people are better able to live comfortably in their community if they have financial resources. These may include salary for part- or full-time work, business profits, money earned from the sale of handicrafts, earned income from services rendered including provision of day-care for others, pensions, savings, unearned income from investments, or money earned through the sale of personal property. Poverty restricts the choice of housing. Unless community, low-income housing for the elderly is provided, the elderly poor will often live in ill-lit, cold, or poorly ventilated single rooms having dangerous or inadequate facilities for cooking. Economic stability

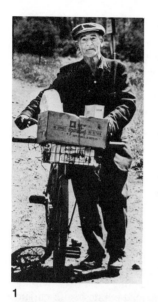
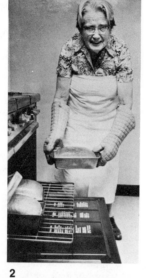

1          2

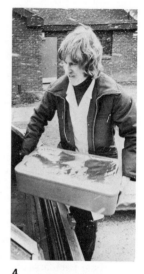

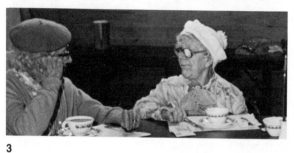

3          4

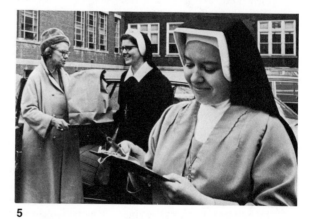

5

FIGURE 1-1    Life Settings of the Elderly

Ability to function well into old age stems from life advantages conferred by good health, motivation to enjoy life, strong social ties, genetic potential for extended longevity, and a prudent diet.

1.    The vigorous man with his bicycle gets good exercise bringing home the groceries.

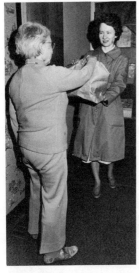

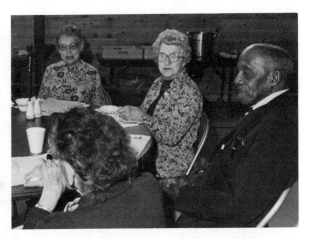

6

7

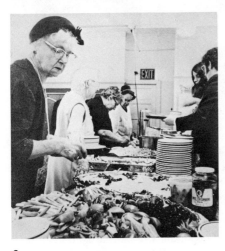

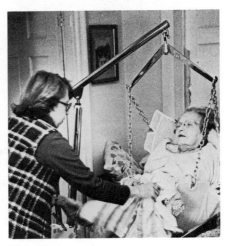

8

9

2. Baking is a pleasure for the lady who cooks for others as well as for herself.

3. Mealtimes for older people are especially pleasurable in a social setting.

4-8. Meal programs for the elderly foster independent living, especially for the disabled or those on meager budgets. Title III provides hot meals in a friendly congregate setting. Hot meals and evening snacks for the homebound are delivered under Title III and Meals-on-Wheels programs.

9. The severely disabled can live at home if there is family commitment, home help, and some aid to mobility.
Independent people who have lost a living companion often choose a domiciliary care facility for relief from loneliness and housekeeping chores.

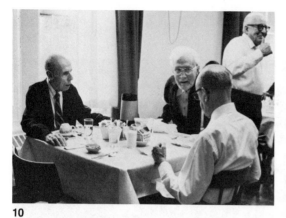

10

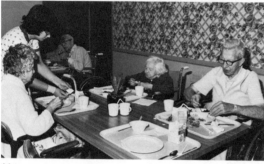

11

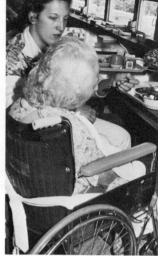

12

**Figure 1-1 (cont.)**

10. The lively men exchanging news at lunchtime obviously still enjoy life.
11. Nursing home patients sometimes lose interest in one another, and meals taken together do not necessarily involve intimacy.
12. Human warmth and a nutritious diet are assured through dedicated nursing and dietary services.

allows a greater choice of foods and an opportunity to purchase different foods of high nutrient value. Financial independence allows an elderly person to obtain domestic help to purchase food and prepare meals, thus freeing the elderly individual from those household chores—an advantage to those who find meal preparation a burden. Financial independence allows elderly people in the U.S. to obtain optimal health care.

The ability of the elderly to lead independent lives is reduced or lost in the following cases:

1. When severe chronic physical illness with permanent disability is present.
2. When the individual is an older, mentally retarded person.
3. When schizophrenia has begun in old age (paraphrenia) with development of a chronic delusional state and disorganized thought process.
4. When paranoid psychosis exists such that the patient is self-abusive or may inflict injury on others.

5. When Korsakoff's psychosis is present—an organic brain syndrome which occurs in chronic alcoholics who are thiamin deficient, leading to disorientation and confusion.
6. When depressive illness is present which does not lift in response to antidepressant drugs. Depressive illness may be due to manic-depressive psychosis or neurosis. The depressed elderly may stop eating.
7. When Alzheimer's disease or other presenile or senile dementia has impaired the ability to fulfill the activities of daily living.
8. When skid row alcoholism has led to eviction or imprisonment.
9. When sight is lost and the individual has adjusted poorly to blindness.
10. When family support and care are not forthcoming.

Major determinants of life setting for the elderly are as follows:

1. Age
2. Motivation
3. Education
4. Job skills
5. Job availability
6. Family support
7. Presence or absence of disabling physical illness
8. Dementia
9. Antisocial tendencies
10. Ability to carry out activities of daily living (ADL)

These determinants are illustrated in Figure 1-2.

Comparative studies of old people have shown that in industrialized societies there is a wide range of physical capacity and functional ability which is independent of culture. In each of several countries studied including the United States, Britain, Denmark, Israel, Poland and Yugoslavia, from 2–4 percent of the elderly are bedridden. The number of elderly people who are housebound varies from 12–24 percent. Four–8 percent of old people living at home and not bedridden need help with simple physical tasks. About 75 percent of the elderly are ambulatory or report only minimal impairment of ability for performance of tasks related to daily living. One quarter of the elderly are in need of medical care and other supportive services in their own homes (Kane and Kane, 1980).

The institutionalized elderly have less support available from community services (including nutritional services) and from family members and friends. They are more impaired in their access to mental health and social resources and are more likely to have had previous need of support or placement. The implications are that expansion of home-care services would reduce the number of elderly in institutions, while mobility and the capacity to live independently is determined by physical, mental, and emotional health.

While health, nutrition, and social services share the goal of helping elderly people remain in the community as long as possible, excessive control

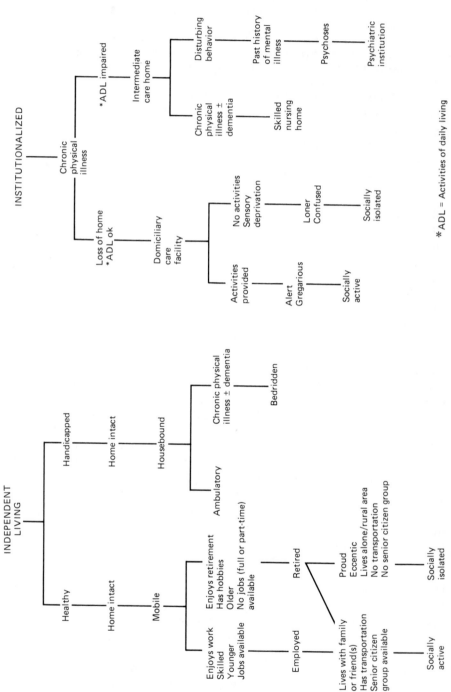

**FIGURE 1-2  Determinants of life setting for the elderly.**

*ADL = Activities of daily living

over the lives of elderly individuals is unacceptable. The problems of elderly people are both medical and social. These problems cannot be solved by providing more nursing homes and clinics or by more efficient placement of the elderly. Health, nutritional and social services should, as far as possible, allow the elderly to make decisions for themselves as to health, nutrition and housing. Even where independent living is no longer feasible and a move to a nursing home is a must, personnel in these geriatric institutions (including dietary service staff) should not make the elderly eat food, play games, or follow routines set up for the convenience of the staff.

Better nutrition for elderly people, whether they live in the community or reside in institutions, requires knowledge of their nutritional needs and wants, as well as provision of food and food services designed to meet their physical, emotional, social, and economic needs.

## QUESTIONS

*Circle letter opposite to all correct answers.*

1. Constraints on independent living for the elderly include
   a) lack of community health care
   b) chronic physical illness with disability
   c) paranoid psychosis
   d) dementia
   e) mental retardation

2. What percent of the elderly are ambulatory?
   a) 25
   b) 25–50
   c) 75

3. The percent of the elderly in industrial societies who are bedridden is
   a) 2–4
   b) 5–10
   c) 10
   d) 20

4. The percentage of elderly in institutions would be decreased by
   a) home visits by a doctor
   b) the expansion of home health care services
   c) the provision of more home delivered meals

5. Attach the correct adjective to these groups of elderly

   | Groups | | Adjectives | |
   |---|---|---|---|
   | i. | institutionalized (in psychiatric institution) | a) | psychotic |
   | | | b) | blind |
   | ii. | housebound (with care at home) | c) | employed |
   | iii. | independently living | d) | healthy |
   | | | e) | physically handicapped |
   | | | f) | homeless |

## REFERENCES

KANE, R.L., and R.A. KANE,  "Long-term care: Can our society meet the needs of its elderly?" *Ann. Rev. Public Health,* 1 (1980), 227–53.

MUIR GRAY, J.A.,  "Do we care too much for our elders?" *Lancet,* 1 (1980), 1289.

*Psychopathology of Aging,* ed. O.J. Kaplan. London and New York: Academic Press, 1979.

SHANAS, E.,  "Health status of older people. Cross-national implications," *Amer. J. Public Health,* 64 (1974), 261–64.

SMYER, M.A.,  "The differential usage of services by impaired elderly," *J. Gerontol.,* 35 (1980), 249–55.

# CHAPTER TWO
# The Physiology
# and Pathology of Aging

## THE AGING PROCESS

It is presently believed that aging is a dual process of progressively impaired self-protection and increased self-destruction (Butler, 1979). Aging is inherent and genetically determined such that within species and between species there is a variability in the time frame of the process. Impaired self-protection is due both to immunodeficiency and loss of chemical protector mechanisms. The self-destruction of cells also occurs because the immune system is deranged and because the reparative functions of cells are lost. Changes in immune function, somatic mutation, hormonal insufficiency, irreversible changes in structural proteins, acquired metabolic error and free radical lipid peroxidation reactions all contribute to aging. The senescence of tissues and organ systems is associated with the loss of cells and a decline in function (Mauderly, 1979).

The rate of the aging process is influenced by the physical and chemical environment. For example, exposure to sunlight ages the skin (Lavker, 1979). Aging within certain organs, such as the pancreas, is increased by chronic intake of food energy beyond the body's needs (Gerritsen, 1976; Andres, 1972). Aging of the lungs is more rapid in smokers (Barnett, 1972). The rate of aging varies between individuals so that at specific ages, different people show different degrees of aging as well as differences in aging between tissues and organ systems.

Pathological changes occur as a result of secondary disease of the elderly, and these may also affect the rate of aging. All components of the aging process are moderated by nutritional factors. Secondary diseases of the elderly can also be prevented or favorably influenced by diet.

## Genetic Components of Aging

The expected duration of life is dependent upon genetic and acquired factors. It is generally accepted that the life span of a warm-blooded animal, including the human, is predestined. Thus the expected life span of a man or woman is about 70 years, whereas the expected life span of a mouse is about two years. It is the predestined component of the prediction of survival which is genetically determined (Hayflick, 1979). Survival at the cellular level implies regenerative activity. The regeneration of cells requires that the genetic material of a cell retain the formula of how to make a cell of the same type as itself. The formula for cell replication is contained in DNA molecules, which must be faithfully duplicated for new cells to be produced having the characteristics of their predecessors. Accurate replication of DNA requires a constant surveillance due to the presence in the cell of repair enzymes (DNA polymerases).

Whereas a low level of DNA error is a condition of life and accounts for evolutionary change, failure to repair DNA is a condition of death. It means either that abnormal cells will be produced and retained, giving rise to cancer, or that the abnormality of the cell is "recognized" by the cellular immune system and deleted.

Aging may result from an accumulation of DNA damage due to a progressive failure of DNA repair. Support for this hypothesis rests in part on the finding that in a rare genetic disease, progeria, which is characterized by premature aging, fibroblasts cannot repair DNA damage induced by ionizing radiation. It has been suggested that in this disease a repair enzyme is missing (Martin, Sprague, and Epstein, 1970). It seems that in normal aging, the DNA repair mechanism may become progressively less efficient and that the rate of decline of DNA repair is genetically determined, leading to different periods of survival. Other genetic determinants of aging reside in the immune system and also in the mixed-function oxidase system, which is responsible for the metabolism of foreign compounds. The ability of cells to activate environmental chemicals to produce cell-damaging metabolites, and the ability of cells to detoxify foreign compounds is related inversely to life span (O'Malley et al., 1971; Vestal, 1980).

## Aging and Immune Function

The efficiency of immune function decreases with age. There are both decreases in immune response and inappropriate responses. Aging is not a passive wearing out of tissue, but rather an active process which is mediated by the immune system. The number of cells responding to antigenic stimulation decreases, and there is also a decline in activity of antigen-stimulated cells. Cellular immune function, rather than humoral immunity, is affected by the aging changes (Makinodan and Adler, 1975; Matzner et al., 1979)

There is also a decreased ability for the body to distinguish self (normal cells) from nonself (foreign or abnormal cells) which is expressed in a destructive process directed or aimed towards cells which are normal components of tissues. Signs of cellular self-destruction, called autoimmune manifestations, are analogous to chronic graft versus host reactions which occur when foreign tissues are introduced into the body. In the adult, prior to aging, potentially autoreactive cell lines (lymphocytic clones) are maintained in a quiescent state by homeostatic mechanisms. With aging, these homeostatic mechanisms are lost (Weksler et al., 1979).

## Change in Hormone Responsiveness

Hormone function requires prior attachment of hormones to specific receptor sites located within cells or on the plasma membrane. Receptors are functionally linked to enzyme systems which mediate hormonal activity. Hormones become reversibly bound to specific receptors forming hormone-receptor complexes. $H + R \rightleftharpoons HR$, where H is the concentration of free hormone, R the concentration of the receptors, and HR the concentration of the hormone-receptor complex. The binding affinity of the receptor may vary with the occupancy of receptor sites by the hormone. Receptor concentration (R) and affinity is influenced by genetic factors, by growth, age and aging, as well as by disease states including "insulin resistant" diabetes.

Altered hormonal responsiveness which occurs with advancing age is related mainly to a change in the concentration of hormone receptors (R). Receptor concentrations decline in many organs and tissues as age advances. Age-related changes in the concentration of hormone receptors (R), and hence, hormone-receptor complexes (HR) vary with hormone, with organ, and ultimately with physiological need for survival.

Decreased receptor concentration is associated with hormone resistance and lack of adaptability to hormone concentration (Gregerman and Bierman, 1974).

## Free Radical Lipid Peroxidation Reactions

Oxidative damage can be induced by oxygen, ozone, hydrogen peroxide, or other environmental oxidants. Cells of the body are normally protected against oxidative damage.

In the process of cellular and membrane aging, lipid peroxidation plays a significant role. Lipid peroxidation involves the formation of semistable peroxides from free radical intermediates by reaction of oxygen and unsaturated lipid. Further reactions occur with the formation of peroxy-, alkoxy-, and hydroxy-free radicals which cause cell damage even in low concentration.

Lipid peroxidation damage occurs mainly in the membranes of subcellular organelles including microsomal, mitochondrial membranes which contain large amounts of polyunsaturated fatty acids. These membranes are key sites for lipid peroxidation because they contain, or are in proximity to, powerful catalysts of the reaction. Fluorescent products of lipid peroxidation which occur in aging cells are ceroid and lipofucsin. Sources of oxidants which trigger lipid peroxidation are contained in the atmosphere and in foreign compounds within the chemical environment.

Free radicals which are generated in lipid peroxidation are important in the development of degenerative diseases associated with aging.

Biological protector systems which prevent oxidant damage to cells include peroxidases and antioxidants. In the membrane portions of cells the antioxidant function of vitamin E is to protect against lipid peroxidation. Within the cytosol and the mitochondria, the selenium-glutathione peroxidase complex can prevent or minimize oxidative damage.

Tissues most vulnerable to damage through free radical lipid peroxidation are the lungs, heart, and brain (Slater, 1972).

### Aging of Connective Tissue

Fibrous elements of connective tissue, including collagen and elastin, undergo qualitative and quantitative changes in the process of biological aging. The relative amounts of different types of collagen in connective tissue are altered. There are also changes in collagen turnover (Chvapil and Hvuza, 1959).

While, in adults, most body collagen is stable, a fraction of the body collagen is continually degraded and replaced. With aging, less of this collagen is degraded and less is synthesized. Changes in cross-linking of collagen occur with aging, but it is not clear that these changes are an integral part of the aging process.

Elastin is a connective tissue component which consists of microfibrils surrounding a nonfibrillar core. In elastogenesis, the microfibrils are formed before the aggregation about the core takes place. With aging, at least in the connective tissue of the skin, there is an increased microfibril formation which may either represent an attempt to replace old elastin with new material or may signify that in older connective tissue there is a loss in functional capacity to produce mature elastin.

There is a progressive loss of elastic recovery of skin after compression stress. Evidence points to changes in the ground substance of the skin as being responsible for the observed change in the mechanical properties of the skin rather than change in the fibrillar components (Daly and Odland, 1979; Prokop et al., 1979).

## Relative Effect of Genetic and Acquired Factors in the Aging Process

The term aging is used to denote irreversible changes in the tissues which develop with time. Implications of the time element are not only that tissues show a progressive loss of repair mechanisms, which is in part genetically determined, but also that tissue changes result from chronic environmental exposure to physical or chemical agents which are damaging. Whether diet can affect molecular changes of aging is not clear. The thermal contractility of tail collagen from rats, maintained on calorie-restricted diets, has been reported to show the characteristics of tail collagen from younger animals on an unrestricted diet (Porta, 1980).

Aging of the skin is highly influenced by ultraviolet light exposure. Persons who develop premature changes of aging in the skin may have genetically determined disorders of DNA repair (Montagna and Carlisle, 1979).

Similarly, aging of other tissues is highly influenced by exposure to environmental toxicants. Aging of the lungs is promoted by air pollutants which cause oxidative damage (Barnett, 1972). Aging of bone leading to osteoporosis is influenced by the toxic effects of chronic alcohol abuse (Albanese et al., 1975). Aging of different tissues occurs at different rates, the time frame of aging in any one tissue being dependent on exposure of that tissue to an environmental damage.

Relationships of aging in different tissues to genetic influences and to the chemical environment are shown in Figure 2-1.

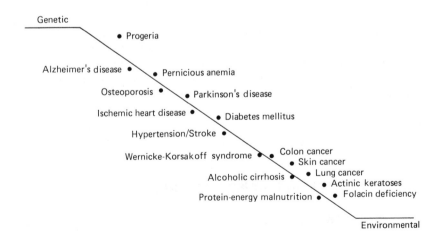

**FIGURE 2-1   Genetic and environmental determinants of geriatric diseases.**

### Cellular Aging

Cellular aging can be studied in human cells which have a short life span and which are easily accessible, such as red blood cells (Ganzoni et al., 1971). They are produced and undergo maturation in the bone marrow. The process of maturation actually is a process of aging in that the cell loses its capability for reproduction by expulsion of the nucleus from the precursor cell, which is called a normoblast. The cell which is the intermediate between the normoblast and the mature red cell (erythrocyte) is the reticulocyte. When the change takes place in which the reticulocyte turns into a mature red cell, intracellular organelles are lost. Reticulocytes retain capability for protein synthesis because they contain the necessary machinery including polyribosomes, messenger RNA, transfer RNA, and the required enzymes for protein synthesis. Protein synthetic activity is important in the reticulocyte but this activity is lost in the red blood cell. Similarly, the reticulocyte contains mitochondria which allow a high rate of oxygen consumption by the reticulocyte. Mitochondria are lost when the reticulocyte becomes a red blood cell.

The mature red blood cell is a biconcave disc with a cell membrane containing enzymes which catalyze processes necessary to physiological function of the cell. New enzyme proteins cannot be produced because the apparatus for protein synthesis no longer exists.

When red blood cells complete their normal life span they are removed by the reticulo-endothelial system. Macrophages or scavenger cells in the reticulo-endothelial system recognize the aging red cell as being no longer needed (aging self) because of biophysical and immunological changes which have taken place in the cell with time. The ability of the cell to undergo reversible changes in shape in order to get through narrow blood vessels is lost.

The density of membrane antigens increases in old red blood cells. There is also a decrease in the surface charge on the aging red blood cell. It is presently believed that the aging red blood cell may be "identified" by the macrophage as having completed its normal life and being ready for destruction by engulfment or phagocytosis both by the change in surface antigens and by the change in surface.

There is evidence that events occurring in the aging of other cells may be analogous to those occurring in red blood cells.

## PHYSIOLOGY OF AGING IN TISSUES AND ORGANS

### The Skin and Its Appendages

The changes in the skin with aging include dryness, wrinkling, mottled pigmentation, loss of elasticity, dilatation of capillaries, particularly on the face, senile purpura (bleeding into the skin in response to minor trauma), and growth of seborrhoeic warts, skin tags, and cherry angiomata which are red vascular lesions having a similar appearance to "blood blisters," but appearing and remaining usually on the abdomen and back.

The skin is divided into the epidermis, or cellular surface layers, and the underlying dermis. The epidermis is anchored to the dermis at the epidermo-dermal junction, characterized by a ridged structure. Aging of the epidermis is associated with flattening of the epidermo-dermal junction and loss of the ridged structure. The epidermis in aged skin is less well anchored to the dermis, and more liable to be torn off or rubbed off by shearing stress. Similarly, it is because of the looser attachment of the epidermis to the dermis in aged skin that blister formation can occur with less trauma than in young skin (Verbov, 1974).

The epidermis retains some of its important functions despite changes in aging. A normal horny surface layer is formed. Barrier function, whereby the epidermis can limit water loss from the body, is also retained. However, increased losses of water from the surface layers of the epidermis occur due to decreased water-holding capacity, and this accounts in large part for the dryness of the aged skin.

The skin also becomes drier because of a decrease in sebaceous (oil) gland activity. However, sebaceous glands enlarge with age in men and in women, and the enlarged glands may be prominent on the nose or on the cheeks, forehead, and temples.

In the dermis, the cells which produce elastic and collagen fibers, the fibroblasts become less active and those that become inactive contain lipofucsin granules. Elastic fibers of the dermis become denser with age, and with time, the elastic fibers shrink and lose their attachment to the epidermis. It is because of these changes in elastic tissue as well as the degenerative changes in the interfibrillar "ground substance" of the dermis, that wrinkling occurs.

Skin capillaries become more fragile, which accounts for bleeding into the skin with very mild trauma in the elderly (purpura). Senile purpura is more common on light-exposed areas such as the forearms. The capillaries also become sparser and functionally less responsive to cold. Coldness is experienced as soon as the ambient temperature begins to fall.

Decline in cellular immune function, which is a general phenomenon of aging, explains in part the greater prevalence of fungal infections in older persons and their increased susceptibility to malignant tumors.

Hair changes include greying of the hair and hair loss. Hair loss in men initially has the distribution of male patterns of baldness with thinning and loss of hair being most prominent over the frontal areas of the scalp. In older men, extensive loss of scalp hair may be accompanied by growth of coarse hair in the nostrils and ears. In women, the scalp hair tends to become sparser over the entire scalp, though thinning of the hair is most noticeable over the vertex. Secondary sex hair on the body decreases in both sexes in the process of aging, and in the female, loss of body hair may begin soon after the menopause.

Changes in the nails include slowed rate of growth, thickening, and deformity (onychogryphosis).

Prematurely aging skin occurs with chronic exposure to sunlight. Aging of the skin occurs earlier and most prominently on light-exposed areas. Changes seen in the skin with actinic skin damage include wrinkling, pigmentary changes, and loss of elasticity, but also the appearance of actinic keratoses which are rough, red areas of the light-exposed skin which, on histological examination, show precancerous changes and which, if untreated, have a strong tendency to develop skin cancer (Montagna and Carlisle, 1979).

Aging of the skin is influenced by genetic factors. Early aging of the skin occurs in light-skinned Caucasians. Premature aging of the skin occurs in general diseases of premature aging, such as progeria. In the very serious skin disorder, xeroderma pigmentosum, DNA of the epidermal cells fails to undergo repair after U.V. (ultra violet) induced injury. Persons with this disease develop skin cancer very early in life, as well as skin changes resembling, in some respects, those seen with aging.

Chronic exposure to sunlight accelerates aging both in the epidermis and in the dermis. In the epidermis, the life span of the keratinocytes (hair-forming cells) is decreased, and in the dermis, collagen fiber synthesis and degradation are slowed.

## Pathophysiology of the Oral Cavity

The flow of saliva is decreased with aging. Dehydration and thinning of the gum tissue occurs and also shrinking of the connective tissue of the mouth. Sensory changes which may occur include impaired taste and glossodynia (pain in the tongue) (Schiffman, 1977).

Masticatory efficiency may be impaired by loss of mobility of the mandibular joint due to osteoarthrosis, periodontal disease, inflammation under a denture, or the edentulous or partially dentulous state. Periodontal disease is common and is associated with inflammation of the gums, loosening of the teeth, and dental abscesses. The bone surrounding the teeth shows rarifaction. It has been suggested that periodontal disease is a calcium deficiency state, but this has not been proven.

Age-related changes in the teeth not associated with periodontal disease include abrasion or wearing down of the crowns, formation of secondary dentine, and resorption of the dental root tips.

Angular cheilitis and/or stomatitis is common, and may or may not be associated with riboflavin deficiency. Frequently both angular cheilitis and stomatitis, i.e. cracks at the corners of the lips or mouth, are associated with deep skin creases and local secondary yeast infection.

Common diseases of the oral mucosa include candidiasis (thrush/yeast infection), leukoplakia (premalignant mucosal changes), cancer of the mouth or oral cavity including the tongue, and xerostomia, associated with Sjogren's syndrome (an auto-immune disease).

Dental caries is uncommon in the elderly, and with age resistance to caries increases. This has generally been explained as being due to maturation of enamel and dentine (Soremark and Nilsson, 1972).

## The Gastrointestinal System

Secretory activity into and within the gastrointestinal tract is reduced with aging. The most marked change in secretory activity is in the stomach, where gastric hydrochloric acid production is diminished. Pepsin and gastric mucus secretion also decline.

In pernicious anemia, a disease which is not uncommon in elderly people, the production of gastric intrinsic factor ceases, and there is also achlorhydria (complete lack of gastric acid production) (Steinberg and Toskes, 1978). Pernicious anemia is an autoimmune disease in which megaloblastic and neurological signs are caused by vitamin $B_{12}$ deficiency. Vitamin $B_{12}$ from the diet cannot be absorbed in the absence of gastric intrinsic factor. The aging process increases the risk of autoimmune disease within the gut.

Physiological decreases in absorptive capacity within the small intestine are moderate. Tolerance of fat is slightly reduced such that with high fat intake, the fat content of the feces is raised. The D-xylose screening test for malabsorption may be used to indicate impairment of absorption, but caution must be used in interpreting the test, which is dependent on retention of normal renal function, a condition which may not be present in the elderly (Stanheber, 1976).

Calcium absorption in the elderly is frequently decreased, and there is also a reduced ability for adaptation to low calcium intake, which may be due to change in vitamin D status.

Constipation is common in the elderly. General causes of constipation in the elderly, as in persons of younger age groups, are 1) delayed transit of feces throughout the colon, and 2) prolonged retention of feces within the rectum. Slowed colonic transit may be due to a low residue diet, semistarvation, drugs (narcotic analgesics), hypothyroidism, laxative abuse, late radiation damage to the gut wall, or chronic intestinal obstruction due to colonic or rectal cancer or inflammatory bowel disease. Slow passage of the colonic contents is associated with dehydration and hardening of the fecal mass. The dehydration of feces occurs when the feces remain longer than normal in the large intestine and more water is extracted because of continued exposure of the feces to the water-absorbing surface of the colon.

In the elderly, constipation is also characterized by fecal hoarding in the rectum due to habitual postponement of defecation or inability to defecate easily.

Habitual postponement of defecation is termed dyschezia. Dyschezia may be due to 1) fear of pain, 2) anxiety and depression, 3) situational factors (inadequate privacy of toilet arrangements), 4) fecal impaction, 5) debility due to chronic disease states or malnutrition of dietary or disease origin, and 6) "loss" of the gastro-colic reflex which initiates propulsive movement of feces from the colon and rectum, producing the desire to defecate. The gastro-colic reflex is normally triggered by intake of warm food or beverages (Berman and Kirschner, 1972).

## The Cardiovascular System

Anatomical changes which take place in the heart with aging include an overall decrease in size, decrease in the size of the cavity of the left ventricle, and increase in the size of the left atrium. The heart valves become more rigid and thickened, and collagen increases in the valves. Calcification occurs in the aortic valve. The heart muscle (myocardium) becomes brownish due to increased lipochrome (lipofucsin) deposition. There is enlargment or hypertrophy of individual muscle fibers of the myocardium, which apparently occurs to compensate for other muscle fibers which are lost. Fat deposition occurs beneath the surface membrane of the heart (pericardium), and thickened whitish plaques appear in the membrane lining the heart (endocardium).

Dilatation of the aorta occurs because of loss of elasticity.

Physiological changes of the heart with aging include decreased myocardial contractility and decreased cardiac output. There is a decreased ability of the heart to utilize oxygen. The aging heart does not tolerate physical stress, such as increase in blood pressure, fever, and strenuous exercise, as well as the younger heart because these stresses can precipitate cardiac failure. While large arteries dilate with aging, there is generally a loss of arterial distensibility with age.

Systolic blood pressure usually increases with age, but changes in diastolic blood pressure are slight (Harris, 1975; Hurst et al., 1974).

## The Respiratory System

Anatomical changes in the lungs with aging include enlargement of the alveoli (air sacs) with weakening of septal membranes and a reduction in the alveolar surface area. Changes in alveolar surface are accompanied by deterioration of elastic properties of the tissue. Decreases in the alveolar surface area are almost linear between the ages of 20 and 80 years, such that by age 80 the surface area is approximately 30 percent of the maximal young adult value.

Changes in the lung elastic tissue are both quantitative and qualitative. The lungs become stiffer and the alveolar tissue less distensible.

Vital capacity decreases with age, and the ability to adapt to exercise is reduced. Maximum breathing capacity and maximum voluntary ventilation of the lungs also decrease with age. The lungs are, of course, the organs of gaseous exchange whereby oxygen enters and carbon dioxide leaves the body. Gas exchange capacity is lowered with aging because of the combined effects of reduced alveolar surface area, increased thickness of alveolar membrane, decreased permeability of the alveoli to respiratory gases, and reduced capillary blood volume (Hook, 1972).

## The Renal System

A morphological change in the kidney associated with aging is a loss of nephrons (renal excretory units). Renal functional changes which occur with aging include a reduction in total renal blood flow, glomerular filtration rate, daily urinary creatinine excretion, sodium conservation, and renal concentrating ability. The renal capacity for reabsorption of glucose declines and the secretory function of the renal tubule is diminished. The physiological adaptation to sodium load, as well as to dietary sodium restriction, is also progressively less efficient with aging. Because of decreased efficiency of sodium handling, the elderly risk developing both hyponatremia and hypernatremia. These abnormalities of sodium homeostases may be life-threatening conditions when elderly people are subjected to physical stress such as injury or infection (Epstein, 1979).

## The Endocrine System

Aging produces marked physiological changes in the endocrine system, but failure of endocrine function is not a generalized phenomenon. Indeed, endocrine dysfunction in the elderly, as in other age groups, is disease-related.

*The Pituitary-Hypothalamic System.* Hypothalamic aging influences endocrine function in the peripheral endocrine system including the pituitary, thyroid, parathyroid, and reproductive glands. Events associated with aging include diminished production of hypothalamic-releasing hormones as well as a lessened sensitivity of the pituitary to the action of hypothalamic-releasing hormones. Decreased growth hormone release occurs in the elderly following the stimulus of hypoglycemia, and this may be explained by loss of growth-hormone-releasing hormone. On the other hand, aging induces impairment in direct renal response to the posterior pituitary antidiuretic hormone (ADH) with less effect of ADH on water conservation or urine concentrating ability. In elderly people, there is also a reducing pituitary response to thyrotropin-releasing hormone.

*Thyroid Glands.* Aging of the thyroid is associated with anatomical alterations in the gland including fibrosis, follicular change, and nodularity. There is no change in plasma levels of thyroxine ($T_4$) in healthy elderly people, but circulating levels of the other thyroid hormone, triodothyronine ($T_3$), are reduced. Aging does not produce hypofunction of the gland.

*Parathyroid Gland.* Aging is associated with slightly decreased blood parathyroid hormone (PTH) levels. The normal PTH drop with age is not seen in osteoporotic individuals. Neither hypoparathyroidism nor hyperparathyroidism is an outcome of aging, though hyperparathyroidism does increase in incidence in older people.

*Reproductive Glands.* Ovarian aging is associated with loss of oocytes (ova/egg producing cells), but this process of oocyte reduction actually begins in infancy and continues throughout life. The cause of human reproductive failure with age is not loss of oocytes. Ova produced by older ovaries are less viable and do not undergo the maturation which occurs in the ova of younger individuals. Estrogen production is reduced in women over about 40 years, and there is a further decrease in estrogen production which occurs after the menopause.

Reduction in plasma total testosterone levels does not occur uniformly with increasing age, and indeed, variability in testosterone production among elderly men is noteworthy. However, physiologically active testosterone is reduced in the elderly male. The loss of libido with age and the impairment of sexual performance is multifactorial. Sterility in the elderly male is commonly disease-related. Disease-related causes of sterility in the elderly male include alcoholism (Gregerman and Bierman, 1974).

*Endocrine Pancreas.* Glucose tolerance decreases with age, and production of insulin is reduced in response to physiological stimulation. Reduced end organ sensitivity to the effects of insulin occurs with obesity, which is common in older people, but end organ sensitivity to insulin is normal in elderly, nonobese individuals (Andres, 1972).

*Adrenal Glands.* Decreased secretion of the sodium-conserving hormone, aldosterone, occurs with age. With sodium restriction older persons, like younger persons, do increase aldosterone production, but the increase is smaller in people over 60. The secretion of renin shows an age-related decrease, which is correlated with the decrease in aldosterone secretion.

Decreased glucocorticoid secretion in response to adrenocorticotrophic hormone (ACTH) may occur in the elderly but is not a uniform finding.

## Physiological Changes in Hemopoiesis

Decreased efficiency of hemopoiesis occurs with aging. In the healthy aged, hemoglobin concentrations are similar to those in younger people. Absorption of available iron sources is also similar in elderly and younger groups. However, the percentage of absorbed iron that is utilized for hemopoiesis is less in the elderly than in the young. In the healthy elderly, iron stores are increased, and it has therefore been assumed that ineffective erythropoiesis is increased. The red cell incorporation of iron decreases with age, and it has been suggested, though it is at present unproven, that in the aged, some absorbed iron may be retained in the liver or in other storage tissues. Both the aged and the young respond to iron deficiency by increased iron absorption. Iron deficiency anemia in the aged is not explained by the change in efficiency of hemopoiesis (Marx, 1979; Matzner et al., 1979).

Limited studies of folacin absorption in the aged suggest that there is a decrease in utilization of ingested polyglutamate forms of folacin derived from foods, but that synthetic sources of folic acid are as well absorbed by the elderly as by the young. Whether or not absorbed folacin is as well utilized for hemopoiesis in the elderly as in the young is currently unknown (Rodriguez, 1978). Present evidence does not suggest that absorption of other B vitamins including vitamin $B_6$, vitamin $B_{12}$, and riboflavin (which are required in hemopoiesis) is decreased with aging. Information is lacking as to whether utilization of any one of these B vitamins for hemopoiesis is decreased in older persons.

## The Central and Peripheral Nervous Systems

Changes in the central nervous system with aging are structural and functional. Aging, independent of disease processes, is associated with a progressive loss of brain cells, particularly in the cortical areas (Brody and Vijayashankar, 1977).

Memory declines but memory losses vary greatly between individuals. While the loss of memory always affects the ability to learn and retain information, those people who are intellectually gifted and continue to be intellectually active and socially stimulated are less likely to show severe impairment. Past skills are retained or may be relearned, provided that the necessary motivation is provided. New skills are acquired with increasing difficulty as aging progresses.

Sensory perceptivity decreases in the elderly. The blunting of sensory perception is related to the special senses; hearing, smell, and taste are less acute. The anguish of pain is lessened.

Sleep is usually unchanged in duration, but sleeping patterns may be reversed so that the elderly tend to sleep more during the day and less at night.

Muscle response to nerve stimulation declines, both because nerve impulses to muscles are conducted more slowly and because of loss of muscle mass.

## The Eye

Aging affects multiple components of the eye concerned with vision. These include (a) the reduction in visual acuity, (b) decline in accommodation, or the loss of ability to focus on near objects, which usually begins in middle life. This is due to an inability of the aging lens to change in curvature in response to the needs of near vision. The loss of the power of accommodation is designated *presbyopia*. (c) Senile cataract, causing opacity of the lens, is due to condensation or an increased density of fibers within the lens. Cataract in the aging eye is classified as cortical and nuclear according to the distribution of the opacity (Weale, 1973). The opacity of the lens limits the usefulness of the lens as a light filter. The development of cataract, even in the early stages, reduces night vision. Approaching lighted objects, such as the headlights of cars, appear fuzzy, and the glare of lights impedes visual judgment. Later cataracts impose a progressive loss of vision which can be relieved by extraction of the lens. The rate of development of cataract usually differs between the two eyes.

With aging, the lens not only becomes rigid and loses translucency, but it also increases in size. This increase in size may lead to impaired drainage of the fluid (the aqueous humor) which is present in the anterior chamber of the eye (in front of the lens). Narrowing the angle between the iris and the cornea occludes drainage of this fluid into the canal of Schlemm. Intraocular pressure builds up with resultant glaucoma, which also imposes a threat to vision because of excessive pressure on the retina or visual membrane. The central area of the retina, called the macula, which is the most sensitive site of visual perception, tends to degenerate in the elderly.

The changes of aging within the eye are subject to wide interperson variability. Important factors which contribute to the early development of these eye changes are familial predisposition (genetic factors), exposure to ionizing radiation (leading to cataract), and diabetes (Passmore and Robson, 1974).

### The Effect of Age on Hearing

Hearing defects of the elderly account for the greatest number of sensori-neural hearing loss disorders. Sensori-neural hearing loss disorders comprise hearing loss arising from impaired function of the inner ear (cochlea) and/or connections of the auditory nerve close to or within the brain.

The hearing disorders of the elderly may result from several factors operating during an individual's life. These factors include genetic determinants of deafness, occupational noise exposure, and chronic middle ear disease. In addition, common health problems associated with hearing loss include Meniere's disease, which increases in incidence with age. Hearing loss in the elderly has been correlated with the extent or severity of athero-sclerosis.

Most elderly people have poorer high-frequency hearing levels. However, chronological age does not determine the rate of decline in hearing (Goldstein and Reichel, 1978).

## PATHOLOGY OF AGING IN TISSUES AND ORGANS

### Skin Diseases of the Elderly

Skin diseases of the elderly should be familiar to the nutritionist for one or more of the following reasons:

1. They may be manifestations of specific forms of malnutrition, e.g. avitami-noses.
2. Healing requires nutritional intervention, e.g. decubitus ulcers.

3. They are indicators of metabolic disease, e.g. diabetes.
4. They cause malnutrition, e.g. systemic sclerosis.
5. They suggest gross personal neglect, e.g. scabies.
6. They are self-induced due to organic brain syndromes or senile psychoses.
7. They require therapy which may compromise nutrition.
8. They are associated with alcoholism.
9. They are due to misuse or abuse of medications.
10. They interfere with food intake.

*Cutaneous Signs of Malnutrition.* In the presence of a *riboflavin deficiency*, seborrhoic dermatitis is present with redness and scaling of the nasolabial folds (skinfold between the nose and the corners of the mouth), and similar scaly lesions of the wrinkles around the eyes may be present. Patients exhibit a dermatitis of the scrotum or vulva. Angular stomatitis is also present (fissures at the corners of the mouth). The tongue is smooth, purplish and sore.

These changes of the skin and mucous membranes disappear when therapeutic doses of riboflavin are given.

Riboflavin deficiency may be secondary to malabsorption or alcoholic liver disease (Sebrell and Butler, 1938).

Skin changes in the elderly which clinically resemble riboflavin deficiency but which do not respond to riboflavin administration are due to causes other than riboflavin deficiency, e.g. intertrigo (Verbov, 1974).

A niacin deficiency, or *pellagra*, is characterized by dermatitis and brownish pigmentation of light-exposed areas of skin. Soreness of the mouth and diarrhea also occur. The patient exhibits signs of an organic brain syndrome characterized by fearfulness, depression, and suicidal thoughts. Cutaneous, gastrointestinal signs of pellagra as well as the characteristic psychoses disappear following niacin administration (Fouts et al., 1937).

*Vitamin $B_6$ deficiency* (pyridoxine) is signalled by dermatitis of the face, ears, trunk, and limbs associated with redness and branny scales, neuritis with complaint of burning feet, depression, confusion or disorientation, and hypochromic anemia. Cutaneous and noncutaneous signs of vitamin $B_6$ deficiency usually clear when therapeutic doses of vitamin $B_6$ are given, but it should be noted that since vitamin $B_6$ deficiency is usually due to chronic intake of drugs such as L-dopa which are vitamin $B_6$ antagonists, change in the dose of the drug or discontinuation of the drug may be necessary to promote resolution of the deficiency.

*Scurvy* is associated with prominence of hair follicles on the limbs and perifollicular hemorrhage into the skin. More widespread purpura may be present. Scorbutic gums which are swollen and bleeding do not occur in elderly people who are edentulous. Signs of scurvy disappear when vitamin C is given in therapeutic doses (Irwin, 1976).

In the presence of a *vitamin A deficiency*, the skin is dry and permanent goose pimples are visible on the limbs. Night blindness is a common complaint. Vitamin A deficiency is very rare in the United States, except in alcoholics or in patients with severe malabsorption syndromes (Steinberg and Toskes, 1978).

Purpura occurs in association with *vitamin K deficiency* (hypoprothrombinemia). The cause is intake of either anticoagulant drugs or other drugs which interfere with vitamin K absorption, e.g. cholestyramine (Roe, 1976).

With an *essential fatty acid deficiency*, the skin shows widespread or generalized scaling and redness. Skinfolds are particularly involved. Other signs include hair loss and poor wound healing. Patients are likely to be receiving semisynthetic enteral or parenteral formulas (Wene et al., 1975).

Cutaneous signs of *zinc deficiency* include dermatitis of the backs of the hands, forearms, and lower legs, which in severe cases becomes generalized. The dermatitis does not respond to any topical medications. Wound healing is impaired. Patients complain of loss of taste. Patients are often alcoholics. Cutaneous and noncutaneous signs of zinc deficiency disappear when zinc supplements are administered (Ecker and Schroeter, 1978).

*Lesions of the Skin Which Require Nutritional Intervention for Optimal Healing.*   Wound healing is dependent on adequate nutrition with respect to protein, B vitamins (niacin, folacin, and riboflavin), ascorbic acid, zinc, and essential fatty acids. The retarded healing of surgical wounds, decubitus ulcers (bed sores), and stasis ulcers (leg ulcers) are associated with deficiency of one or more of these nutrients. Scar formation with deposition of collagen requires vitamin C. Epithelialization (surface closure) of wounds and ulcers requires optimum B vitamins and zinc nutrition. Wound edema, associated with protein deficiency, retards healing (Steffee, 1980).

*Cutaneous Signs of Metabolic Disease.*   *Gout* is a disorder of purine metabolism associated with hyperuricemia. Cutaneous signs of gout include chalky deposits of urate around finger and toe joints and also on the ears. In acute gouty attacks, local redness, swelling, and tenderness of the tophi occurs (Verbov, 1974).

Cutaneous signs of *diabetes* are fat atrophy at the sites of insulin injections, widespread fungus and yeast infections of the skin involving primarily the feet and legs, ulcers and abscesses of the feet with diabetic neuropathy, recurrent boils and carbuncles, other recurrent pyodermas (bacterial infections of the skin), gangrene (usually of the toes or feet), and necrobiosis lipoidica diabeticorum (NLD). NLD consists in oval areas of thinned skin over the shins in which small underlying blood vessels are clearly visible. Dermatitis of skinfolds (*intertrigo*) is common in obese patients with maturity-onset diabetes (Passmore and Robien, 1974; Verbov, 1974).

Signs of *atherosclerosis* include xanthomata, which are yellow skin nodules around the elbows and knees, on the hands, and along the Achilles tendon consisting of deposits of cholesterol, and cholesterol esters in the skin. They are present in patients with genetically determined hyperlipopro-teinemias. Many patients with these lesions (Type IIA, IIB, III and IV) do not survive to be senior citizens because of predisposition to atherosclerotic heart disease in early or middle life. Xanthelasma, which is a variant of xanthoma-tous lesions, consists in unilateral or bilateral small, yellow plaque-like lesions in or below the lower eyelids. They are more common in the elderly. Half of the patients with xanthelasmas have elevated serum cholesterol values (Verbov, 1974).

*Hemochromatosis* is an iron-storage disorder, sometimes primary, due to genetically determined hyperabsorption of iron or secondary to alcoholism or certain hematological diseases such as thalassemia. Signs appear in middle life or later. The skin is greyish in color due to deposition of iron. Loss of secondary sex hair is usual. Patients with this disease have cirrhosis and diabetes mellitus (Braverman, 1970).

*Cutaneous Diseases Which Cause Malnutrition.* *Systemic sclerosis* is a progressive connective tissue disease leading to hardening of the skin and progressive impairment of upper and lower gastrointestinal function. Decreased pulmonary and renal function are also common. Signs related to the skin are Raynaud's phenomenon (blanching of the fingers in response to cold), and ulceration of the fingers and toes.

Dysphagia and regurgitation of food occur with upper GI tract involvement. Intestinal malabsorption is found in a high percentage of cases. The combination of poor food retention and malabsorption leads to malnutrition.

*Bullous pemphigoid* and *pemphigus* are both generalized blistering eruptions of the skin. Bullous pemphigoid is mainly seen in people over 60 years of age, whereas pemphigus is more common in younger age groups. Loss of serum proteins from the skin due to blistering can cause protein malnutrition in both of these diseases.

In *exfoliative dermatitis*, the whole skin surface (or most of it) is red, dry, and peeling. Exudation of serum may be present and edema is common. Nails and hair are often lost. In many cases, itching is intense. Common causes are adverse drug reaction, psoriasis, Norwegian scabies, neuro-dermatitis, and lymphomas. A severe loss of protein from the skin occurs as epidermal keratin and serum. Malnutrition is a result of low food energy intake associated with anorexia and protein loss. Folacin deficiency may occur because of an increased rate of turnover of epidermal cells.

*Cutaneous Indicators of Neglect.* Gross personal neglect in the elderly is strongly suggested by the presence of infestation. Common parasitic skin diseases in the elderly are (1) pediculosis corporis due to infestation with body lice and (2) scabies due to infestation with the scabies mite. Generalized scabies with exfoliation is called Norwegian scabies. Malnutrition due to a faulty diet and infestation associated with lack of personal hygiene occur together in socially isolated elderly people.

*Self-Induced Skin Lesions.*    *Delusions of parasitosis* occur when elderly people become convinced that they are infested (Verbov, 1974). They scratch themselves obsessionally and will bring to the doctor's office containers of skin fragments and/or small bits of thread which they insist are insects which are infecting them. Patients with this obsession are usually paranoid. Obsessions may not be limited to skin parasites but frequently extend to food. Ideas that certain foods are poisonous or poisoned may also be present.

With *factitial dermatitis*, self-inflicted skin lesions including self-inflicted thermal or chemical burns may occur. Patients are psychotic and associated psychoses include organic brain syndromes. Patients who burn or mutilate their own skin may also rub feces into the wound and develop severe infections which can compromise nutritional status.

*Chemotherapy and Radiation Therapy of Cutaneous Disease.* Cancer and lymphomas of the skin may require either radiation therapy or chemotherapy for curative or palliative treatment. Basal and squamous cell cancers of the skin are treated by radiation therapy as well as by surgery. Cutaneous diseases which require chemotherapy include Kaposi's sarcoma and mycosis fungoides.

Both radiation therapy and chemotherapy are likely to cause nausea and anorexia, which diminish food intake and can be responsible for protein-energy malnutrition, which in turn diminishes tolerance for treatment (Bergevin, 1976).

*Dermatoses Associated with Alcoholism.*    Elderly people are unlikely to give an accurate account of their drinking habits to a dietitian or clinical nutritionist, especially if they are alcoholics.

Skin diseases and disorders which are commonly associated with alcohol abuse and may offer presumptive evidence of alcoholism in the elderly are rosacea (a red and bulbous nose), raindrop-like pigmentation of the shoulders and upper back, dilated capillaries (''spiders'') over the face, back and chest, and light sensitivity appearing in later life due to porphyria (porphyria cutanea tarda). See also the discussion of grey skin pigmentation in hemochrometosis (Braverman, 1976).

*Eruptions Caused by Medications.*    The elderly are common drug users. Laxative abusers are found particularly among older people, and secrecy about the habit may be maintained. Malnutrition with potassium depletion and fat malabsorption can result from laxative abuse or a particularly high intake of phenolphthalein containing preparations. Phenolphthalein may cause a fixed drug eruption which consists in reddish hyperpigmented circular skin lesions, which become very red when the drug is ingested. The finding of a fixed drug eruption in elderly people can lead to discovery of laxative abuse, though fixed drug eruptions are also associated with intake of drugs other than phenolphthalein (Verbov, 1974).

*Dermatoses Which Interfere with Food Intake.* Dermatoses which interfere with food intake include those which cause intractable itching (such as exfoliative dermatitis) or pain (such as herpes zoster, or shingles), those which are skin manifestations of internal cancer, those which require radiation or chemotherapy, as well as dermatoses which may also involve the mucous membrane of the mouth and throat (such as pemphigus and avitaminoses) and those which are associated with disease of the esophagus (such as systemic sclerosis) (Wormsley, 1964).

# COMMON DISEASES OF THE ORAL CAVITY IN THE ELDERLY

## Ulceromembranous stomatitis *(Vincent's angina)*

Multiple painful greyish ulcers occur with this condition, involving the mouth and, most commonly, the pharynx. The mouth has a foul odor, and swallowing is difficult. The lymph glands in the neck are enlarged, and there may be a fever. Patients are frequently malnourished, and resistance to infection is often impaired. Vincent's organisms, which normally live within the mouth without causing infection, become pathogenic.

## Candidiasis

Yeast infections of the mouth are frequently seen in the elderly. Whitish patches are present on the mucous membranes of the mouth. Localization may be to the tongue, gums, or lips, but it is not unusual to see generalized candidiasis infections of the mouth. Malnutrition and poor oral hygiene accompany this disease.

## Black Hairy Tongue

Here, the upper surface of the tongue appears blackish in color, the pigmentary development on the tongue being due to proliferation of pigment-producing microorganisms. Factors which promote development include prolonged intake of antibiotics and poor oral hygiene.

### Glossitis

Glossitis may be nutritional or non-nutritional in origin. Common nutritional causes are iron deficiency, riboflavin deficiency, and folacin deficiency. Pellagra is now a very uncommon cause of glossitis in the United States. All nutritional disorders which cause glossitis are associated with loss of the projections on papillae normally occurring on the surface of the tongue.

Geographic tongue is a benign condition of the tongue in which irregular areas on the upper surface of the tongue become denuded of papillae. The disorder may be accompanied by soreness when hot food is eaten or hot beverages drunk.

### Leukoplakia

Leukoplakia causes whitish, persistent thickened patches or streaks on the lips and on the mucous membrane within the mouth. The lesions, if untreated, are sites of cancer development.

### Plummer-Vinson Syndrome (Sideropenic Dysphagia)

This syndrome is characterized by dysphagia, angular stomatitis, atrophic tongue (denuded of papillae), brittle and/or spoon-shaped nails and a pharyngeal or esophageal web. The patients are mostly women and are all chronically iron deficient. A high percentage of patients with this condition develop cancer of the pharynx or esophagus.

### Cancer (Squamous Cell Carcinoma)

Cancer of the lips, tongue, and the mucous membrane lining the buccal cavity is most likely to develop in areas of leukoplakia. Cancers may appear as a lump or ulcer. With early lesions pain is often absent. Spread to a regional (neck) gland occurs. More advanced lesions are extremely painful and cause dysphagia such that food intake by mouth becomes difficult or virtually impossible (Shaw and Sweeney, 1980).

## DISEASES OF THE GASTROINTESTINAL TRACT IN THE ELDERLY

Diseases of the gastrointestinal tract encountered in the elderly fall into one or the other of two categories:

1.   Diseases that are age related.
2.   Diseases that are not age related.

In the first category, there are three subgroups:

a.  Diseases which occur as complications of aging in the gut, e.g. diverticulitis.
b.  Diseases which are due to systemic degenerative disease which is progressive with age, e.g. mesenteric infarction, that is, a block of the mesenteric artery causing gangrene of the gut, which is secondary to generalized atherosclerosis.
c.  Diseases due to previous chemical or physical insult characterized by slow development, e.g. colon cancer, radiation enteritis.

In the second category are diseases which can occur at any age. Subgroups are

a.  Diseases of long duration, e.g. gluten sensitive enteropathy.
b.  Diseases of short duration, e.g. peptic ulcer.

Diseases of the gastrointestinal tract found in the elderly are commonly classified (as in Table 2–1) by location. Common symptoms of serious disease of the GI tract in the elderly are dysphagia or difficulty in swallowing, gastrointestinal bleeding, change in frequency of defecation (diarrhea or constipation), abdominal pain, and jaundice. In the elderly, it is often difficult to differentiate symptoms of minor disorders of the GI tract from symptoms of serious disease (Berman and Kirschner, 1972).

**TABLE 2-1  Diseases of the Gastrointestinal Tract Classified by Site of Involvement**

| SITE | DISEASE |
|---|---|
| Mouth (including tongue) | Nutritional stomatitis (niacin, riboflavin, folacin, ascorbic acid deficiencies) |
| | Candidiasis (thrush-yeast infection) |
| | Leukoplakia (precancerosis) |
| | Pemphigoid |
| | Cancer |
| | Sjogren's syndrome |
| | Mixed salivary tumors |
| Salivary glands | Mixed salivary tumors |
| | Cancer |
| Pharynx | Pharyngitis |
| | Pharyngeal paralysis |
| | Cancer |
| Esophagus | Zenker's diverticulum |
| | Esophageal varices |
| | Esophageal stricture |
| | Peptic esophagitis |
| | Plummer-Vinson syndrome |
| | Progressive systemic sclerosis |
| | Achalasia of the esophagus |
| | Cancer |

**TABLE 2-1** (continued)

| SITE | DISEASE |
|------|---------|
| Stomach | Hiatus hernia |
| | Gastric ulcer |
| | Acute gastritis |
| | Chronic gastritis |
| | Giant hypertrophic gastritis |
| | Post-gastrectomy syndrome |
| | Pyloric stenosis |
| | Zollinger-Ellison syndrome |
| | Cancer |
| Duodenum | Duodenal ulcer |
| Exocrine pancreas | Acute pancreatitis |
| | Chronic pancreatitis |
| | Cancer |
| Small intestine | Tropical sprue |
| | Acute enteritis |
| | Gluten-sensitive enteropathy |
| | Progressive systemic sclerosis |
| | Whipple's disease |
| | Intestinal lymphagiectasia |
| | Crohn's disease (Regional enteritis) |
| | Malignant lymphomas |
| | Carcinoid tumors |
| | Radiation enteritis |
| | Amyloidosis |
| | Mesenteric arterial insufficiency and infarction |
| Large intestine | Crohn's disease |
| | Ulcerative colitis |
| | Diverticulosis |
| | Diverticulitis |
| | Appendicitis |
| | Ischemic colitis |
| | Colonic polyposis |
| | Cancer of the colon or rectum |

Adapted from I.A.D. Bouchier, *Gastroenterology*, 2nd Ed. (London: Bailliere Tindall, 1977).

## Dysphagia

Pharyngeal and esophageal diseases are recognized by dysphagia. Progressive dysphagia in the elderly is most frequently due to cancer. Dysphagia with or without nasal regurgitation of food is common in cerebrovascular disease involving the medulla such as bulbar palsy. A list of diseases which most often cause dysphagia is given in Table 2-2.

TABLE 2-2   Diseases of the Elderly Associated
with Dysphagia

| | |
|---|---|
| *Acute* | Pharyngitis ⎫ due to infection, drugs, radiation |
| | Stomatitis  ⎭ |
| | Pharyngeal abscess |
| | Foreign body |
| | Trauma, including surgery |
| | Esophagitis |
| *Chronic* | Neurological disorders* |
| | Oropharyngeal tumors |
| | Xerostomia |
| | Plummer Vinson syndrome |
| | Esophageal strictures |
| | Reflux esophagitis |
| | Systemic sclerosis |
| | Esophageal ulcer |
| | Esophageal cancer |
| | Zenker's diverticulum |

*Commonly late effects of cerebrovascular accidents,
amyotrophic lateral sclerosis or Alzheimer's disease.

Adapted from J. Loren Pitcher, "Dysphagia in the elderly:
causes and diagnosis," *Geriatrics,* 28 (1973), 64-69.

## Gastrointestinal Bleeding

Severe or chronic gastrointestinal bleeding is associated with iron deficiency
anemia (an otherwise unusual condition in the elderly) and the lowering of
blood pressure, most dramatic in people with previous hypertension. Upper
gastrointestinal bleeding, which if massive may be associated with hema-
temesis or vomiting of blood, is most often silent except for a gradual onset of
anemia. Upper GI bleeding is characteristic of disease of the esophagus and
particularly the stomach. Common causes in the elderly are listed in Table 2-3.

TABLE 2-3   Causes of Upper GI
Bleeding in the
Elderly

Gastritis due to aspirin
Esophageal varices associated
with alcoholic cirrhosis
Gastric or duodenal ulcer
Esophageal tear
Esophagitis
Cancer of the esophagus or
stomach

Adapted from E. L. Rogers,
"Emergency management of
gastrointestinal bleeding," *Geriatrics,* 35 (1980), 35-40.

Rectal bleeding with blood in the stool may be due to colon or rectal cancer. Other common causes are diverticulosis and ischemic (atherosclerotic) colonic diseases.

## Diarrhea

Causes of diarrhea can be divided into causes of acute and of chronic diarrhea. Acute (or short duration) diarrhea occurs in the presence of bacterial gastroenteritis, pseudomembranous colitis (due to drugs), and laxative abuse. Chronic diarrhea is characteristic of inflammatory bowel disease including regional enteritis and diseases of the small intestine which lead to maldigestion or malabsorption. Maldigestion occurs in diseases shown in Table 2-4. Malabsorption occurs in diseases shown in Table 2-5.

In the elderly, when diarrhea is associated with abdominal pain, acute ischemic colitis is a common cause. Frequent, very small stools occur with fecal impaction.

## Constipation

Constipation is related to low dietary fiber ingestion and debility. Misuse of laxatives as well as diverticular disease causes intermittent constipation. Constipation of short duration is usually due to colon pathology including colon cancer. Chronic constipation occurs in hypothyroidism, early ischemic colitis, and with drugs including narcotic analgesics.

---

**TABLE 2-4  Causes of Maldigestion of Fat in the Elderly**

Due to decreased production, activity, release or contact with:
  Pancreatic lipase
  Chronic pancreatitis
  Cancer of the pancreas
  Gastric surgery (partial or total gastrectomy)
  Zollinger – Ellison syndrome
  Neomycin therapy

Due to decreased quantity of bile acids:
  Obstructive jaundice
  Hepatocellular disease
  Ileal resection
  Cholestyramine therapy
  Crohn's disease
  Bacterial overgrowth in the small intestine due to blind loops,
    diverticula, progressive systemic sclerosis, diabetes, partial
    obstruction, fistulae or amyloidosis.

---

Adapted from W. M. Steinberg and P. P. Toskes, "A practical approach to evaluating maldigestion and malabsorption," *Geriatrics,* 33 (1978), 73-85.

TABLE 2-5   Causes of Malabsorption in the Elderly

Decreased number of absorptive cells due to intestinal resection.

Mucosal and submucosal disease or damage including tropical sprue, gluten-sensitive enteropathy, progressive systemic sclerosis, blind loop syndrome (bacterial overgrowth in small intestine), amyloidosis, ischemic bowel disease, drugs including neomycin, colchicine and methotrexate.

Decrease in lymphatic drainage due to:
Intestinal lymphangiectasia
Lymphoma
Congestive heart failure
Constrictive pericarditis
Abdominal tuberculosis
Whipple's disease
Crohn's disease

Transfer defect
Pernicious anemia
Alcohol abuse

Causes of malabsorption unknown
Drug-associated, laxatives and cathartics
Hormonally mediated—carcinoid, hypoparathyroidism, and hyperthyroidism
Addison's disease, mast cell disease
Parasitic diseases, e.g. giardiasis

Adapted from I.A.D. Bouchier, *Gastroenterology,* 2nd. Ed. (London: Bailliere Tindall, 1977), p. 84.

## Abdominal Pain

Common causes of acute abdominal pain are the following:

Intestinal obstruction (due to cancer, volvulus, or appendicitis)
Acute myocardial infarction
Cardiac failure
Lung disease plus pleural involvement
Disease of the urinary tract
Acute cholecystitis
Acute pancreatitis
Acute mesenteric infarction
Dissecting aneurysm

A common cause of chronic or recurrent abdominal pain is cancer of the pancreas.

It should be remembered that causes of abdominal pain in the elderly may be local or referred and may be from disease of the GI tract or disease of other organs.

## DISEASES OF THE CARDIOVASCULAR
## SYSTEM IN THE ELDERLY

Atherosclerosis is a progressive degenerative condition of the arteries, characterized by appearance of fatty streaks (cholesterol deposits), fibrous plaques, and raised lesions as deep as and involving the inner arterial lining. Complications involving the raised lesions are ulceration, calcification, and thrombosis. Thrombosis of an arteriosclerotic artery leads to occlusion, which results in partial or complete loss of arterial blood supply to tissues normally receiving blood from this vessel (Hurst et al., 1974).

Atherosclerotic changes in the arteries begin in childhood, but clinical signs of atherosclerosis do not usually appear until later in life. An exception is when a kindred or individuals have antecedent hypercholesterolemia due to inborn errors of lipoprotein metabolism.

Risk factors for the development of atherosclerotic vascular disease are genetic factors, male sex, high intake of cholesterol and saturated fat, hypercholesterolemia, cigarette smoking, diabetes, hypertension, possibly oral hypoglycemic agents, and stress-related and/or type A behavior pattern. (Type A behavior indicates excessive competitiveness, aggressiveness, restlessness, haste, and impatience [Friedman and Rosenman, 1959].) Softness of the drinking water has also been associated with mortality due to atherosclerotic heart disease (Vavrik, 1974).

Factors conditioning the distribution of atherosclerotic lesions within the cardiovascular system include the internal diameter of the artery and multiple factors related to local blood flow and blood pressure.

Manifestations of atherosclerotic vascular disease are myocardial infarction (heart attack), angina pectoris, cerebral thrombosis and cerebral hemorrhage (both commonly designated as strokes), cerebrovascular ischemic episodes (minor strokes), atherosclerotic leg ulcers, and gangrene and uremia due to atherosclerosis of the renal vessels.

Morbidity and mortality from specific atherosclerotic vascular diseases is influenced by factors which directly or indirectly affect atherosclerotic development in particular organs. For example, strokes are the end results in hypertensives of atherosclerosis of the arteries of the brain and particularly of the middle cerebral artery.

Proximate causes of death in people with atherosclerotic vascular disease are:

Heart attack
Cardiac failure
Respiratory failure
Stroke
Hemorrhage or shock from auto accidents sustained during heart attacks
Carbon monoxide poisoning

## COMMON RESPIRATORY DISEASES OF THE ELDERLY

*Chronic bronchitis* has been so defined on the basis of symptoms including chronic cough and sputum production. Etiological factors include smoking, air pollution, and recurrent respiratory infection. The disorder consists in obstructive inflammation of the smaller air passages. Patients with chronic bronchitis are at particular risk of developing pneumonia.

*Pulmonary emphysema* occurs with aging, but is far more extensive in elderly people who are or have been smokers. Both chronic bronchitis and emphysema cause progressive reduction in pulmonary function. Associated breathlessness may cause the patient to reduce food intake (Barnett, 1972).

The *pneumonias* are acute or chronic diseases of the lungs, characterized by "consolidation" of the alveoli or a filling up of these air sacs with inflammatory cells and fluid. Pneumonia may be due to bacterial, viral, fungus, or mold infection, or due to inhalation of vomited food or inert substances, such as mineral oil. Despite the availability of antibiotics, pneumonias are life-threatening to the elderly, and more especially to those whose immune function is compromised by malnutrition or cancer chemotherapeutic drugs.

*Influenzal pneumonia* is particularly serious in the aged, and particularly in elderly people with pre-existing cardiac and respiratory disease, in whom it is likely to lead to respiratory failure. High fever, cough, malaise, and chest pain due to accompanying pleurisy reduce food intake. Low intake of food and the catabolic effects of the disease can rapidly lead to protein-energy malnutrition (Hook, 1972).

The development of *carcinoma* or *cancer of the lung* has been clearly associated with cigarette smoking. Cancer is more likely to develop in emphysematous lungs than in nonemphysematous lungs. Occupational exposure to carcinogens (such as occurs in men working for a long time around coke ovens) can also cause lung cancer. Peak incidence is in the sixth decade of life, but occurrence in the elderly is also common. Early stages of lung cancer are asymptomatic. Symptoms include cough, chest pain, hemoptysis (coughing up of blood), and symptoms of pneumonia. Systemic manifestations include fever, phlebitis, and most importantly for the nutritionist, anorexia and rapid weight loss. With metastatic lung cancer, particularly when liver metastases are present, the sense of smell is often perverted so that meat tastes rotten. Tolerance of cancer chemotherapy or radiation therapy is related to nutritional support (Pool, 1972; Bergevin, 1976).

## RENAL DISEASE OF THE ELDERLY

The physiological decline in functional capacity of the kidney is symptom-free and does not per se cause renal failure, because of its normal functional reserve (Epstein, 1979).

Renal disease of the elderly is commonly chronic. Chronic diseases of the kidney in the elderly include conditions arising in later life as well as end stages of pre-existing disease. Common to many diseases of the kidney are the signs of chronic renal failure (uremia), including polyuria (passage of large volumes of dilute urine), neurological signs such as headache, convulsions, tremor, and coma, and bleeding episodes. Secondary bone disease may occur both because of impaired metabolic synthesis of the active form of vitamin D in the kidney and because of secondary hyperparathyroidism. Anemia may be due to the bleeding episodes, but a more common cause is failure of the diseased kidney to produce erythropoietin, a hormone-like substance which normally stimulates red cell production and output from the bone marrow into the blood stream. General signs of uremia include nausea, anorexia, and vomiting. Low output of urine (oliguria) and failure of urinary output (anuria) may occur terminally. Renovascular hypertension is a major complication of chronic renal disease.

Laboratory data indicative of renal disease in the elderly include elevation of the blood urea and blood urea nitrogen. Increased serum creatinine is present, but levels are less indicative of renal failure than in younger patients because of diminished production of creatinine by the elderly.

Diseases of the elderly which commonly lead to chronic renal failure are chronic nephritis, chronic pyelonephritis, and renovascular disease which may be associated with diabetes. Other causes of renal failure in the elderly are lupus nephritis and renal complications of systemic sclerosis. Pyelonephritis (inflammatory disease of the kidney) may be secondary to obstructive renal disease (kidney stones). Acute renal failure in the elderly is most often due to an adverse drug reaction.

Causes of oliguria in the elderly male include prostatic enlargment due to simple hypertrophy or cancer causing obstruction to urine outflow, and urinary retention can be due to prostatic disease or disease of the bladder (Rosen, 1976).

## DIABETES IN THE ELDERLY

Diabetes in the elderly may be insulin-dependent or insulin-insensitive. When diabetes develops in later life, it is commonly of the insulin-insensitive type (maturity-onset diabetes). Glucose tolerance decreases with age, and there is a decreased response of the beta cells of the Islets of Langerhans of the pancreas to a rise in blood sugar. However, the glucose uptake of the tissues in response to insulin does not appear to be age-related. When a glucose load is given to older people, their blood sugar (glucose) levels increase more than in younger persons, and the return of the blood glucose to preload levels is slower.

Risk factors for the development of glucose-insensitive diabetes include genetic predisposition, prolonged excessive food-energy intake, obesity, and genetically determined hyperlipoproteinemias. The assumption that diabetes of this type is related to high carbohydrate intakes now seems untenable, unless the high carbohydrate intake is also associated with high total food-energy intake. It has been shown that approximately 75 percent of patients with maturity-onset diabetes are obese at the time that diabetes is diagnosed (Gerritsen, 1976). Reduction in energy expenditure and increase in food intake may account for the increased prevalence of diabetes in developing societies within and outside the United States. Plasma insulin levels are high in maturity-onset diabetes, but the level decreases when weight reduction is achieved. In the elderly, reduction in body weight alone may be sufficient to control the diabetes.

Whereas diabetes in the elderly is usually of the insulin-insensitive type, insulin-dependent or insulin–requiring diabetes may also be found among older people. Older people with insulin-dependent diabetes are 1) those who have had this form of diabetes since early or middle life and 2) those who have developed insulin-insensitivity (maturity-onset diabetes) and in whom the diabetic state has changed over time. It has been postulated that in the obese with maturity-onset diabetes, overfunctioning of the pancreas with hyperproduction of insulin can lead to a state of exhaustion of the beta cells of the pancreas. While this theory is not generally accepted, it is true that with time, some patients who have not previously required insulin may alter their diabetic state such that they require insulin for glucose homeostasis and control of the diabetic state.

Older diabetics without complications of the disease show few, if any, physical signs of a specific nature. Complaints and physical findings which should alert the physician to investigate for the presence of the disease are

1. *Generalized or local itching.* The itching is frequently localized to the scalp, though it may involve the hands, feet, or legs.
2. *Dermatitis.* The diabetic may develop dermatitis in areas which are persistently scratched due to intractable itching. Dermatitis in skinfolds (intertrigo) is common, and infections in these areas are usually caused by yeasts or fungi. Severe mycotic infection of the feet and legs is common (athlete's foot). The athlete's foot may show moist macerated lesions between the toes and blisters on the feet, as in the classic form, but more often lesions are dry and scaly and may extend both over the feet and up the legs. Involvement of the toenails with the fungus infection is also very common. This leads to a distortion and thickening of nail growth.
3. *Boils and abscesses.* Recurrent boils that are slow to heal as well as carbuncles (infection of multiple hair follicles with cellulitis) are common to diabetics. "Silent infections" of the feet, with large collar stud abscesses, occur in diabetics who have sensory loss in the feet. They are unable to feel the pain from stepping on small objects, resulting in injury to the sole of the foot which, if untreated, may infect and produce a large abscess in the deep tissues of the sole.
4. *Neuropathies.* Elderly people may complain of pain in the legs, particularly the lower legs, which is often burning in character and may only occur at night.

The pain is usually associated with unpleasant sensations in the feet and lower legs including prickling, excessive or abnormal perception of heat, cold, pain or touch, and/or a feeling that he/she is walking on cotton.

5. *Failing vision.* Failing vision is a common complaint of elderly diabetics. The condition may be due to cataract or to diabetic retinopathy. Diabetic retinopathy is associated with obliterative changes occurring in the retinal arterioles. Retinal ischemia occurs as well as micro-aneurysms, hemorrhage, and exudates. This ischemic retinal disorder can lead to blindness, which may be unilateral or bilateral.

Frequently in the elderly the classical symptoms of diabetes, including excessive thirst and excessive urination, do not occur. Excessive thirst is uncommon in elderly diabetics; excessive urination (polyuria) may occur but is frequently confused by the elderly patient with frequency of urination associated with increasing age.

Common complications of diabetes in the elderly include cardiovascular accidents. High risk factors in the development of atherosclerotic cardiovascular disease are diabetes, hypertension, and hypercholesterolemia. Arterial disease is the most common cause of death in diabetics over the age of 50, and the mortality rate for these diseases is much higher than in nondiabetic persons. Ischemic heart disease and peripheral arterial disease are particularly common. Peripheral arterial disease is the precursor of gangrene. Because elderly diabetics often have poor eyesight and impaired sensation in the feet (due to neuropathy) as well as an increased susceptibility to cutaneous infection (due to the presence of glucose in sweat), trivial injuries to the feet are common and these are very likely to become infected. The infection is often neglected and may progress to tissue necrosis, and this, together with the impaired circulation to the foot, leads to a gangrenous state which may progress to a ''wet'' gangrene, requiring amputation.

Diabetic retinopathy, as described above, may lead to blindness and is indeed the most important ocular complication of diabetes which can result in loss of eyesight.

While vascular complications are particularly common in elderly diabetics having the insulin-insensitive form of the disease, in insulin-requiring diabetics, diabetic ketoacidosis may develop. Prognosis is poor in severe diabetic ketoacidosis in the elderly unless treatment is prompt. Insulin reactions may also occur due to hypoglycemia. Diabetic nephropathy leading to end-stage renal failure is more likely to occur in diabetics of the insulin-requiring type (Passmore and Robson, 1974).

## ANEMIAS IN THE ELDERLY

Anemias in the elderly, as in other age groups, may be nutritional or nonnutritional in origin. Common types of anemia and etiological factors are summarized in Table 2-6.

**TABLE 2-6**   **Classification of Anemias of the Elderly and Common Etiological Factors**

| TYPE OF ANEMIA | ETIOLOGY |
|---|---|
| *Microcytic hypochromic anemia* | |
| Iron deficiency | a. Low iron intake |
| | b. Intake of foods/beverages which decrease iron absorption |
| | c. Blood loss due to disease or drugs |
| Vitamin B$_6$ deficiency | a. Drugs, alcohol |
| *Macrocytic hyperchromic anemia* | |
| Folacin deficiency | a. Low folacin intake |
| | b. Malabsorption due to disease or drugs |
| | c. Intake of folate antagonists |
| | d. Intake of drugs which increase catabolism of folacin |
| Vitamin B$_{12}$ deficiency | a. Pernicious anemia |
| | b. Vegan diet |
| | c. Ileal resection or disease |
| | d. Postgastrectomy anemia |
| *Hemolytic anemia* | a. Drugs ± glucose-6-phosphate dehydrogenase deficiency (G6PD deficiency) |
| *Aplastic anemia* | a. Drugs, radiation to bone marrow, cancer, leukemia |
| *Hypoplastic anemia* | a. Erythropoietin deficiency in end-stage renal disease |

Adapted from B. A. Brown, *Hematology: Principles and Procedures* (Philadelphia: Lea & Febiger, 1973), p. 191.

Iron deficiency anemia may be due to low iron intake, which is particularly likely when the daily diet is low in food energy and consists of foods which are of low total iron content. Inadequate intake of heme iron may also contribute to iron deficiency, since heme iron is better utilized than non-heme iron. Other factors of dietary origin which increase the risk of iron deficiency anemia are low intake of ascorbic acid and high intakes of foods or beverages which contain non-nutrient substances. Iron absorption is decreased by high intake of tea (due to formation of iron tannates), oatmeal (due to formation of iron phytates), and bran (due to adsorption of iron on fiber particles). In the elderly, chronic blood loss is a frequent cause of anemia. The major route of chronic blood loss is the gastrointestinal tract. Causes of blood loss via the gastrointestinal tract are 1) high and prolonged intake of aspirin or indomethacin, 2) hemorrhage from colonic or diverticular polyps, and 3) hemorrhage from colon or rectal cancer. Blood loss from leaking esophageal varices may cause iron deficiency anemia in alcoholics with cirrhosis.

Nutritional macrocytic anemia in the elderly is most commonly due to inadequate intake of dietary folacin. Low intake of foods rich in folacin like raw and cooked green, leafy vegetables and liver is particularly likely with advanced age. Also, the aged, because of lack of familiarity with or dislike of fortified cold breakfast cereals, may not obtain synthetic folic acid from this source. Folacin malabsorption occurs in elderly people who are alcoholics, and also in those with gastrointestinal disease including systemic sclerosis, mesenteric vascular insufficiency, tropical sprue, gluten-sensitive enteropathy, chronic radiation enteritis, and intestinal resection. Drugs contributing to the production of folacin deficiency in the elderly include diphenylhydantoin, barbiturates, glutethimide, and folate antagonists, including methotrexate and triamterene. In the elderly, folacin deficiency has also been associated with congestive heart failure and with chronic liver disease, whether or not this is alcoholic cirrhosis.

Vitamin $B_{12}$ deficiency in the elderly is most commonly due to pernicious anemia. Pernicious anemia results from an autoimmune process, whereby a gastric intrinsic factor is no longer produced or is produced in inadequate amounts, causing insufficient vitamin $B_{12}$ absorption. Pernicious anemia is particularly liable to occur in Caucasians of Northern European origin. Patients may show signs of dyspnea due to severe anemia, weakness, loss of balance, and sensory changes including parasthesias in the lower limbs. Vitamin $B_{12}$ deficiency occurs less commonly in the elderly as a late complication after partial or total gastrectomy or after ilial resection. A rare cause of vitamin $B_{12}$ deficiency is prolonged adherence to a totally vegetarian (vegan) diet.

Sideroblastic anemia due to vitamin $B_6$ deficiency may occur in elderly alcoholics or may be due to intake of drugs which are vitamin $B_6$ antagonists, including isonicotinic acid hydrazide or hydralazine.

Hemolytic anemias may occur in older people, usually due to ingestion of drugs which carry a risk of immunologically determined hemolysis. The drug methyldopa is a cause of a hemolytic anemia of this type. In the elderly, as in younger people, susceptibility to drug-induced hemolytic anemia is markedly increased if they carry the genotype of glucose-6-phosphate dehydrogenase deficiency.

Aplastic anemia in the elderly may be drug-induced or may follow chronic radiation to long bones for the treatment of cancer. Metastatic involvement of bone marrow by cancer can also lead to aplastic anemia, and chronic leukemia can lead to aplasia of normal cells of the hemopoietic system.

Anemia is commonly present in elderly people with end-stage renal disease because of inadequate synthesis and release of the renal hormone, erythropoietin.

Studies of elderly anemic patients have indicated that anemia was secondary to underlying disease in about 50 percent of the cases. Patients with anemia due to underlying disease, rather than to an inadequate intake of nutrients required in hemopoiesis, may fail to respond to hematinics including iron and folic acid. In elderly hospitalized patients, severe anemias with very low hemoglobin values have been most commonly found in patients with gastrointestinal bleeding, chronic renal disease, pernicious and hemolytic anemia, and also hypothyroidism. Elderly patients with metastatic cancer as well as those with chronic infections, i.e. tuberculosis or recurrent infections including those of the urinary tract, may exhibit anemia. Causes of anemia in cancer and in infection include inadequate intake of iron and folacin, increased or decreased life span of red blood cells, block in the release of iron from storage sites, or a combination of these factors. Blood loss is a common cause of anemia in cancer patients (Kalchthaler and Tan, 1980).

## ORGANIC BRAIN SYNDROMES IN THE ELDERLY

The term ''organic brain syndrome''is used to denote a group of disorders associated with loss of mental function, a known pathology, as well as absence of manic-depressive psychosis and other psychiatric illnesses. Organic brain syndromes now include Alzheimer's disease, senile dementia, and other diseases of the brain which disturb cerebration and other brain functions. Table 2-7 gives a classification of organic brain syndromes grouped according to type and cause.

**TABLE 2-7   Classification of Organic Brain Syndromes in the Elderly**

| CLASSIFICATION | SYNDROMES | CAUSE |
|---|---|---|
| Nutritional | Korsakoff's syndrome | Thiamin deficiency in alcoholics |
| | Pellagrous psychosis | Niacin deficiency |
| | Pernicious anemia (mental changes in) | Vitamin $B_{12}$ deficiency |
| | Nutritional dementia | Folacin deficiency |
| Metabolic | Myxedema | Hypothyroidism |
| | Uremia | End stage renal disease (e.g. chronic nephritis) |
| Toxic | Drug-induced encephalopathies | Alcohol Morphine Barbiturates Phenothiazines |
| Vascular | "Stroke" [atherosclerotic brain atrophy] | Cerebrovascular atherosclerosis + hypertension |
| Neoplastic | "Brain cancer" | Primary or secondary malignant brain tumor |
| Infective | General paralysis of the insane | Syphilis |
| Degenerative | Alzheimer's disease | Unknown |
| | Senile dementia | Unknown |

Adapted from A. McGee Harvey, R. J. Johns, V. A. McKusick, A. H. Owens, and R. S. Ross, *The Principles and Practice of Medicine,* 20th. Ed. (Englewood Cliffs, N.J.: Prentice-Hall, Inc., 1980), p. 1193.

## Alzheimer's Disease

Alzheimer's disease is a progressive, degenerative condition of the brain which always causes dementia. The disease can be considered to represent a cerebral form of premature aging, though in syndromes of premature aging such as Werner's syndrome, signs of Alzheimer's disease are absent. Alzheimer's disease is often familial. The disease appears first from middle age (40–45 years) onwards. Three stages are defined. In the first stage, which may last from 2–4 years, there is loss of memory, spatial disorientation, and a lack of spontaneous emotional response. The second stage is characterized by progressive dementia with peculiar focal signs, including inability to identify or interpret familiar sounds (including the spoken word), sights, or smells. In the third stage, seizures develop and speech is lost. The patient is indifferent to his or her environment. Compulsive eating may occur, with consumption of inedible objects, but more commonly all interest in food is lost, and when the patient is fed, food is pushed out of his or her mouth by tongue movement.

Autopsy examination reveals atrophy of the brain, a reduction in brain weight, loss of cortical neurons and widespread neurofibrillary tangles. The cause of Alzheimer's disease is unknown (Sowrander and Sjogren, 1970).

## Senile Dementia

This disease, or group of diseases, presently called senile dementia, resembles Alzheimer's disease in many of its clinical manifestations. Differences are the later age of onset, and the absence of focal signs related to sensory perception and interpretation. Undoubtedly many cases previously labeled as senile dementia were in fact cases of Alzheimer's disease. Other cases of so-called senile dementias are organic brain syndromes, having a specific nutritional or metabolic etiology, or resulting from vascular disease or tumors. Diagnosis of senile dementia must follow exclusion of these other organic brain syndromes (many of which are amenable to treatment) and Alzheimer's disease. Still unclear is whether senile dementia is a specific entity.

Signs of senile dementia include memory loss, repetition of stories, songs and poems from the past, disinterest in personal appearance and hygiene, ataxia, nausea, and repeated falls.

Memory loss may be masked, as for example when the patient claims that money or other belongings have been stolen, when in fact they were put away in a drawer and forgotten. Sentence forms are shortened and complexities of speech disappear. Depression may follow memory loss, because the patient is aware of his or her declining intellectual function. Disorientation may cause the patient to wander and to get lost both outside and inside the home. Abnormal sleep patterns are common, with nocturnal wakefulness and frequent naps throughout the day.

Incontinence of urine, and later of urine and feces, occurs with advancing dementia. The patient loses the ability to dress, undress, bathe, and eat unaided. The patient finally loses interest in surroundings and becomes unable to recognize family, friends, or nursing staff of the nursing home or hospital where she or he resides.

### Organic Brain Syndromes and Nutrition

Organic brain syndromes may be nutritional in origin, due to thiamin, niacin, folacin, or vitamin $B_{12}$ deficiencies. Reversibility of these syndromes may be possible, but nutritional therapy is not always successful, because of irreversible brain changes. Organic brain syndromes always result early in diminished ability to obtain and prepare food. In the later stages, intake of food is severely reduced. Patients have to be fed, and even then food is frequently not swallowed and may be pushed out of the mouth (Roth, 1978).

## CHRONIC NEUROLOGICAL DISEASE OF THE ELDERLY

Parkinson's disease is a degenerative condition of the basal ganglia of the brain in which production of the neurotransmitter, dopamine, is greatly reduced. The disease is characterized by slowness of movement (*brady-kinesia*), rigidity, tremor, and loss of facial expression. Treatment is with levo-dopa (L-dopa) given in combination with a peripheral decarboxylase inhibitor (McGee Harvey et al., 1980; Yahr, 1975).

## GERIATRIC DISEASES OF THE MUSCULOSKELETAL SYSTEM

Diseases of the musculoskeletal system which are commonly seen in older people may begin in later life or may develop in youth or middle age and be progressive or more disabling with age. The relationship of joint and bone diseases of the elderly to the aging process is popularly accepted, but except in the case of osteoporosis, this theory remains largely unproven. Genetic as well as acquired factors determine the occurrence of musculoskeletal diseases in the elderly as well as localization of the disease process, severity, complications, and disability.

Common musculoskeletal diseases which begin in middle or later life include osteoarthrosis, pseudogout, osteoporosis, Paget's disease, infectious arthritis, and rheumatic polymyalgia. Characteristics of these diseases are summarized in Table 2-8. Whereas these diseases all occur in both sexes, osteoporosis and osteomalacia are more common to women.

Diseases of muscle, connective tissue, joints, and bone which usually start in early life but are seen as major causes of disability in older people include polymyositis, progressive systemic sclerosis, rheumatoid arthritis, ankylosing spondylitis, psoriatic arthropathy, and alveolar bone loss with periodontal disease (Brenenstock and Fernanto, 1976).

**TABLE 2-8  Characteristics of Common Musculoskeletal Diseases in the Elderly**

| DISEASE | USUAL AGE OF ONSET | PATHOLOGY | SYMPTOMS | COMPLICATIONS AND DISABILITY | ETIOLOGY/RISK FACTORS |
|---|---|---|---|---|---|
| Osteoarthrosis | 50 or above | Cartilage degeneration<br>Bony outgrowths | Pain on motion<br>Stiffness after rest | Limp<br>Deformity<br>Muscle wasting | Preexisting disease of the joints<br>Trauma<br>Obesity<br>Acromegaly<br>Gram toxin<br>Intracellular corticosteroids<br>Aging(?) |
| Pseudogout (Chondrocalcinosis) | 60 or above | Calcium pryophosate in joint fluid<br>Acute recurrent or chronic arthritis | Pain<br>Joint swelling | Intermittent or progressive lameness | Diabetes<br>Parathyroid disease<br>Hypothyroidism<br>Aging(?) |
| Osteoporosis | 40 or above | Progressive reduction in skeletal mass | None except with fractures | Fracture of femoral neck<br>Compressed fracture vertebra | Aging<br>Menopause<br>Disuse<br>Alcoholism<br>Low calcium intake |

**TABLE 2-8** (continued)

| DISEASE | USUAL AGE OF ONSET | PATHOLOGY | SYMPTOMS | COMPLICATIONS AND DISABILITY | ETIOLOGY/RISK FACTORS |
|---|---|---|---|---|---|
| Osteomalacia | 70 | Decalcification of bone<br>Incomplete fractures | Bone pain<br>Bone tenderness<br>Muscle weakness | Deformities of spine,<br>chest, pelvis, and legs | Vitamin D deficiency<br>Lack of sunlight<br>Low intake vitamin D<br>Drug intake (barbiturates,<br>diphenylhydantoin) |
| Paget's disease | 40<br>or<br>above | Disorganized bone<br>structure<br>Sarcoma as<br>complication | Bone pain<br>Girdle pain | Deformity of long bones<br>Enlargement of head | Unknown |
| Infectious<br>arthritis | 60<br>or<br>above | Joint infection<br>staph. strep.<br>pneumococcus<br>G-ive organism | Pain<br>Fever | Joint destruction | Diabetes<br>Cancer<br>Alcoholism<br>Uremia<br>Pneumonia<br>Subacute bacterial endocarditis |
| Rheumatic<br>polymyalgia | 50<br>or<br>above | Tuberculosis<br>Fungi<br>Giant cells<br>Arteritis | Shoulder or<br>pelvic stiffness<br>and pain<br>Morning stiffness<br>Fatigue | Intermittent claudication<br>Raynaud's phenomena<br>Headache<br>Loss of vision | Unknown |

Adapted from McGee Harvey et al., 1980, p. 1165.

## CANCER IN THE ELDERLY

The increased incidence of cancer and other malignant diseases in the elderly has three main causes:

1. Long-term exposure to environmental carcinogens including diet-related carcinogens, smoking, ultraviolet light, and industrial chemicals.
2. Failure of cellular immune defense mechanisms against cancer, usually age-related.
3. Inadequate treatment of precancerous conditions, e.g. Plummer-Vinson syndrome associated with chronic iron deficiency, or other precancerous conditions including actinic keratoses and leukoplakia. Diagnosis of cancer in the elderly may be missed because symptoms are confused with those of other diseases common in the elderly.

Common forms of cancer in the elderly are 1) cancer of the breast, 2) cancer of the colon and rectum, 3) cancer of the lung, 4) cancer of the pancreas, 5) cancer of the uterus, 6) cancer of the prostate, 7) cancer of the bladder, and 8) cancer of the skin (Pool, 1975; Bergevin, 1976). Common symptoms and/or signs which point to cancer of one or the other of these organs are summarized in Table 2-9, which also indicates the nutritional significance of particular clinical indicators of these cancers.

TABLE 2-9  Symptoms and Signs of Common Forms of Cancer in the Elderly with Their Nutritional Significance

| SITE OF CANCER | PRESENTING SIGNS | NUTRITIONAL EFFECT (early) |
|---|---|---|
| Breast | Mass<br>Nipple discharge | |
| Colon and Rectum | Change in bowel habit<br>Rectal bleeding<br>Reduction in blood pressure | Iron deficiency anemia |
| Lung | Cough, wheeze, sputum<br>Fever, chest pain | Loss of weight |
| Pancreas | Jaundice | |
| Uterus | Vaginal bleeding | Iron deficiency anemia |
| Prostate | Difficulty in urination<br>Urinary retention | |
| Bladder | Blood in the urine<br>Painful urination | Iron deficiency anemia |
| Skin | "Spot," "mole," nodule or<br>ulcer that does not heal | |

Adapted from M. E. Shils, "Nutritional problems induced by cancer," *Med. Clin. N. Amer.*, 63 (1979), 1011.

TABLE 2-10  **Paraneoplastic (Ectopic Hormone) Syndromes and Their Adverse Nutritional Effects**

| ENDOCRINE DISORDER | TUMOR ASSOCIATION | ADVERSE NUTRITIONAL AND METABOLIC EFFECTS |
|---|---|---|
| ACTH syndrome | Ca. lung<br>Ca. pancreas | Weakness<br>Hypokalemia |
| Inappropriate antidiuretic hormone secretion | Ca. lung | Urinary sodium wastage<br>Hyponatremia |
| Ectopic parahormone secretion | Ca. kidney<br>Ca. lung | Hypercalcemia |
| Ectopic insulin production | Ca. liver<br>Ca. adrenal | Hypoglycemia |
| Serotonin hyperproduction | Carcinoid | Pellagra |

Adapted from McGee Harvey et al., 1980, p. 592.

Paraneoplastic syndromes may develop in patients with cancer and are either due to secretion of hormones or other biologically active compounds by the tumor cells or represent auto-immune phenomena. Some of these syndromes have adverse nutritional effects (see Table 2-10). These syndromes are usually resolved with effective or temporarily suppressive therapy of the underlying cancer.

## Leukemia

Recent mortality statistics indicate a rise in deaths from leukemia in the elderly. Whether this represents a true increase in the incidence of leukemia has been questioned. An alternate and plausible explanation of the increased reported deaths from leukemia in older age groups is improved diagnosis, whereby more cases of leukemia are identified.

Acute leukemia occurs most frequently in two groups: children under 5 years old and adults over 60. Chronic myeloid leukemia is most common in people over 50. Chronic lymphatic leukemia is essentially a disease of the elderly, with the incidence increasing with age.

Signs of leukemia may include 1) profound and progressive weakness, 2) weight loss, 3) breathlessness (due to anemia), 4) hemorrhage, 5) enlargement of the abdomen (due to progressive increase in the size of the spleen and/or lymphatic masses), and 6) susceptibility to infection.

Chronic lymphatic leukemia is frequently asymptomatic in the elderly. Symptoms which may be present in this disease include breathlessness associated with anemia, cardiorespiratory embarrassment, jaundice due to hemolysis, bleeding into the skin or from mucous membranes due to thrombocytopenia, and pain due to intestinal obstruction or glandular masses pressing on nerves. Weight loss and profound weakness also occur. Treatment of leukemia is by chemotherapy and/or radiation therapy. Decision to treat chronic lymphatic leukemia in the elderly is based on the presence or absence of symptoms such as anemia, hemorrhage, glandular masses, or weight loss (Gibson, 1974).

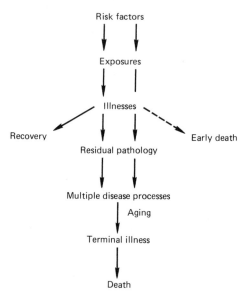

FIGURE 2-2    Development and outcome of disease processes in the elderly.

## INTERRELATIONSHIPS OF DISEASE PROCESSES IN THE ELDERLY

Disease processes which are found in life or at autopsy of the elderly may be of recent origin (acute), or they may be of long standing (chronic). Acute diseases such as pneumonia may be superimposed on chronic disease and may be the immediate cause of death (Hook, 1972). The process of aging predisposes elderly persons to certain diseases including cancer, maturity-onset diabetes, osteoporosis, and autoimmune diseases such as pernicious anemia. On the other hand, chronic disease in the elderly may be the end result of disease which has developed over many years but which was originally independent of the aging process. Examples of such disease are congestive heart failure due to rheumatic heart disease and chronic nephritis following long-term use of the drug phenacetin (Vavrik, 1974; Rosen, 1976). Widespread atherosclerosis in the elderly is the end result of a disease which developed slowly over many years. Malnutrition may develop in the elderly as a result of inadequate diet, disease, drugs, or a combination of these factors. Further, the elderly who are conspicuous users of medications and have a diminished drug tolerance are prone to develop adverse drug reactions which contribute to organ pathology and may be the proximal cause of death (Caranases et al., 1974).

In the elderly, disease processes are often of complex origins, as for example strokes (cerebral hemorrhage or cerebral thrombosis), which are the end result of hypertension and atherosclerosis of the arteries of the brain. Diseases are also commonly multiple and it is not unusual to find several related or unrelated diseases in any one elderly person (Baker and Baker, 1975). Origin, course, and outcome of disease processes of the elderly are illustrated in Figure 2-2.

## QUESTIONS

*Instructions: Circle all correct answers (there may be more than one correct answer to each question).*

1. What are the consequences of failure of DNA repair?
   a) Production of abnormal cells
   b) Regeneration of cells
   c) Death of cells
   d) Evolutional changes
   e) Premature aging

2. Which of the following contribute to the process of aging?
   a) Autoimmune cell destruction
   b) Atherosclerosis
   c) Free radical lipid peroxidation reactions
   d) Chronic exposure to sunlight
   e) Not using a skin moisturizer

3. Identify which of the following statements is correct.
   a) The aging heart tolerates physical stress badly.
   b) Vital capacity decreases with age.
   c) Aging causes nightblindness.
   d) Glucose tolerance decreases with age.
   e) Calcium absorption is increased in the elderly.

4. In the elderly, chronic constipation is commonly due to
   a) not taking a laxative
   b) depression
   c) debility
   d) low residue diet
   e) obesity

5. Which of the following geriatric diseases are influenced by diet?

   a) Alzheimer's disease     d) Colon cancer
   b) Osteoporosis     e) Lung cancer
   c) Diabetes mellitus

6. Which of the following are *NOT* risk factors for the development of atherosclerotic heart disease?
   a) Hypercholesterolemia
   b) High intake of cholesterol
   c) Diabetes mellitus
   d) Daily intake of alcoholic beverages
   e) Tuberculosis

## REFERENCES

ALBANESE, A.A., A.H. EDELSON, E.J. LORENZE, M.L. WOODHULL, and E.H. WEIN, "Problems of bone health in elderly; ten-year study," *New York J. Med.* 75 (1975), 326–36.

ANDRES, R., "Aging and carbohydrate metabolism," in *Nutrition in Old Age*, Symp. Swedish Nutrition Foundation, ed. L.A. Carlson. Uppsala: Almqvist and Wiksell, 1972, pp. 24–31.

BAKER, A.B., and L.H. BAKER, eds., *Clinical Neurology*. New York: Harper and Row, 1975.

BAKER, H., S.P. JASLOW, and O. FRANK, "Severe impairment of dietary folate utilization in the elderly," *J. Amer. Geriat. Soc.*, 26 (1978), 218–29.

BARNETT, T.B., "Chronic bronchitis and pulmonary emphysema," Vol. 2, in *Bronchopulmonary Diseases and Related Disorders*, eds. C.W. Holman and C. Muschenheim. New York: Harper and Row, 1972, pp. 632–64.

BERGEVIN, P.R., "The increasing problem of malignancy in the elderly. New concepts in diagnosis and management," *Med. Clin. N. Amer*, 60, no. 6 (1976), 1241–51.

BERMAN, P.M., and J.B. KIRSCHNER, "The aging gut. II. Diseases of the colon, pancreas, liver and gall bladder. Functional bowel disease and iatrogenic disease," *Geriatrics*, 27 (1972), 117–24.

BRAVERMAN, I.M., *Skin Signs of Systemic Disease*. Phila., London, Toronto: W. B. Saunders Co., 1970, p. 344.

BRENENSTOCK, H., and K.R. FERNANTO, "Arthritis in the elderly," *Med. Clin. N. Amer.*, 60 (1976), 459–1211.

BRODY, H., and N. VIJAYASHANKAR, "Anatomical changes in the nervous system," eds. C.E. Finch and L. Hayflick, *Handbook of the Biology of Aging*. New York: Van Nostrand, 1977, pp. 241–61.

BUTLER, R.N., "Overview of the biology of aging," Chairman, a symposium programmed by the Gerontological Society and The American Physiological Society and presented at the 62nd Annual Meeting of the Federation of American Societies for Experimental Biology, Atlantic City, NJ, April 10, 1978. *Fed Proc.*, 38 (1979), 1955–71.

CARANASES, C.J., R.B. STEWART, and L.E. CLUFF, "Drug–induced illness leading to hospitalization," *J. Am. Med. Assoc.*, 228 (1974), 713–17.

CHVAPIL, M., and Z. HVUZA, "The influence of aging and undernutrition on chemical contractility and relaxation of collagen fibers in rats," *Gerontologia*, 3 (1959), 241–52.

DALY, C.H., and G.F. ODLAND, "Age-related changes in the mechanical properties of human skin," *J. Invest. Dermat.*, 73 (1979), 84–7.

ECKER, R.I. and A.L. SCHROETER, "Acrodermatitis and acquired zinc deficiency," *Arch. Dermatol.*, 114 (1978), 937–39.

EPSTEIN, M., "Effects of aging on the kidney," *Fed. Proc.*, 38 (1979), 168–71.

FOUTS, P.J., O.M. HELMER, S. LEPKOVSKY, and T.H. JUKES, "Treatment of human pellagra with nicotinic acid," *Proc. Soc. Exp. Biol. Med.*, 37, 405–7.

FRIEDMAN, M., and R.H. ROSEMAN, "Association of specific overt behavior pattern with blood and cardiovascular findings: Blood cholesterol level, blood clotting time, incidence of arcus senilis, and clinical coronary artery disease," *J. Am. Med. Assoc.*, 169 (1959), 1286–96.

GAIN, S.M., "Bone loss and aging," in *The Physiology and Pathology of Human Aging*, eds. R. Goldman, M. Rockstein, and M.L. Sussman. New York: Academic Press, Inc., 1975, pp. 39–57.

GANZONI, A.M., R. OAKES, and R.S. HILLMAN, "Red cell aging in vivo," *J. Clin. Invest.*, 50 (1971), 1373–78.

GERRITSEN, G.C., "The role of nutrition to diabetes in relation to age," in *Nutrition, Longevity, and Aging*, eds. M. Rockstein and M.L. Sussman. New York: Academic Press, Inc., 1976, pp. 229–52.

GIBSON, I.I.J.M., "Advances in the treatment of leukemia," in *Geriatric Medicine*, eds. W. Ferguson-Anderson and T.G. Judge. London and New York: Academic Press, Inc., 1974, pp. 184–90.

GOLDSTEIN, S., and W. REICHEL, in *Clinical Aspects of Aging*, ed. W. Reichel. Baltimore: Williams and Wilkins Co., 1978, pp. 429–33.

GREGERMAN, R.I., and E.L. BIERMAN, "Aging and hormones," in *Textbook of Endocrinology*, 5th ed., ed. R.H. Williams. Philadelphia: W.B. Saunders Co., 1974, pp. 1059–69.

HARRIS, R., "Cardiac changes with age," in *The Physiology and Pathology of Human Aging*, eds. R. Goldman and M. Rockstein. New York: Academic Press, 1975, pp. 109–22.

HAYFLICK, L., "Cell biology of aging," *Fed. Proc.*, 38 (1979), 1847–50.

HOOK, E.W., "The pneumonias and viral respiratory infections," Vol. 1 in *Bronchopulmonary Diseases and Related Disorders*, eds. C.W. Holman and C. Muschenheim. New York: Harper and Row, 1972, pp. 279-340.

HURST, J.W., R.B. LOGUE, R.C. SCHLANT, and N.K. WENGER, eds., *The Heart, Arteries and Veins*, 3rd Ed. New York: McGraw-Hill, 1974.

IRWIN, M.I., "A conspectus of research on vitamin C requirements of man," *J. Nutr.*, 106 (1976), 821–97.

KALCHTHALER, T., and M.E.R. TAN, "Anemia in institutionalized elderly patients," *J. Amer. Geriat. Soc.*, 28 (1980), 108–13.

LAVKER, R.M., "Structural alterations in exposed and unexposed aged skin," *J. Invest. Dermat.*, 73 (1979), 59–66.

MAKINODAN, T., and W.H. ADLER, "The effects of aging on the differentiation and proliferation of cells of the immune system," *Fed. Proc.*, 34 (1975), 153–58.

MARTIN, G.M., C.A. SPRAGUE, and C.J. EPSTEIN, "Replicative life-span of cultivated human cells: effects of donor's age, tissue and genotype," *Lab. Invest.*, 23 (1970), 86.

MARX, J.J.M, "Normal iron absorption and decreased red cell iron uptake in the aged," *Blood*, 53 (1979), 204–11.

MATZNER, Y., S. LEEVY, N. GROSSOWICZ, G. IZAK, C. HERSHKO, "Prevalence and causes of anemia in elderly hospitalized patients," *Gerontology*, 25 (1979), 113–19.

MAUDERLY, J.L., "Effect of age on preliminary structure and function of immature and adult animals and man," *Fed. Proc.*, 38 (1979), 173–77.

MONTAGNA, W., and K. CARLISLE, "Structural changes in aging human skin," *J. Invest. Dermat.*, 73 (1979), 47–53.

O'MALLEY, K., J. CROOKS, E. DUKE, and I.H. STEVENSON, "Effect of age and sex on human drug metabolism," *Brit. Med. J.*, 3 (1971), 607–9.

PASSMORE, R., and J.S. ROBSON, eds., *A Companion to Medical Studies*, Vol. 3. Part I. Oxford, London, Edinburgh, Melbourne: Blackwell Sci. Publ., 1974, pp. 23.74–23.101.

POOL, J.L., *Carcinoma of the Lung and Trachea in Bronchopulmonary Diseases and Related Disorders,* eds. C.W. Holman and C. Muschenheim. Hagerstown, MD: Harper and Row, 1972.

PORTA, E.A., "Nutritional factors and aging," in *Advances in Modern Human Nutrition,* eds. R.B. Tobin and M.A. Mehlman. Park Forest South, IL: Pathotox Publ. Co., 1980, pp. 65–119.

PROCKOP, J.D., and others, "The biosynthesis of collagen and its disorders," Part 2. *New Eng. J. Med.*, 301 (1979), 77–85.

RODRIGUEZ, M.S., "Conspectus of research on folacin requirements of man," *J. Nutr.*, 108 (1978), 1983–2103.

ROE, D.A., *Drug-Induced Nutritional Deficiencies.* Westport, CT: AVI Publ. Co., 1976, pp. 36–38.

ROSEN, H., "Renal disease in the elderly," *Med. Clin. N. Amer.*, 60 (1976), 1105–19.

ROTH, M., "Diagnosis of senile and related forms of dementia," in *Alzheimer's Disease: Senile Dementia and Related Disorders* (Aging, vol. 7), eds. R. Katzman, R.D. Terry, and K.L. Bich. New York: Raven Press, 1978, pp. 71–85.

SCHIFFMAN, S.S., "Food recognition by the elderly," *J. Gerontol.*, 32 (1977), 586–92.

SEBRELL, W.H. and R.E. BUTLER, "Riboflavin deficiency in man," *Public Health Rep.*, 53 (1938), 2282.

SHAW, J.H. and E.A. SWEENEY, "Nutrition in relation to dental medicine," in *Modern Nutrition in Health and Disease*, 6th Ed., eds. R.S. Goodhart and M.E. Shils. Philadelphia: Lea & Febiger, 1980, pp. 886–90.

SLATER, T.F., *Free Radical Mechanisms in Tissue Injury.* London: Pion Ltd., 1972.

SMITH, R., "Bone disease in the elderly," *Proc. Roy. Soc. Med.*, 69 (1976), 925–26.

SOREMARK, R., and B. NILSSON, "Dental status and nutrition in old age," in *Nutrition in Old Age*, Symp. Swedish Nutrition Foundation, ed. L.A. Carlson. Uppsala: Almqvist and Wiksell, 1972, pp. 147–66.

SOWRANDER, P., and H. SJOGREN, "The concept of Alzheimer's disease and its clinical implications," in *Alzheimer's Disease and Related Conditions*. London: J. & A. Churchill, 1970, pp. 11–32.

STEFFEE, W.P., "Nutrition intervention in hospitalized geriatric patients," *Bull. N.Y. Acad. Med.*, 56 (1980), 564–74.

STEINBERG, W.M., and P.P. TOSKES, "A practical approach to evaluating maldigestion and malabsorption," *Geriatrics*, 33 (1978), 73–85.

STEINHEBER, F.U., "Interpretation of gastrointestinal symptoms in the elderly," *Med. Clin. N. Amer.*, 60 (1976), 1141–57.

VAVRIK, M., " 'High risk' factors and atherosclerotic cardiovascular diseases in the aged," *J. Amer. Geriat. Soc.*, 22 (1974), 203–7.

VERBOV, N.J., *Skin Diseases in the Elderly.* London: Wm. Heinemann Med. Books Ltd., 1974, p. 187.

VESTAL, R.E., "Methodological problems associated with studies of drug metabolism in the elderly," in *Clinical Pharmacology and Therapeutics.*, Proc. First World Conf. Clin. Pharmacol. Therap., London, Aug 3–9, 1980. London and Basingstroke: Macmillan Publ. Co., 1980.

WEALE, R.A., "The effects of the ageing lens on vision," in *The Human Lens in Relation to Cataract*, Ciba Foundation Series 19. Amsterdam, New York, London: N.S. Elsevier, Excerpta Med., North Holland Assoc. Sci. Publ., 1973, pp. 5–20.

WEKSLER, M.E., J.E. INNES, and G. GOLDSTEIN, "The role of the thymus in the senescence of the immune response," in *Aging and Immunity*, eds. S.K. Singal, N.R. Sinclair, and C.R. Stiller. New York: Elsevier/North Holland, 1979, pp. 165–72.

WENE, J.D., W.E. CONNOR, and L. DENBENSTEN, "The development of essential fatty acid deficiency in men fed fat-free diets intravenously and orally," *J. Clin. Invest.*, 56 (1975), 127–34.

WORMSLEY, K.G., *The Skin and Gut in Disease*. London: Pitman Medical Publ. Co. Ltd., 1964.

YAHR, M.D., "Levodopa," *Ann. Intern Med.*, 83 (1975), 677–82.

# CHAPTER THREE
# The Nutritional Status of the Elderly

In the last fifteen years, several studies have been conducted to investigate the nutritional status of elderly populations in industrialized countries. Prior assumptions have been that there might be a high incidence of malnutrition among elderly people because of constraints on their ability to obtain a nutritious diet, because of the adverse nutritional effects of chronic disease, because therapeutic drugs might impair nutritional status, or because of interactive or additive effects of these variables. Surveys that have been performed have either examined the nutritional status of independently-living elderly or the nutritional status of geriatric patients in institutions. Major questions asked in the surveys have been whether the elderly have too little to eat, whether they exhibit clinical signs of nutritional disease, and whether they show hematological or biochemical evidence of subclinical nutritional deficiencies. Another survey goal has been to determine, by repeated surveys of the same population, whether nutritional status deteriorates with advancing age. Longitudinal studies have also looked at changes in anthropometric measurements and body composition with age. Findings have been that the nutrition of the elderly varies according to chronological age, sex, health status, and living situations (O'Hanlon and Kohrs, 1978).

Difficulties have been encountered in obtaining reliable estimates of food-energy and nutrient intakes. Most surveys have found a low prevalence of clinical signs which could be proven to be due to nutritional deficiency. Severely malnourished persons among the independently-living sample populations have been eccentric, socially isolated, and lacking in interest in their own well-being (Clark et al., 1975). Severely malnourished institutionalized patients have chronic severe physical and mental disorders including dementias. Biochemical evidence of the presence of one or more vitamin deficiencies has been common, especially among persons over 75 years of age (Exton-Smith, 1972; Kalchthaler and Tan, 1980; Steffee, 1980). Change in body composition with age has been found with increase in body fat in certain age groups.

## SURVEYS OF INDEPENDENTLY-LIVING ELDERLY POPULATIONS

Longitudinal nutrition studies of the elderly have been conducted in the United Kingdom by Exton-Smith and his coworkers. The first extensive survey by this group was conducted from 1967–68. The study population consisted in independently-living people over the age of 65 living in four areas of England and two areas in Scotland (Exton-Smith, 1979). The survey, published in 1972, showed differences in nutrient intakes between men and women, between people of different age groups, and also between the different study areas. For the most part, differences in nutrient intake reflected variations in total food-energy consumption. Malnutrition was diagnosed in 3 percent of the total study population of 879 persons. For the most part, malnutrition was associated with disease, but in about 2 percent of those who were malnourished, no obvious medical cause was found, nor could malnutrition be attributed to dietary inadequacy on the basis of poverty. The incidence of subclinical malnutrition was difficult to assess because normal ranges of biochemical indices of nutritional status for the older-age groups are unknown.

A subsample of the same study population agreed to participate in another nutritional survey in 1972–73. This subsample were still living in their own homes. The 1979 report by Exton-Smith's group describes findings in 365 subjects who participated fully in both surveys. It was found that in the total group, men and women aged 80 years or over had lower mean daily intakes of food-energy than younger persons. However, the healthy persons who were 80 years or over had mean daily food-energy intakes that were not significantly different from those of persons less than 80 years of age. It was therefore assumed that lower intakes of food-energy were in those who were not in good health. Housebound men and women had lower food-energy intakes than those who were mobile. Men had higher food-energy intakes than women. Food-energy intakes were not statistically greater in obese subjects, but were greater in taller men and women and in men with larger arm muscle measurements, which may reflect total muscle mass. Tentative explanation of this finding was that physical activity, which would be reflected in large muscle mass, is an important determinant of food-energy intake.

The nutrient density of the diet was similar for both men and women. Twenty-six (7.1 percent) of the 365 participants were considered to be clinically malnourished. Malnutrition was more than twice as common in subjects of 80 years or more than in subjects under that age. Malnutrition included scurvy, osteomalacia, and nutritional anemias. Several people had multiple nutritional deficiencies. Diets of the malnourished were of poor nutritional quality. Medical factors related to malnutrition were history of partial gastrectomy, chronic bronchitis and emphysema, depression, dementia, difficulty in swallowing, and non-use or nonavailability of dentures. Housebound individuals were more likely to be malnourished. The housebound had lower nutrient intakes. There was an association between lower nutrient intakes of the housebound elderly and the presence of chronic disease. It was inferred that lower nutrient intakes of the housebound elderly could also be related to decreased physical activity and poorer choice of food. The housebound had less satisfactory vitamin D status, which was probably due to lack of sunlight exposure.

A gerontological survey was carried out in the city of Göteborg, Sweden, in which food-energy and nutrient intakes, meal habits, body composition, and laboratory tests of the nutritional status of 70-year-old men and women were observed (Göteborg study, 1977). In Sweden the life expectancy for males is 73 years and for females, 77 years. The study was started in 1971/72 with an investigation of a representative sample of about three-tenths of the 70 year olds in the city population. Only about 3 percent of these 70 year olds had handicaps or diseases for which institutionalization was required. The physical and mental condition of the subjects was generally good.

The dietary habits of a subsample of 191 males and 199 females were studied and among these, 182 males and 188 females took part in the complete dietary interview. In this population the dietary history method gave a better estimate of food intake than 24-hour recalls. On an average, 1.8 hot meals and 0.9 light meals of a beverage and a sandwich were consumed daily. Intakes of energy and nutrients were variable, but generally satisfactory. Significant associations were found between sources of intake of energy and nutrients. Subjects with an education beyond elementary school showed a higher proportion of energy intake from protein than other subjects. Males who lived alone had lower iron intakes than other males.

In a comparison between this study and a study of middle-aged women in Göteborg, it was shown that energy intakes and body composition were similar in the two groups.

Body composition studies were carried out on a subsample of 49 males and 56 females. Average values for body weight were 76.2 kg for males and 66.3 kg for females. Males at the age of 70 years had a higher relative body cell mass than females and slightly more extracellular water, but their body fat mass, as calculated, was little over half that of the females (Table 3-1).

Biochemical indicators of nutritional status showed inter-subject variability but no consistent differences between men and women. Hemoglobin levels were lower in females than in males.

**TABLE 3-1   Body Composition of Elderly Men and Women
in the Göteborg Study**

|  | MALES | | FEMALES | |
|---|---|---|---|---|
|  | MEAN | SD | MEAN | SD |
| Height (cm) | 173 | 5.9 | 160 | 6.0 |
| Body weight (kg) | 76.2 | 11.1 | 66.3 | 12.4 |
| Absolute values (kg) | | | | |
| BCM | 28.1 | 3.5 | 20.3 | 2.7 |
| ECW | 26.5 | 5.0 | 20.0 | 4.3 |
| BF | 12.5 | 6.5 | 18.1 | 7.2 |
| Relative values (percent of BW) | | | | |
| BCM | 37.1 | 4.0 | 30.9 | 4.0 |
| ECW | 34.9 | 5.6 | 30.2 | 4.9 |
| BF | 16.1 | 7.0 | 26.6 | 6.7 |

Adapted from B. Steen et al., "Body composition in 70-year-old males and females in Göteborg, Sweden, a population study," *Acta Med. Scand.*, Suppl. 611 (1977), p. 97.

Anthropometric data and information on body composition were also obtained for women living in Göteborg (Noppa et al., 1980). The women were initially studied in 1968 and 1969, and again from 1971–75. Body height was found to decrease with age. The reduction in body height was greater at higher ages. Body weight increased with age, the change however was partly a cohort effect and partly a time effect of age. Arm muscle mass decreased with age. The increase in subcutaneous fat with age was both in the arm and in the trunk. However, between the initial study and the follow-up, body fat did not change significantly.

A recent study of the nutritional status of apparently healthy, independently-living elderly people in Corvallis, Oregon included dietary and biochemical assessment (Yearick et al., 1980). The total sample consisted in 100 persons (75 women and 25 men). Calcium, vitamin A, and thiamin were the dietary nutrients most likely to be low, particularly in women. Nutrient supplements taken were frequently inappropriate and often excessive. The mean biochemical indices of nutritional status were within acceptable limits.

In a randomly selected subsample of 20 persons, 11 subjects had serum folacin below an acceptable level of 6 ng/ml, and of these, three had values in the deficiency range. Mean calculated intake of folacin for this group was very low, but the author would caution interpretation because of missing and inaccurate values in food composition tables.

## NATIONAL NUTRITION SURVEYS
## IN THE UNITED STATES

The Ten-State Nutrition Survey 1968–70 was limited to Washington, California, Texas, Louisiana, South Carolina, Kentucky, West Virginia, Michigan, Massachusetts and New York, including a separate survey of New York City (DHEW Publ. 72-8131; 72-8133; 72-8134). The primary interest in each of these states was the evaluation of malnutrition among the poor. Sampling procedures used are believed to have produced a representative sample of low income families but higher income families, also included in the sample, are not thought to have been representative of middle and high income families.

The evaluation of nutritional status involved 40,000 individuals. High-risk subgroup populations included in the sample were persons over 60 years of age.

The total survey included more than 86,000 individuals (23,846 families) of which 10.9 percent were 60 years of age or more. According to the survey report, these people consumed less food than was needed to meet nutrient standards for their age, sex, and weight. However, the reliability of the data is in some doubt, because of dependence on 24-hour recalls in all states surveyed except Missouri, where a dietary history was obtained. Limiting nutrients were protein, iron, vitamin A, and calcium in older men. There was no strong relationship between dietary intake and income. Dietary intakes were positively related to biochemical findings. Although there was a high incidence of obesity in the total adult population sample studied, the mean triceps skinfold thickness was lower in females and (more strikingly) in males over 60 years.

The First Health and Nutrition Examination Survey (HANES I) was conducted between 1971–1974 (O'Hanlon and Kohrs, 1978). The population sample for HANES I was meant to be a representative sample of the U.S. population. In fact, it was a stratified probability sample of the noninstitutionalized population between the ages of 1 and 74 years. Dietary information was obtained from a 24-hour recall and a food frequency interview. In the preliminary report of HANES I, low intakes of iron were prevalent in the low income older group.

O'Hanlon and Kohrs (1978) point out that it is difficult to compare nutritional surveys which include or focus on the elderly because of differences in dietary methodology and standards.

## COMPARISON OF INDEPENDENTLY-LIVING
## AND INSTITUTIONALIZED ELDERLY

The nutritional status of institutionalized and independently living elderly has been studied in Belfast, Northern Ireland (Vir and Love, 1979). There were 196 subjects over 65 years of age who were either in hospital geriatric units, in sheltered living facilities, or in residential accommodation. All subjects were grouped according to whether they did or did not take multivitamin supplements.

Three-day weighed diet records were obtained, clinical examination was undertaken, and there was biochemical assessment of nutritional status. Energy intake of females in the geriatric units and in sheltered dwellings was considered to be "comparatively low." The energy intakes of these institutionalized groups were lower than the noninstitutionalized group.

Dietary nutrients which were least often adequate in amount were potassium, magnesium, vitamin D, and vitamin $B_6$. Clinical signs of malnutrition were rare. According to the definition of anemia used (<13.0 g/dl hemoglobin for males and <12.0 g/dl for females), 18.6 percent of the sample were anemic. Of the subjects not on multivitamin preparations, 91.3 percent had some biochemical evidence of nutritional deficiency, and among subjects who were receiving multivitamin preparations, 64.3 percent had biochemical evidence of a vitamin or mineral deficiency.

The authors conclude that although intake of multivitamin preparations may help to alleviate subclinical deficiencies, vitamin A requirements were not met by these preparations. The question to be asked is whether patients took the nutrient supplements regularly.

The prevalence and causes of anemia in the elderly have been studied. A study was carried out by Matzner et al. (1979) in Jerusalem of 104 patients over 60 admitted to a general ward. In males and females, mean hemoglobin levels were approximately 1g less than healthy younger persons. Of the patients who had hemoglobin values of less than 11 g/dl, none could be identified as having a primary nutritional anemia. Most common causes of anemia were chronic renal failure, metastatic carcinoma, gastrointestinal bleeding, and infection.

Major areas needing further research include

1. Food-energy needs of sedentary and bedridden nursing home patients.
2. Nutrient needs of these same patients.
3. The means to best carry out nutritional screening and assessment of geriatric patients in these facilities.
4. The interpretation of clinical, anthropometric, hematological, and biochemical indices of nutritional status in chronically sick elderly patients with or without skin disease, with or without disease-related muscle wasting, with or without anemia which may be multifactorial, and with or without renal failure which will influence blood levels and urinary levels of nutrients.
5. The responsiveness of patients showing one or more indices of malnutrition to nutrient supplementation.
6. Acceptable values for nutritional status indicators in nursing home patients.

It is necessary to develop and carry out a national survey of geriatric patients in institutions in the United States, as well as of homebound individuals.

Constraints on performance of major nutritional surveys of institutional-ized geriatric patients are

1. Lack of planning
2. Inadequate methodology
3. Need for informed consent of participants
4. Lack of funds
5. Lack of commitment

## QUESTIONS

1. Are the following statements true or false?
   a) Nutrition of the elderly varies with chronological age.
   b) Differences in nutrient intake frequency reflect change in food-energy consumption.
   c) Malnutrition is usually associated with disease.
   d) Normal ranges for biochemical indices of nutritional status for the elderly are not known.

2. Medical factors related to malnutrition in the Exton-Smith survey were (circle all correct answers):
   a) history of partial gastrectomy
   b) chronic bronchitis and emphysema
   c) dementia
   d) blindness
   e) deafness

3. Common causes of anemia in elderly hospitalized patients are (circle all correct answers):
   a) low intake of liver
   b) chronic renal failure
   c) gastrointestinal bleeding
   d) low iron absorption
   e) anticoagulant therapy

4. Malnutrition in the elderly may be related to one or more causes. Separate the causes into two groups, specifying which causes are more likely to occur in 1)independently living and 2) institutionalized (or hospitalized) patients.
   a) Social isolation
   b) Dementias
   c) Psychoses
   d) Lack of self-interest
   e) Chronic renal failure

5. Are the following statements true or false?
   a) The nutritional status of patients in nursing homes in the U.S. is known from a recent national survey.
   b) Most patients in nursing homes in the U.S. are malnourished.
   c) In several independent studies of nursing home patients there has been a high prevalence of anemia.

# REFERENCES

CLARK, A.N.G., G.D. MANKIKAR, and I. GRAY, "Diogenes syndrome, a clinical study of gross neglect in old age," *Lancet*, 1 (1975), 366–68.

EXTON-SMITH, A.N., "Physiological aspects of aging: relationship to nutrition," *Amer. J. Clin. Nutr.*, 25 (1972), 853–59.

The Gerontological and Geriatric Population Study in Göteborg, Sweden. *Acta Med. Scand.*, Suppl. 611 (1977), 3–112.

KALCHTHALER, T., and M.E. RIGOR TAN, "Anemia in institutionalized elderly patients," *J. Amer. Geriat. Soc.*, 28 (1980), 108–13.

MATZNER, Y., S. LEVY, N. GROSSOWICZ, G. IZAK, and C. HERSHKO, "Prevalence and causes of anemia in elderly hospitalized patients," *Gerontology*, 25 (1979), 113–19.

NOPPA, H., M. ANDERSSON, G. BERGTSSON, et al., "Longitudinal studies of anthropometric data and body composition. The population study of women in Göteborg, Sweden." *Amer. J. Clin. Nutr.*, 33 (1980), 155–62.

*Nutrition and Health in Old Age.* The cross-sectional analysis of the findings of a survey made in 1972/3 of elderly people who had been studied in 1967/8. Report by the Committee on Medical Aspects of Food Policy, Department of Health and Social Security Report on Health and Social Subjects #16. Her Majesty's Stationery Office, London, 1979.

O'HANLON, P., and M.B. KOHRS, "Dietary studies of older Americans," *Amer. J. Clin. Nutr.*, 31 (1978), 1257–69.

*Reports on Health and Social Subjects #3*, A nutrition survey of the elderly. Department of Health and Social Security. Her Majesty's Stationery Office, London, 1972.

STEFFEE, W.P., "Nutritional intervention in hospitalized geriatric patients," *Bull. N.Y. Acad. Med.*, 56 (1980), 564–74.

Ten-State Nutritional Survey 1968–70. Highlights. DHEW Publ. No. (HSM) 72-8134.

Ten-State Nutritional Survey 1968–70. III. Clinical; Anthropometry; Dental. DHEW Publ. No. (HSM) 72-8131.

Ten-State Nutritional Survey 1968–70. V. Dietary. DHEW Publ. No. (HSM) 72-8133.

VIR, S.C., and A.H.G. LOVE, "Nutritional status of institutionalized and non-institutionalized aged in Belfast, Northern Ireland," *Amer. J. Clin. Nutr.*, 32 (1979), 1934–47.

YEARICK, E.S., M-S. L. WANG, and S.J. PISIAS, "Nutritional status of the elderly: Dietary and biochemical findings." *J. Gerontol.*, 35 (1980), 663–71.

# CHAPTER FOUR
# Nutritional Requirements

## FOOD ENERGY AND NUTRIENT NEEDS

While there is evidence that the nutritional needs of most adults are qualitatively the same, quantitative requirements differ with age. Quantitative differences in energy and nutrient requirements vary with physiological and pathological conditions. It has been shown that nutritional requirements may change with age because of an alteration in the amount of physical activity, a change in the weight and composition of the body, or a decrease in muscular efficiency (Durnin, 1964).

The total energy production per square meter of body surface falls progressively with advancing age. The average reduction in energy production is about 12 calories/meter$^2$ per hour between the ages of 20 and 90 years. These decrements may be due to a loss of metabolizing tissue. The reduction in the energy metabolism of older people is related both to a decrease in physical activity, which becomes most pronounced after the age of 75, and to tissue loss (Exton-Smith, 1972).

Decreased nutrient absorption and increased nutrient losses will increase nutrient requirements. Nutrient absorption may decrease with aging. In catabolic states associated with injury or surgery or with acute or certain chronic diseases of the elderly, negative nitrogen balance occurs, implying that nitrogen losses exceed usual dietary nitrogen intake. In these conditions, protein deficiency can be averted if proteins of high biological value are fed at a level to meet the increased nitrogen requirements. However, there is no sound scientific evidence that, in the absence of catabolic states or states of malabsorption (when fecal nitrogen losses are high) the nitrogen requirements of the elderly are greater than those of younger persons. Since muscle mass decreases with age, it might be anticipated that protein requirements would decrease. Healthy elderly subjects have not been found to require more protein per unit of body weight than younger subjects studied under similar conditions.

In defining the individual protein or nitrogen requirements of the elderly, several factors need to be considered. Physiological changes that occur with aging which could alter protein requirement include reduced daily synthesis of body protein and reduction in lean body mass (Winterer et al., 1976; Forbes and Reina, 1970). However, there is no good evidence that these factors reduce protein requirements, perhaps because aging is also associated with a reduced efficiency of protein utilization (Zanni et al., 1979). There is a decline in renal function related to aging, and further chronic renal disease is common in the elderly. The work of the kidney is increased by the need to excrete nitrogenous end products of dietary protein when intake is high. Further reduction in renal function and retention of toxic nitrogenous waste are a result. When elderly patients have impaired renal function, total protein in the diet should be restricted but proteins supplied should be of high biological value (Exton-Smith and Overstall, 1979).

On the other hand, in considering the protein needs of the elderly, it has to be remembered that animal protein foods are rich sources of heme iron, calcium, vitamins A and D, riboflavin, niacin, and vitamin $B_{12}$ (Smith, 1965). Further prevention of protein deficiency with attendant hypoalbuminemia is most important in the elderly when protein-bound drugs are being taken. In the presence of hypoalbuminemia, less of the drug is bound to albumin and therefore more of the drug will reach receptor sites which can result in drug toxicity. Dietary protein deficiency also increases the risk of certain hepatotoxic drugs (Vestal, 1980).

Nutrient requirements are dependent on many environmental factors, including drug intake and exposure to sunlight. Drugs can increase nutrient requirements because of drug-induced malabsorption or malutilization of nutrients. Dietary requirements for vitamin D increase if the level of ultraviolet light exposure is reduced so that less of the vitamin is synthesized in the skin. Vitamin D requirements are also increased by intake of certain drugs, e.g. phenobarbital and diphenylhydantoin (Dilantin). Development of osteomalacia in elderly, housebound people is related to lack of adjustment upwards of the dietary intake of vitamin D when the patient is no longer exposed to sunlight and when the patient is taking drugs that affect vitamin D needs (Roe, 1976).

There is a lack of agreement as to whether the elderly have a high requirement for selected nutrients (Munro, 1980). The assumption is that if the nutritional requirements of elderly persons are in the same range as those of younger people, then, at similar levels of intake, nutritional status measurements would be similar. The logic of this approach would be satisfactory if we could be assured that our present means of determining nutritional adequacy are rational in that they determine functional adequacy. Currently we are concerned that it may be necessary to compute nutritional adequacy differently in the elderly than in younger persons. Correlations have been found in the elderly between dietary intake of specific nutrients and biochemical measurements of nutritional status. These relationships can be assessed in elderly persons of above average health. However, the relationship between dietary intake of nutrients and functional nutritional normalcy may be altered by disease or by drugs. Needs for specific nutrients may be increased by progressive loss of tissue function attendant upon aging. In a British nutritional survey of the elderly and of younger people, none of the hematological indices of nutritional status showed significant differences between age groups (Nutrition and Health in Old Age, 1979). On the other hand, mean values for serum iron, folacin, vitamin $B_{12}$, and pyridoxine concentration were lower for subjects in the survey who were above 65 years of age (Exton-Smith and Overstall, 1979). Considerations at present are:

1. Can we attempt dietary recommendations which mitigate against development of aging changes in body composition?
2. Since aging results in the accumulation of disease such as osteoporosis, atherosclerosis, and cancer, which are at least in part age-related, can we offer guidelines for the diets of younger people to be continued throughout life which will protect them from the development of these diseases?
3. What are the criteria which we should be employing in order to understand the nutrient needs of the old?

Age-related changes in body composition, reduction in cardiac, respiratory, hepatic, and renal function as well as the decline in capacity for sustained exercise may influence nutritional needs. Further, in the elderly a slowed rate of homeostatic regulation and enzyme induction may affect nutrient requirements. Whereas we do have good evidence that the energy needs of the elderly are reduced, we do not as yet have any good basis for recommending that nutrient requirements of the healthy elderly are different from those of the young, unless disease is present or drugs are being taken which increase specific nutrient needs (Harper, 1978). To reduce energy intakes in the elderly and to maintain nutrient intakes at levels which are optimal for health in young persons, the elderly will need to consume diets of higher nutrient-to-energy ratios.

It has been suggested that one way to determine needs of the elderly for particular nutrients could be by incremental addition of that nutrient to the basal diet while sequential tests of nutritional status are performed. This approach presupposes that it is possible to demonstrate a change in functional efficiency with nutrient intake. Our capabilities in this area are limited and, further, it is very possible that optimum nutrition for one physiological function, e.g. erythropoiesis (formation of red blood cells) is not the same as optimum nutrition for another function, e.g. metabolism of foreign compounds such as therapeutic drugs.

As we move towards a better definition of the nutritional needs of the elderly, two concepts must be born in mind. First, our goal is to provide guidelines for nutrient intakes by the elderly which will allow the best health protection of the most people in different age ranges 65 years and over and, second, we must obtain more precise information about the long-term diets of very old people who have remained healthy until an advanced age. It is well documented that patterns of eating laid down in early life are generally maintained through the life span. Therefore, if particular patterns of food and nutrient consumption are correlated with extended longevity, a sensible recommendation might be to use such a diet as a guideline for nutrient needs of the elderly. Limitations of this approach are twofold: first, the diet of the long-lived healthy person may, for its desired effect, have to be maintained over a period of years and not suddenly imposed in later life, and second, it must be remembered that all persons are not alike, and that nutrient requirements for health maintenance are influenced by genetic as well as by environmental factors (Munro and Everett, 1981).

## RECOMMENDED DIETARY ALLOWANCES FOR THE ELDERLY

In the 1980 Recommended Dietary Allowances (Table 4-1), it is proposed that "energy allowances for persons between 51 and 75 years of age be reduced to about 90 percent of the amount required as a young adult and for persons beyond 75 years about 75–80 percent of that amount." The Food and Nutrition Board of the National Academy of Sciences based their recommendation on studies of the adult population which showed that body composition changes through life with the proportion of fat increasing, that with increasing age, metabolically active tissues are slowly reduced, and that physical activity declines with age. In making this recommendation for reduced food energy needs for elderly people, caution is requested by the Food and Nutrition Board, lest with reduction in food intake, amounts of essential nutrients fall below desirable levels.

For people 50 years and over, it is recommended that at least 12 percent of calories should be provided by protein to ensure protein needs for maintenance of nitrogen balance in health and in convalescence from recurring diseases requiring repletion of body protein (Young et al., 1976).

Since it is desirable that elderly people consume diets of high nutrient density, the Food and Nutrition Board suggests that a different computation of nutrient requirements for the elderly as unit weight of that nutrient per 1000 kilocalories should be used; that is, the elderly need more of certain nutrients per 1000 kcal than younger people.

TABLE 4-1  Recommended Dietary Allowances
for the Elderly[a]

|  | MALES | FEMALES |
|---|---|---|
| Age | 51+ | 51+ |
| Weight (kg) | 70 | 55 |
| (lb) | 154 | 120 |
| Height (cm) | 178 | 163 |
| (in) | 70 | 64 |
| Protein (g) | 56 | 44 |
| Vitamin A ($\mu$g RE)[b] | 1000 | 800 |
| Vitamin D ($\mu$g)[c] | 5 | 5 |
| Vitamin E (mg $\alpha$-TE)[d] | 10 | 8 |
| Vitamin C (mg) | 60 | 60 |
| Thiamin (mg) | 1.2 | 1.0 |
| Riboflavin (mg) | 1.4 | 1.2 |
| Niacin (mg NE)[e] | 16 | 13 |
| Vitamin $B_6$ (mg) | 2.2 | 2.0 |
| Folacin ($\mu$g)[f] | 400 | 400 |
| Vitamin $B_{12}$ ($\mu$g) | 3.0 | 3.0 |
| Calcium (mg) | 800 | 800 |
| Phosphorus (mg) | 800 | 800 |
| Magnesium (mg) | 350 | 300 |
| Iron (mg) | 10 | 10 |
| Zinc (mg) | 15 | 15 |
| Iodine ($\mu$g) | 150 | 150 |

[a] The allowances are intended to provide for individual variations among most normal persons as they live in the United States under usual environmental stresses. Diets should be based on a variety of common foods in order to provide other nutrients for which human requirements have been less well defined.

[b] Retinol equivalents. 1 retinol equivalent = 1 $\mu$g retinol or 6 $\mu$g $\beta$ carotene.

[c] As cholecalciferol. 10 $\mu$g cholecalciferol = 400 IU of vitamin D.

[d] $\alpha$-tocopherol equivalents. 1 mg *d-$\alpha$* tocopherol = 1$\alpha$-TE.

[e] 1 NE (niacin equivalent) is equal to 1 mg of niacin or 60 mg of dietary tryptophan.

[f] The folacin allowances refer to dietary sources as determined by *Lactobacillus casei* assay after treatment with enzymes (conjugases) to make polyglutamyl forms of the vitamin available to the test organ.

Adapted from Food and Nutrition Board, National Academy of Sciences, *National Research Council Recommended Daily Dietary Allowances,* Revised 1980 (9th Ed., Washington, D.C.).

Specific recommendations for higher nutrient requirements for the elderly are not given in the 1980 RDA Handbook, since present knowledge does not justify such recommendation. Megadoses of vitamins are not required by the elderly and such intakes may impose specific health risks. Pharmacological intakes of niacin are strongly discouraged because of the high incidence of cardiac arythmias, abnormal biochemical findings, and gastrointestinal problems. Pharmacological doses of vitamins C and E are not recommended because of lack of evidence that healthy elderly persons benefit from these nutrient supplements. Intake of vitamin D above the recommended allowance is not recommended for the healthy elderly because of potential toxicity.

## RELATIONSHIPS BETWEEN FOOD AND NUTRIENT INTAKE

Patterns of food intake determine nutrient intake. The diversity or variety of foods consumed has a profound influence on the nutrient quality of the diet. It can be generalized that a broad selection of foods from different food groups provides assurance against dietary deficiency of essential nutrients. Food groups that are generally recognized are 1) dairy products, 2) the ''meat'' group or other protein-rich foods, 3) vegetables and fruits, and 4) cereal products. Elderly people should eat two servings daily of dairy products, one to two servings of the meat group, four servings of vegetables and fruits (which may include fruit juices), and four servings of cereals. Table 4-2 indicates foods which elderly adults should eat daily from the different food groups. Justification of this approach to dietary adequacy is that foods from the various food groups complement one another in supplying needed nutrients. Food sources of specific nutrients are indicated in Table 4-3. When elderly people consume less than the recommended number of servings of food from the different food groups, the risk is that one or more nutrients may be consumed in less than optimal amounts. For example, elderly individuals who do not eat or drink dairy products are likely to consume too little calcium, vitamin D, and riboflavin for their needs.

Those who do not eat green vegetables or fruits may be at risk of not obtaining enough folacin, vitamin C, beta carotene, and potassium for their needs.

While omission of dairy food, green vegetables, and fruit from the daily diet can be accepted as an index of a poor quality diet, alternate means of satisfying nutrient needs are now available. One may take vitamin-mineral mixtures in physiological doses or a formula-type nutrient supplement. If an elderly individual will drink a small volume of milk per day, important nutrient requirements can be supplied by eating one to two servings of fortified

**TABLE 4-2    Recommended Daily Foods from the Four Food Groups**

| GROUP | FOOD | SERVINGS | HOUSEHOLD MEASURE |
|-------|------|----------|-------------------|
| Dairy | Milk, skim | 2 | 16 oz. |
|       | -or- | | |
|       | American cheese + | 1 | 1 slice |
|       | Ice cream | 1 | 1/2 cup |
| Meat  | Chicken + | 1 | 3 oz. |
|       | Peanut butter | 1 | 1 tbsp. |
|       | -or- | | |
|       | Lean beef, lamb, or veal + | 1 | 3 oz. |
|       | Peas | 1 | 1/2 cup |
| Vegetables | Broccoli + | 1 | 1/2 cup |
| and Fruits | Tomatoes + | 1 | 2 medium |
|       | Orange juice | 2 | 1-1/2 cups |
|       | -or- | | |
|       | Carrots + | 1 | 1/2 cup |
|       | Spinach + | 1 | 1/2 cup |
|       | Canteloupe + | 1 | 1/2 |
|       | Orange juice | 1 | 3/4 cup |
| Breads and | Bread, enriched + | 3 | 3 slices |
| Cereals | Cold cereal, fortified | 1 | 1/2 cup |
|       | -or- | | |
|       | Bran muffin + | 2 | 2 |
|       | Rice, enriched + | 1 | 1/2 cup |
|       | Bread, enriched whole wheat | 1 | 1 slice |

**TABLE 4-3    Food Sources of Specific Nutrients**

| FOOD | NUTRIENTS |
|------|-----------|
| Milk | Protein, vitamins A, D, $B_2$, $B_{12}$, calcium |
| Cheese | Protein, vitamins $B_2$ and $B_{12}$, calcium |
| Ice cream | Vitamin $B_2$, calcium |
| Chicken | Protein, niacin, vitamin $B_{12}$, iron |
| Peanut butter | Protein, fat |
| Fish | Protein, iron |
| Peas | Protein, vitamin $B_1$, niacin, zinc |
| Broccoli | Pro-vitamin A, vitamin C, folacin, potassium |
| Tomatoes | Vitamin C |
| Orange juice | Vitamin C, potassium |
| Carrots | Pro-vitamin A |
| Spinach | Pro-vitamin A, vitamin C, folacin, vitamin K, iron, potassium |
| Canteloupe | Vitamin C, potassium |
| Bread, enriched whole wheat | Carbohydrate, vitamins $B_1$, $B_2$, niacin, magnesium |
| Cereals, fortified | Carbohydrate, vitamins A, C, $B_1$, $B_2$, niacin, folacin, $B_6$ (+ fiber) |
| Bran muffins | Carbohydrate, B vitamins (+ fiber), vitamins $B_1$, $B_2$, niacin, magnesium |
| Rice, enriched | Carbohydrate, thiamin |

**TABLE 4-4  Alternate Means of Supplying Daily Nutrient Needs**

| A. LOW CALORIE MENU OF MANY NUTRIENT-RICH FOODS | B. HIGH CALORIE MENU WITH FEW NUTRIENT-RICH FOODS |
|---|---|
| RECOMMENDED | NOT RECOMMENDED |

*Breakfast*

| | |
|---|---|
| Orange juice, 1 glass | Apple juice, 1 glass |
| Cereal, 3/4 oz. | Frozen waffles, 2 |
| Milk, skim, 1 glass | Syrup, 2 tbsp. |
| | Margarine, 2 tsp. |
| | Whole milk, 1 cup |

*Lunch*

| | |
|---|---|
| Grilled cheese sandwich, 1 | Chicken noodle soup, 1 can |
| (whole wheat bread, 2 slices, | Saltine crackers, 8 |
| American cheese, 1 slice) | Cake, marble, 1 slice |
| Banana, 1 | |

*Dinner*

| | |
|---|---|
| Chicken, 3 oz. | Beef pot pie, 1 |
| Spinach, 1/2 cup | Broccoli, 1/2 cup |
| Potato, baked, 1 small | Sherbet, 1/2 cup |
| Margarine, 1 tbsp. | Cookies, 5 |
| Orange, whole, 1 med. | |

*Snack*

| | |
|---|---|
| Milk, skim, 1 glass | Salted roast peanuts, 1/4 cup |
| | Milk chocolate bar, 2 oz. |
| | Whole milk, 1 cup |

*Number of foods*

| | |
|---|---|
| 10 | 14 |

*Total Kcal*

| | |
|---|---|
| 1200 | 2600 |

*RDA*

| | |
|---|---|
| Meets or exceeds in all specified nutrients if cereal is fortified. | Low in protein, vitamins A, D, C, $B_1$, $B_2$, niacin, folacin, calcium, and potassium if milk and broccoli are omitted. |
| | High in sodium. |

**C. SEMISYNTHETIC LIQUID DIET**

Full liquid diets containing nutrients $\geq$ RDA can be supplied by Ensure (Ross), formulated to give 2000 kcal in 2 quarts. Indications for use of Ensure as a total liquid diet are when solid food cannot be swallowed. Single cans of Ensure can be given as a nutritional supplement when the diet is inadequate to meet nutrient requirements.

TABLE 4-5  Stability(S) and Lability(L) of Vitamins

| TREATMENT | PROA | RETINOL | D | E | K | C | B$_1$ | B$_2$ | NIA | FOL* | B$_6$+ | B$_{12}$ |
|---|---|---|---|---|---|---|---|---|---|---|---|---|
| | | | | | | | VITAMIN | | | | | |
| Heat | L | S | S | L | S | L | L | S | S | L | L | S |
| Light Exposure | S | L | L | S | L | S | S | L | | L | L | L |
| pH↑ | S | S | S | S | S | L | L | S | S | S | S | L |
| pH↓ | S | S | S | S | S | S | S | S | S | S | S | S |
| Dehydration | L | S | S | S | S | S | S | S | S | S | S | S |
| Oxygen | S | S | L | S | S | S | S | S | S | S | S | S |
| Sulfite | S | S | S | S | S | S | L | S | S | S | S | S |
| Leaching | S | S | S | S | S | S | S | S | L | L | L | S |

*Microwave cooking.

+Autoclaving.

cereal with the milk. A caution for dietitians advising the elderly on intake of foods fortified with folic acid: such foods should not be recommended until the elderly person has had a complete blood count with measurement of red cell indices. If a macrocytic anemia is discovered, serum vitamin B$_{12}$ should be determined. No elderly person should be receiving daily folic acid supplements unless vitamin B$_{12}$ deficiency (due to pernicious anemia) has been excluded.

Alternate means of supplying nutrient requirements to the elderly to meet the RDA are shown in Table 4-4. The aim of this table is to demonstrate that nutrient needs can be supplied by carefully selected nutrient-rich foods or by semisynthetic formula foods, but that when foods included in the diet have a low nutrient-to-calorie ratio, more foods and more food items are required to cover nutrient needs.

Particular risks associated with unwise food selection, storage, and preparation by the elderly are:

1. Too few different foods selected to supply nutrient needs
2. Food energy intake unrelated to actual needs
3. Destruction of vitamins due to prolonged food storage, light exposure, prolonged cooking of foods in a large volume of water, addition of soda, microwave cooking, and overcooking for soft texture
4. Low fiber intake

Stability and lability of vitamins with specific pre- and postpurchase treatments are shown in Table 4-5.

## QUESTIONS

*Circle correct answers.*

1. Food energy needs are reduced with advancing age. The major reason is that
   a) old people cannot digest much food
   b) old people conserve body heat better than young people
   c) sick older people recover more quickly on a restricted diet
   d) if a person is taking medicines, he or she should eat less food
   e) decreased physical activity is associated with decreased energy production

2. Needs for vitamin D are increased by
   a) frequent colds
   b) decreased sunlight exposure
   c) consumption of a low cholesterol diet
   d) decreased physical activity
   e) intake of certain drugs

3. In 1980, Recommended Dietary Allowances were given for specific age ranges among the elderly for
   a) zinc
   b) vitamin D
   c) folacin
   d) thiamin
   e) food energy

4. Protein requirements could change with age. Present evidence indicates that the protein requirements of healthy elderly are
   a) less than those of younger persons
   b) equal to those of young persons
   c) greater than those of younger persons

5. Prevalent conditions among the elderly which we know can alter nutrient needs are
   a) decline in renal function
   b) congestive heart failure
   c) malabsorption
   d) chronic intake of medications
   e) dryness of the skin

## REFERENCES

DURNIN, J.V.G.A., "Dietary intake of the elderly," in *Current Achievements in Geriatrics*, eds. W.F. Anderson and B. Isaacs. London: Cassell, 1964.

EXTON-SMITH, A.N., "Physiological aspects of aging: relationship to nutrition," *Amer. J. Clin. Nutr.*, 25 (1972), 853–59.

EXTON-SMITH, A.N., and P.W. OVERSTALL, *Geriatrics*. Lancaster, England: M.T.P. Press, Ltd. Internat. Med. Publ., 1979.

FORBES, G.B., and J.C. REINA, "Adult lean body mass declines with age: Some longitudinal observations," *Metabolism*, 19 (1970), 653–63.

HARPER, A.E., "Recommended Dietary Allowances for the elderly," *Geriatrics*, 33 (1978), 73–80.

MUNRO, H.N., "Major gaps in nutrient allowances. The status of the elderly," *J. Amer. Dietet. Assoc.*, 76 (1980), 137–40.

MUNRO, H.N., and A.V. EVERETT. Introduction to mini-symposium on nutrition and aging. Nutrition in Health and Disease and International Development. Proc. Symp. XII Internat. Congr. Nutr., Aug., 1981, San Diego, eds. A.E. Harper and G.K. Davis. New York: Alan R. Liss, Publ., 1981, pp. 677–85.

*Nutrition and Health in Old Age*. The cross-sectional analysis of the findings of a survey made in 1972/3 for elderly people who had been studied in 1967/8. Report by the Committee on Medical Aspects of Food Policy, Department of Health and Social Security Report on Health and Social Subjects #16. Her Majesty's Stationery Office, London, 1979.

*Recommended Dietary Allowances*, 9th Revised Ed. Committee on Dietary Allowances, Food and Nutrition Board, NRC/NAS, Washington, D.C., 1980.

ROE, D.A., *Drug-Induced Nutritional Deficiencies*. Westport, CT: AVI Publ. Co., 1976, pp. 99–100.

SMITH, E.L., *Vitamin $B_{12}$*, 3rd Ed. New York: John Wiley and Sons, 1965, p. 180.

VESTAL, R.E., "Methodological problems associated with studies of drug metabolism in the elderly," *Proc. First World Conf. Clin. Pharmacol. and Therap.*, London, Aug. 3–9, 1980, ed. P. Turner. London: Macmillan Publ. Ltd., 1980.

WINTERER, J.C., W.P. STEFFEE, W.D.A. PERERA, R. UANY, N.S. SCRIMSHAW, and V.R. YOUNG, "Whole body protein turnover in aging men," *Exp. Gerontol.*, 11 (1976), 79–87.

YOUNG, V.R., W.D. PERERA, J.C. WINTERER, et al., "Protein and amino acid requirements of the elderly—an overview," in *Nutrition and Aging*, ed. M. Winick. New York: John Wiley & Sons, 1976, pp. 77–118.

ZANNI, E., D.H. CALLAWAY, and A.Y. ZEZULKA, "Protein requirements of elderly men," *J. Nutr.*, 109 (1979), 513–24.

# CHAPTER FIVE
## Factors Determining Food Intake

## FOOD HABITS

### Food Preferences

*Cultural Factors.*   In the elderly as in younger people, food preferences are to a great extent determined by family traditions, by ethnicity, and by religious or traditional beliefs (Le Gros Clark, 1968).  Foods that are familiar are liked best, and even the elderly whose food intake is limited by health problems prefer dishes which they have enjoyed since early life. Regional foods are appealing if they are considered to be staples, essential components of a "good meal," or a meal accompaniment.  In the United States, an example of regional staples would be corn bread and corn meal muffins, which are commonly eaten in the Southern states. "Essential" components of meals include eggs and toast for breakfast, soup and a sandwich for lunch, and meat or fish for dinner. The elderly may prefer dinner foods in the middle of the day. Appropriate accompaniments to meals include tea, coffee, and jam for breakfast, milk for lunch, and potatoes and gravy for dinner.

With aging, rigidity of food habits usually increases, and the familiar food pattern is much sought after. Ethnicity will determine food habits if the traditions of the foods have been preserved. The elderly working-class Italians usually want their pasta, as well as the zuppa or polenta which remind them of a secure family life. When an elderly person has always eaten foods of his or her country of origin, it is very difficult to win them away from these foods, and they will become particularly unhappy if such foods are denied them when they are in the hospital or in an extended-care facility.

Religious custom may determine food choice. For example, the Orthodox Jew believes that only kosher food may be eaten. Food choice may also be determined by season, whether the season is religious or climatic (fish during Lent and soup in the winter). Prestigious foods might be selected whether or not they are appropriate to the person's health and needs; for example, white bread is usually preferred over whole wheat or rye. Folklore and tradition may determine the choice of food for invalids and it is for this reason that the ailing elderly may want chicken broth, which is "strengthening."

*Social Factors.*    Food preferences are highly influenced by education. As previously indicated, elderly people usually prefer familiar foods. Uneducated people are likely to have only had the experience of a relatively small number of different foods, and their food choices are among the foods that they know well. More educated people are likely to have experienced many different foods and therefore may have broader ranges of likes and dislikes.

The desire to try new foods in later life is a reflection of cultural experience in earlier years. Elderly people, however disabled, will enjoy unusual foods if they have done so during their earlier years. The university professor who is 90 and has lived in France may prefer ripe Brie cheese over processed cheese, whereas a 90-year-old ex-factory worker who has neither education nor the experience of foreign travel might dislike Brie intensely and would select the processed cheese.

Nutrition education affects food choice in that elderly people who have a knowledge of the caloric value of foods and also of the nutrient composition of foods may prefer to eat foods that have a high nutrient-to-calorie ratio. Many people who want to adhere to a special diet, either self-imposed or prescribed by a physician, will follow the diet more closely if they have a knowledge of nutrition and are able to read and comprehend food labels.

*Situational Factors.*    In the elderly, situational factors have a large bearing on food preference and choice. If an elderly person has limited financial resources, food choice will be from cheaper foods. If the person lives a long distance from a store or has no transportation, and the store has no delivery service, then preference is for foods that can be easily carried and that can be stored without refrigeration. If there are no cooking arrangements, or if cooking arrangements in the individual's residence are inadequate, then food choice will be from among items that do not require cooking or which only require a simple preparation. If the individual is living alone or with one other person of a similarly advanced age, then food preference is for items that are sold in small packages. When larger packages are purchased, usually part of the package has to be thrown away or the purchaser has to eat the same food, perhaps a vegetable, on several nights in succession. If an elderly person is disabled, then constraints on food choice and preference are multiple, resulting in a need to select from foods that do not require preparation, do not have to be removed from cans, and need not be cooked in any way which requires special manual dexterity.

Food availability determines the food choice of elderly people who live in domiciliary care facilities or nursing homes. In these situations food choice is from the menu supplied as well as from the diet prescribed.

While food preferences of the elderly may be similar to those of the young, people who are undertaking geriatric care often believe that their elderly charges want only certain foods which they deem appropriate. Nursing personnel in facilities for the elderly will commonly state that the residents or patients ''won't eat salad or raw fruit'' when, in fact, they have not made the experiment of directly presenting these items in an attractive form.

*Medical Factors.*    When unpleasant symptoms are associated with the intake of specific foods or beverages, these tend to be avoided. For example, if milk, cereal products, or fats induce diarrhea, then selection will be from among other types of food. Taste loss or perversion of taste and smell which occur in certain elderly people may determine avoidance of some foods and preference for others. Iatrogenic (doctor-prescribed) diets limit food choice, and if these are used additively by patients, food choice may be limited to a very few items, to an extent that may contribute to malnutrition (Clarke and Wakefield, 1975)

## DETERMINANTS OF FOOD INTAKE

### Hunger and Appetite

*Hunger* comprises the physiological sensations that indicate a need for food. *Repletion* is the term for the visceral sensations associated with having eaten enough to satisfy hunger. *Appetite* indicates the desire for food including hunger, but also includes the appeal of food whether hunger is present or not. *Satiety* indicates that enough food has been eaten to satisfy both hunger and the desire for food. Often satiety is also associated with indicators of having had enough such as distension or abdominal bloating.

Appetite may be disturbed or reduced by 1) food aversions, and 2) anorexia.

*Food Aversion.*    Reduction in food intake by the elderly may occur when the eating situation is unpleasant or when eating causes distressing symptoms. Circumstances which reduce the desire to eat include:

1.  *Unattractive surroundings.* Eating is less attractive when the surroundings are dark because the food cannot be seen; when the room is noisy because of the

distracting effect of noise; when the room is cold, because the person is preoccupied with the need to get warm; when the room is excessively hot, because of a feeling of faintness; and when the room is dirty or unkempt, because this suggests that the hygiene of the food may be in doubt and also because the appeal of food is always reduced if it is served in an unattractive manner.

2. *Unpleasant company.* An elderly person is less likely to eat if others present including family, household members, home health aides, nurses' aides or nurses are silly, impatient, inattentive, abusive, or, in the hospital situation, when other patients are noisy or psychotic.

3. *Bad food service.* The elderly will eat less if food is monotonous, if portions are too small or too large, if hot dishes are served cold, if vegetables are not drained, if food is not fresh, if food arrives late, if food ordered is not available, if food is unattractive in appearance, if foods on the menu are disliked, if dishes are unfamiliar, if no provision is made for special diets, and if food taboos are not recognized.

4. *Disturbances during meals.* Less food will be eaten if meals are served at unaccustomed times or are interrupted. In hospitals, meals may be interrupted when procedures are scheduled at mealtimes.

Food aversion is a term which denotes antipathy to one or more foods, unwillingness to eat, or dislike of eating. Food aversions arise under the following circumstances:

1. When food or the process of eating food produces an unpleasant sensation.
2. When the sight or thought of certain foods or the taste or smell of certain foods evokes the memory of something unpleasant.
3. When foods are believed to have some unpleasant property.

In the elderly, the following food-related symptoms evoke food aversion:

1. Gastric distension leading to breathlessness, as it occurs in patients with congestive heart failure.
2. Abdominal pain and gassy diarrhea as found in patients with secondary lactose intolerance associated with malabsorption syndromes.
3. Dysphagia (pain on swallowing) associated with cancer of the mouth, pharynx, or esophagus, operative conditions of the mouth, pharynx, or esophagus, radiation therapy involving the pharynx or neck, and cancer chemotherapy (e.g. methotrexate) which can cause oral ulceration.
4. Distortion of taste or smell, usually associated with metastatic or widespread cancer and/or radiation therapy or cancer chemotherapy employed in the treatment of cancer.
5. Nausea with or without vomiting, related to radiation therapy or chemotherapy, is likely to lead to food aversion. It is to be emphasized that food aversions arise when foods are associated with these unpleasant events, though eating those foods no longer in fact induces unpleasant sensations. Thus, for example, if chocolate chip ice cream has been eaten at a time when intravenous cancer chemotherapeutic drugs are or have just been administered, then chocolate chip ice cream will forthwith be disliked because of its association with severe nausea which was actually the result of the bolus drug administration (Shils, 1979; Carter, 1981).

Eating aversion in the elderly may indicate severe psychiatric disturbance. Causes include:

1. Psychotic depression causing a complete disinterest in food.
2. Confusional states, where the patient is unaware of time or place.
3. Paranoia, where patients believe the food is poisoned.
4. Dementia (e.g. Alzheimer's disease), where patient is unwilling to swallow or has developed a gagging reflex (Exton-Smith, 1973).

Elderly patients, particularly those with severe chronic disabilities or terminal illnesses, may stop eating as an unspoken signal that they do not wish to go on living.

The feeding of patients who rebel against eating should be approached with great caution, because it is not uncommon for patients under these circumstances to inhale pieces of food that have been fed to them by an overzealous relative, attendant, or nurse.

*Anorexia.*     Anorexia in the elderly is usually associated with acute or chronic physical disease. Acute diseases associated with anorexia are febrile conditions such as pneumonia (bacterial or viral) and gastroenteritis. Chronic diseases associated with anorexia are:

1. Gastrointestinal disease, whether or not it is associated with jaundice, e.g. alcoholic liver disease, primary or secondary carcinoma of the liver, or carcinoma of the head of the pancreas.
2. Cardiovascular diseases, e.g. congestive heart failure.
3. Respiratory diseases, e.g. emphysema with pulmonary decompensation.
4. Chronic renal disease, e.g. chronic nephritis with uremia.
5. Cancer. In the elderly, the most common cause of severe anorexia in a patient who has previously had a good appetite is cancer. When anorexia develops in the elderly without obvious cause, the physician should carry out full oncological screening. If a patient complaining of loss of weight is seen by the nutritionist and loss of appetite is admitted, it is necessary for this to be reported immediately to the M.D., in order that the patient can be investigated to find out whether or not cancer is present.

Other conditions associated with anorexia are:

1. Intake of marginal diets (diets low in protein or thiamin).
2. Malnutrition. Avitaminoses including deficiences of thiamin, niacin, folacin, and vitamin $B_6$ are associated with anorexia. Zinc deficiency as may occur in elderly patients with alcoholic cirrhosis causes anorexia in association with loss of taste.
3. Postgastrectomy syndromes. Elderly patients who have had partial or total gastrectomies frequently are anorectic and/or may display early satiety. Reasons for this include vitamin deficiencies which are the result of combined low intake and malabsorption, dumping syndrome (which causes a fear of eating rather than true anorexia), and an early feeling of fullness because of the small size of the gastric remnant (Floch, 1981).

4. Drugs. Therapeutic drugs used in short- and long-term therapy can induce severe anorexia. Anorexia may be inevitable, as with certain cancer chemotherapeutic drugs, and may be associated with high drug dosage as with high levels of digoxin, or may be associated with drug toxicity, i.e. hepatotoxicity or nephrotoxicity (Roe, 1979). (See discussion of the effects of drugs in the elderly in Chapter 9.)

Causes of reduced food intake in the elderly are summarized in Table 5-1.

TABLE 5-1   Major Causes of Reduced Food Intake
            in the Elderly

| | |
|---|---|
| Unattractive surroundings | Cirrhosis |
| Unpleasant company | Congestive heart failure |
| Bad food service | Pulmonary insufficiency |
| Mealtime disturbances | Chronic renal disease |
| Breathlessness | Cancer |
| Gastric distension | Malnutrition |
| Abdominal pain | Postgastrectomy syndromes |
| Gassy diarrhea | Incoordination |
| Dysphagia | Paralysis |
| Taste or smell perversion | Arthritis |
| Nausea and vomiting | Loss of consciousness |
| Depression | Drugs, e.g. digoxin or cancer |
| Confusion | chemotherapeutic agents |
| Paranoia | Restricted diets |
| Dementia | Alcohol abuse |

## DISEASES ASSOCIATED WITH DECREASED INTAKE OF FOOD

Diseases that are not associated with anorexia can nevertheless cause the patient to take in very little food (Floch, 1981). Reasons are:

1. The patient cannot open the mouth or cannot open it adequately.
2. The patient cannot swallow.
3. The patient cannot retain food due to vomiting or regurgitation.
4. Food cannot be given by mouth because the patient is unconscious or consciousness is disturbed.

A summary of diseases which lower food intake is indicated in Table 5-2.

TABLE 5-2   Geriatric Diseases Which Lower Food Intake

| DISEASE | MECHANISM |
|---|---|
| Congestive heart failure | Food-related breathlessness |
| Scleroderma | Mouth cannot be fully opened |
| Cancer of the esophagus | Painful swallowing and regurgitation |
| Stroke | Unconsciousness |

## DISABILITIES WHICH REDUCE FOOD INTAKE

Severely disabled elderly people have reduced food intake unless they can obtain assistance with food preparation and/or with eating (Exton-Smith, 1973). Types of disability associated with low food intake are paralyses (as in stroke patients), dementia (as in patients with Alzheimer's disease), crippling (as in patients with arthritis), incoordination (as in patients with Parkinson's disease), and blindness, particularly if the loss of vision has developed in later life.

## DENTAL STATUS AND FOOD INTAKE

Elderly people who are edentulous and without dentures, as well as some who have dentures, experience difficulty in chewing certain foods (Posner, 1979; Kohrs et al., 1978). Dietary habits of denture wearers are influenced by the age at which the denture was acquired, the condition of the denture, the presence or absence of oral mucosal damage due to an ill-fitting denture, and motivation to eat. Many healthy denture wearers and edentulous older people eat foods which we believe require mastication. It appears that loss of masticatory ability can be tolerated in these people without health risk. Foods such as roast meat may be swallowed in larger pieces or may be cut up before it is eaten. Swallowing unchewed pieces of meat does not result in seriously impaired digestion.

A more significant problem with respect to the quality of the diet of edentulous or partially edentulous patients with or without dentures is that less motivated individuals will deliberately avoid meats, crisp vegetables, raw fruits and even crisp bread rolls because they complain that they cannot chew these foods and therefore cannot eat them. The physical, mental, and emotional health of these people should be evaluated. Health professionals should be aware that food avoidance in the elderly may be a sign of depression, even if absence of teeth or unserviceable dentures have previously been blamed for change in food habit.

Elderly patients who are in nursing homes and who are not afforded adequate opportunities for oral hygiene after meals, may deliberately avoid foods which stick to their teeth or to their dentures.

## SPECIAL DIETS

Just as the elderly are the chief drug users, so they are the chief users of special diets. Their diets may be:

1.  Obtained by physician's order, either in the medical office or in an acute care hospital or in a nursing home.
2.  On the advice of a physician by telephone call or by home visit.
3.  From a dietitian.
4.  From a community nutritionist.
5.  From a public health nurse.
6.  From another health paraprofessional such as an EFNEP (Expanded Food and Nutrition Education Program) aide.
7.  From family or friends.
8.  Self-prescribed.
9.  From newspapers or magazines.
10. From other media, including TV and radio.

Common ailments and prescribed special diets are:

1.  Congestive heart failure—low sodium diet.
2.  Atherosclerotic heart disease—low cholesterol diet.
3.  Hypertension—low sodium diet.
4.  Obesity—low calorie diet.
5.  Diabetes—low calorie, low sugar diet.
6.  Renal failure—low protein diet.
7.  Cirrhosis—low protein, low sodium diet.
8.  Diverticulosis/diverticulitis—low fat diet.
9.  Constipation—high fiber diet.
10. Hiatus hernia—low bulk diet.
11. Cholecystitis and cholelithiasis—low fat and cholesterol diet.
12. Colostomy—low fiber diet.

Since chronic diseases of several different organ systems frequently coexist in the elderly, diets may be superimposed. Superimposition of diets either on the advice of a physician or other health professional, as a result of lay advice from one or more people, or due to the individual's own conviction of need is a major cause of low food intake and dietary inadequacy.

Special diets are a major cause of malnutrition in the elderly. Special diets can be nutritionally inadequate when:

1.  Food-energy intake is too low.
2.  The number of food sources of essential nutrients is too limited.
3.  The diet is too unpalatable to be consumed.
4.  Foods excluded contain nutrients not included in foods permitted.
5.  The adverse nutritional effects of the diet add to nutritional deficiencies due to disease and/or drugs.

## DRUGS AND FOOD INTAKE

Drugs may be hyperphagic, producing increased food intake, or hypophagic, causing decreased food intake (Roe, 1979). With certain drugs or drug groups, effects on appetite are highly influenced by situational factors.

### Hyperphagic Agents

*Antihistamines.* The appetite in debilitated elderly people can be stimulated by giving cyproheptadine hydrochloride (Periactin, Merck, Sharp and Dohme), which is both an antihistamine and a serotonin antagonist. Increased hunger with the administration of cyproheptadine occurs mainly when anorexia previously existed. However, cyproheptadine may produce unwanted sleepiness as a side effect.

*Psychotropic Agents.* Appetite-promoting effects of psychotropic drugs have been recognized, particularly in older psychiatric patients on prolonged high dosage therapies. Phenothiazines such as chlorpromazine (Thorazine, Smith, Kline and French) improve appetite in agitated patients. Benzodiazepines including chlordiazepoxide (Librium, Roche) and diazepam (Valium, Roche) stimulate appetite and increase food intake in certain older people. Although the tranquilizers given to disturbed psychotic patients often cause a marked increase in food intake so that patients become obese, these same drugs given to geriatric patients may have an opposite effect. When phenothiazines or benzodiazepines are given in high dosage to elderly patients whose rate of drug metabolism is slowed, somnolence and disinterest in food is common and may be responsible for lowered food intake.

*Tricyclic Antidepressants.* Specific drugs in this class are recognized as having a marked effect on the desire for food. Amitriptyline (Elavil, Merck, Sharp and Dohme) increases appetite and food intake and may cause marked weight gain. Patients receiving these drugs may have a craving for sweets. Combined tricyclic and monamine oxidase inhibitor antidepressants have been found to induce weight gain in patients with depressive illness. It is to be noted, however, that for the elderly, use of antidepressant drugs may cause severe behavioral problems, and trycyclic antidepressants sometimes cause agitation which may interfere with eating.

### Hypophagic Drugs

*Cancer Chemotherapeutic Agents.* Cancer chemotherapeutic agents may induce anorexia because of their effects on the gastrointestinal tract. The effects on food intake are usually related to associated nausea and vomiting.

Drugs which at the time of administration commonly cause anorexia are dox-orubicin hydrochlor (Adriamycin, Adria), asparaginase (Elspar, Merck, Sharp and Dohme), cyclophosphamide (Cytoxan, Mead Johnson), daunorubicin (Cerubidine, Ives), carmustine (BICNU, Bristol), methotrexate (Lederle) and mithramycin (Mithracin, Miles).

Anorexia associated with the administration of these drugs may be of brief duration, or may be prolonged due to effects of the drug on the gastrointestinal tract. The anorexia associated with cancer chemotherapeutic agents can and frequently does markedly reduce food intake such that weight loss occurs (Johns, 1979).

*Chelating Agents.*   D-Penicillamine (Cuprimine, Merck, Sharp and Dohme) is used in the elderly for the treatment of rheumatoid arthritis. The drug can produce loss of taste due to drug-associated zinc and copper deficiency. Penicillamine forms complexes with these metals which then are excreted in the urine.

### Alcohol

Alcohol abuse in the elderly can cause anorexia (Roe, 1979). Causes of anorexia in elderly alcoholics are inebriation, gastritis, lactose intolerance, pancreatitis, hepatitis, cirrhosis, ketoacidosis, alcoholic brain syndromes, and withdrawal syndromes. Anorexia in alcoholics can also be due to thiamin, zinc, or protein deficiencies. It has been found that among the elderly, those who are drinkers may tend to have lower food intake than age-matched non-drinkers, even in the absence of alcohol abuse.

### Cardiac Glycosides

Digitalis and other related cardiac glycosides, in high dosage, cause anorexia which is usually associated with nausea (Banks and Nayab, 1974). Vomiting may also occur. Digitalis cachexia can result from chronic digitalis over-dosage, and the marked weight loss found in this condition can imitate cancer cachexia. Return of appetite occurs rapidly when the drug dosage is appropriately adjusted.

### QUESTIONS

1. True or false:
   a) Rigidity of food habits usually increases with aging.
   b) The elderly in nursing homes will not eat salads.
   c) Food preferences are influenced by food experiences.
   d) Appetite and hunger are synonymous.

2. True or false:
   a) People on cancer chemotherapy may develop food aversions.
   b) People on cancer chemotherapy may develop anorexia.
   c) Anorexia is associated with cancer.
   d) Anorexia is associated with cancer cure.
   e) Anorexia explains weight loss in the cancer patient.

3. Cross out the incorrect word(s) "do" or "do not" in the following sentences:
   a) Diseases associated with anorexia *do/do not* cause elderly patients to consume very little food.
   b) Edentulous elderly people who enjoy roast meat *do/do not* eat meat.
   c) Food avoidances in the elderly *do/do not* signify depression.
   d) Diets low in thiamin *do/do not* cause anorexia.
   e) Diets high in thiamin *do/do not* cause anorexia.

4. The two lists indicate special diets and their medical indications. Pair correctly:

   a) low cholesterol              i. cirrhosis
   b) low sodium                   ii. congestive heart failure
   c) low protein                  iii. diabetes
   d) low protein, low sodium      iv. atherosclerotic heart disease
   e) low calories, low sugar      v. renal failure

5. Malnutrition may arise from special diets which restrict the following foods. Circle letters opposite correct answers.
   a) cookies
   b) calories
   c) number of foods
   d) cholesterol
   e) protein

## REFERENCES

BANKS, T., and A. NAYAB, Letter. Digitalis cachexia. *New Eng. J. Med.*, 290 (1974), 746.

CARTER, S.K., "Nutritional problems associated with cancer chemotherapy," in *Nutrition and Cancer: Etiology and Treatment*, eds. G.R. Newell and N.M. Ellison. New York: Raven Press, 1981, pp. 303–17.

CLARKE, M., and L.M. WAKEFIELD, "Food choices of institutionalized vs. independent-living elderly," *J. Am. Dietet. Assoc*, 66 (1975), 600–604.

EXTON-SMITH, A.N., "Nutritional deficiencies in the elderly," in *Nutritional Deficiencies in Modern Society*, eds. A.N. Howard and I. McLean Baird. London: Newman Books Ltd., 1973, p. 86.

FLOCH, M.H., *Nutrition and Diet Therapy in Gastrointestinal Disease*. New York: Plenum Publ. Corp., 1981, pp. 151–61.

JOHNS, M.P., *Drug Therapy and Nursing Care*. New York: Macmillan Publ. Co., Inc., 1979, pp 263–92.

KOHRS, M.B., R. O'NEAL, A. PRESTON, D. EKLUND, and O. ABRAHAMS, "Nutritional status of elderly residents in Missouri," *Amer. J. Clin. Nutr.*, 31 (1978), 2186–97.

LE GROS CLARK, F.,   *Food habits as a practical nutrition problem.* World Rev. Nutr. Dietet., 9, (1968), Basel/New York: Karger, 56–84.

POSNER, B.M.,   *Nutrition and the Elderly.* Lexington, Mass.: Lexington Books, D.C. Heath and Co., 1979.

ROE, D.A.,   *Alcohol and the Diet.* Westport, CT: AVI Publ. Co., 1979, pp. 27–41.

ROE, D.A.,   "Interactions between drugs and nutrients," *Med. Clin. N. Amer.,* 63 (1979), 985–1007.

SHILS, M.E.,   "Nutritional problems induced by cancer," *Med. Clin. N. Amer.,* 63 (1979), 1009–25.

# CHAPTER SIX
## Assessment of Nutritional Status

**DIETARY ASSESSMENT IN THE COMMUNITY**

The purpose of assessment is to find out what an individual is eating now, what he or she has eaten in the past, recent changes in the diet, and how many nutrients are consumed. Dietary assessment may involve qualitative or quantitative methods. Qualitative methods include a) a short dietary quiz, and b) a food frequency questionnaire.

Qualitative methods are used to screen the diets of independently living elderly for possible nutritional deficiencies or excesses and to determine their pattern of food intake. Information can be obtained on what foods are eaten or not eaten, how often particular foods are consumed, and how many foods are consumed. Food frequency questionnaires can also be used to examine the diversity of the diet. In the elderly the quality of the diet is directly related to the number of different foods eaten or to the diversity of the diet. Semiquantitation of food frequency questionnaires can be achieved, e.g. when questions are asked on how often a *glass* of milk is drunk, or a *slice* of bread is eaten. Examples of qualitative and semiquantitative food frequency questionnaires appropriate for use in the elderly are shown in Figures 6-1 and 6-2.

In the elderly, food frequency questionnaires are best administered by either a dietitian or other nutritionist, or by a health professional such as a physician or nurse.

The advantages of using food frequency questionnaires are that they do not require recordkeeping, that they do not require an extended time commitment, and that they can be administered by a non-nutritionist.

**FIGURE 6-1**    Qualitative food frequency questionnaire.

| FOOD ITEM | FREQUENCY* | USUAL METHOD OF PREPARATION USED** |
|---|---|---|
| Milk | Examples: 1 | f dried, reconstituted |
| Cheese | 3 | b |
| Yogurt | 0 | |
| Ice cream | 0 | |
| Eggs | 3 | b |
| Dried beans | 0 | |
| Peas | | |
| Peanut butter | | |
| Meat | | |
| Fish | | |
| Poultry | | |
| Liver | | |
| Bread | | |
| Rice | | |
| Pasta | | |
| Tortillas | | |
| Cereal < Hot Cold | | |
| Potatoes | | |
| Vegetables < Green Yellow | | |
| Citrus fruit and Fruit juices | | |

*0 = never  
 1 = once a day or more  
 2 = several times a day  
 3 = once a week  
 4 = once a month  

**a = raw  
 b = cooked  
 c = fresh (fruit/vegetable)  
 d = frozen  
 e = canned  
 f = other (state)

    The information given is not useful, however, unless the respondent retains memory of food intake and is truthful and cooperative. Another disadvantage is that actual intake levels of food-energy and nutrients are not obtained.

    A diet questionnaire or short diet quiz is shown in Figure 6-3. Diet questionnaires or short diet quizzes examine the pattern of food intake and find out

**FIGURE 6-2** Semiquantitative food frequency questionnaire.

| FOOD ITEM | FREQUENCY* | AMOUNT EATEN** | USUAL METHOD OF PREPARATION USED*** |
|---|---|---|---|
| Example: Milk | 1 | 6 oz. cup | canned, diluted |
| Bread | 2 | 1 slice | f toasted |
| | | | |
| | | | |

| | | |
|---|---|---|
| *0 = never<br>1 = once a day or more<br>2 = several times a day<br>3 = once a week<br>4 = once a month | **Glass<br>(size)<br>Cup<br>Slice<br>Number | ***a = raw<br>b = cooked<br>c = fresh (fruit/vegetable)<br>d = frozen<br>e = canned<br>f = other (state) |

what foods are omitted from the diet. Diet quizzes are essential when it is necessary to prescribe a regime of medication using drugs which may be influenced by intake of food or beverages. Diet questionnaires which address the pattern of food intake are also appropriately used in situations when therapeutic diets are being prescribed or modified.

The advantages of short dietary questionnaires are that they can be administered by non-nutritionists, that they require only moderate patient cooperation, that they require only limited memory, and that the patient does not have to keep records. The disadvantages are that no information is obtained on amounts of food consumed, that information given may be misleading if the patient provides false information because of a desire to please the questioner or in self-defense, e.g. when an alcoholic indicates that he or she has a good diet.

Quantitative dietary assessment may be made using:

1. 24-hour recall of food intake
2. Diet record
3. Diet history
4. Individual or household survey
5. Observation of actual food consumed
6. Diet analysis (analysis of diet replicates)

*Recalls.* Twenty-four hour diet recalls have been widely used in individual and group dietary assessment. Food intake may be recorded on a form such as that illustrated in Figure 6-4. Use of 24-hour food records to evaluate the diet of an aged person is seldom advisable because valid information requires excellent memory, responsibility of the respondent for her or his own food preparation, or cooperation from a household member or home helper who has been responsible for the preparation of the respondent's food and has actually been able to observe what has been consumed.

**FIGURE 6-3    A sample dietary questionnaire.**

|  | Yes | No |
|---|---|---|
| Do you drink milk? | ☐ | ☐ |

| | |
|---|---|
| If yes, whole milk | ☐ |
| 2% milk | ☐ |
| skim milk | ☐ |
| other | ☐ |

Specify _____

_____

Please indicate which of the following foods you eat and how often.

|  | never or hardly ever (less than once a week) | sometimes (not daily but at least once a week) | every day or nearly every day |
|---|---|---|---|
| Cheese, yogurt, ice cream | ☐ | ☐ | ☐ |
| Eggs | ☐ | ☐ | ☐ |
| Dried beans, peas, peanut butter | ☐ | ☐ | ☐ |
| Meat, fish, poultry | ☐ | ☐ | ☐ |
| Bread, rice, pasta, grits, cereal, tortillas, potatoes | ☐ | ☐ | ☐ |
| Fruits or fruit juices | ☐ | ☐ | ☐ |
| Vegetables | ☐ | ☐ | ☐ |

If you eat fruits or drink fruit juices every day or nearly every day, which ones do you eat or drink most often? (Not more than three.)

_____

_____

If you eat vegetables every day or nearly every day, which ones do you eat most often? (Not more than three.)

_____

_____

*Diet Records.*    Three-, five-, and seven-day diet records are an excellent means of obtaining dietary information from very cooperative elderly patients who have been fully instructed on how to make these records. Usually in the elderly, diet diaries that exceed three days' length are not dependable. If the weekend diet differs from that of other days, it is appropriate to use a weekend day as well as week days in the diet record. In all diet records, the respondent is requested to write down the time of day when a food or beverage

**FIGURE 6-3    (cont.)**

|  | Yes | No |
|---|---|---|
| Do you usually eat anything between meals? | ☐ | ☐ |

If yes, name the 2 or 3 snacks (including bedtime snacks) that you have most often.

_____

_____

|  | Yes | No |
|---|---|---|
| Do you or the person who prepares your meals have use of a |  |  |
| working stove | ☐ | ☐ |
| refrigerator | ☐ | ☐ |
| piped water | ☐ | ☐ |
| Do you take vitamins or iron? | ☐ | ☐ |

If yes, how often? _____

What kind? _____

Do you take other nutrient supplements?

Sustacal    ☐

Ensure    ☐

Wheat germ    ☐

Bone meal    ☐

Kelp    ☐

Other (state) _____

Are you on a special diet?      Yes _____ No _____    If yes, what is the reason?

low salt; specify type of diet    ☐ _____

weight reduction; specify type    ☐ _____

diabetic; specify type of diet    ☐ _____

Other; specify reason for diet and type of diet    ☐ _____

Who recommended the diet? _____

Do you eat meals in a congregate meal site?    Yes ____ No ____ If yes, no. meals/wk. ____

Do you have meals delivered to your home?    Yes ____ No ____ If yes, no. meals/wk. ____

is consumed, the name of that food or beverage, its composition, and the amount eaten or drunk. A representative set of instructions for keeping a diet diary and a recording sheet are shown in Figures 6-5a and 6-5b.

Interpretation and analysis of information supplied in the diet record has to be done by a trained nutritionist or dietitian. However, it is necessary that

**FIGURE 6-4    24-hour food recall.**

We want you to tell us all you have eaten or have drunk for the last 24 hours.
Start by telling us what you ate most recently.

| DATE | TIME | FOOD/BEVERAGE ITEM | AMOUNT | DESCRIPTIONS* |
|---|---|---|---|---|
| SAMPLE: | | | | |
| 9/9/82 | 8 am | Coffee, doughnut | 1 coffee,<br>1 doughnut | Black with sugar |
| 9/8/82 | 10 pm | Cookies<br>Ginger ale | 3<br>1 glass | Chocolate chip<br>Canada Dry |
| 9/8/82 | 6 pm | Soup<br><br>Toast | 1 cup<br><br>2 slices | Campbell's chicken<br>noodle<br>Pepperidge Farm,<br>white |
| 9/8/82 | Noon | Coffee<br>Waffles<br>Syrup<br>Butter | 2 cups<br>2<br>2 tbsp.<br>2 tsp. | Black<br>Frozen<br>Vermont Maple |
| | | | | |
| | | | | |

*Columns may be added for "where eaten" and "who prepared."

the nutritionist give oral instructions to the person making the diet record on exactly how the record should be prepared. The use of food models is also advised in demonstrating to the individual how to indicate amounts of food by household measures. When the diet record is handed in, it has to be checked for completeness and the respondent may be questioned when it seems likely that meals or parts of meals have been omitted, or where detail on the amount of food has been omitted. Completed diet records are analyzed using food composition tables such as USDA Handbook 8 or 456, or by using computerized food composition data bases such as the Ohio State Data Base (Watt and Merrill, 1963; Adams, 1975; Herzler and Haever, 1977). When each day's food intake has been analyzed for food energy content and content of those nutrients which are of specific interest and importance, then an average may be taken of each day's food energy and nutrient content, and this is then expressed as a percent of RDA (RDA = Recommended Dietary Allowances, Food and Nutrition Board, National Academy of Sciences, 1980).

In the elderly, advantages of the diet record as a means of nutritional assessment include the fact that more than one day's food intake is obtained and also the diet record can be used as a means to obtain information on intake and regularity of intake of nutrient supplements including vitamins, minerals,

**FIGURE 6-5a   Three-day food diary instructions.**

INSTRUCTIONS FOR RECORDING 3-DAY FOOD DIARY

1. This diary is to be kept for three consecutive days (e.g., Tuesday, Wednesday, Thursday).

2. Please write down everything that you put in your mouth (food, drink, nutrient supplements, vitamins, etc.). For each day use a separate sheet—you may need more than one sheet for the same day.

3. Record under the headings provided:

   Time—approximate time of day food is eaten

   Where Eaten—was it at home, dining hall, daughter's house, etc.

   Food Item—a detailed description of foods eaten

   List name of food or beverage
      brand name whenever possible
      type—fresh, canned, dried, frozen
      list approximate ingredients and amounts in mixed dishes (e.g. stews)

   Amount Eaten—approximate measure—
      by cup (or portion of a cup, e.g., one-half cup)
      and/or by tablespoon or teaspoon
      and/or dimensions (size), in inches

    Use the measuring cups and spoons and ruler to help you here.

   Method of Preparation—please indicate how the foods were prepared/cooked, i.e., boiled, steamed, fried, poached, broiled, toasted, grilled, baked, microwaved, or fresh/raw.

   Who Prepared—Did you prepare the meal? (self) or a friend, family member, etc?

   Do not forget to measure and record added milk, cream, and sugar, and also any alcohol-containing beverages, i.e. brandy, whiskey, wine, beer, etc.

or mineral-vitamin mixtures, as well as alcoholic beverages and medications. Records of alcoholic beverage consumption are commonly underestimated in patients who are alcohol abusers. The disadvantages of the diet record method in the elderly are that it is necessary that the respondent be responsible for food preparation or that the food preparer keep the diet record. The quality of diet records is related to education. Diet records necessitate writing capability and/or understanding of the use of a tape recorder. The diet record method cannot be utilized unless a nutrition professional is available to interpret the data supplied.

*Diet Histories.*   Diet histories must be obtained by a trained dietitian. These histories give information on long-term dietary habits and current diet (Burke, 1947). Qualitative and quantitative data are obtained. The elderly individual must be fully cooperative and have an intact memory. Diet histories can be of use in the home or in a domiciliary care facility.

*Individual or Household Survey.*   Foods available to the individual or household can be determined by interview coupled with examination of foods

FIGURE 6-5b    Example of three-day food diary.

NAME    *Jane Brown*

DAY _2_

DATE    *August 3, 1982*

| TIME | WHERE EATEN | FOOD ITEM | AMOUNT EATEN | METHOD OF PREPARATION | WHO PREPARED |
|---|---|---|---|---|---|
| 12:30 PM | home | Roast beef sandwich w/Milbrook white bread | 2 slices | toasted | self |
| " | " | Roast beef | 3 slices; about 3 oz. | roasted | " |
| " | " | iceberg lettuce | 1 leaf | fresh | " |
| " | " | Kraft mayonnaise | 1 tsp. | | " |
| " | " | Low fat milk | 1 cup | | |
| " | " | peach, fresh | 1 med. | fresh | |
| 6 PM | daughter's house | chicken thigh | 1 thigh | fried | daughter |
| " | " | white rice | 1/2 cup | boiled | " |
| " | " | carrots, frozen | 1/2 cup | boiled | " |
| " | " | lettuce salad: romaine lettuce | 2 leaves | fresh | " |
| " | " | cucumber slices | 3 slices 1/4 in. thick | " | " |
| " | " | red wine | 1/2 cup | | homemade |
| " | " | Saralee chocolate cake, frosted | 2" slice | bought | bought |
| 8:30 PM | home | whole milk with brandy: milk | 8 oz. milk | warmed | self |
| | | brandy | 2 tbsp. | | |
| " | " | Lorna Doone cookies | 3 whole | bought | |

present in the home. The usefulness of this method depends upon the identification of the nutritional risk to the elderly of a limited quantity or low quality of food. If an elderly individual is living with other family members or household members, examination of foods available in the home will not necessarily provide insight into the food available to or consumed by the elderly individual. On the other hand, when an elderly person is living alone or with another elderly person, survey of food in the home can offer important information on foods available to and eaten by that individual. It is of course important to ascertain from the interview whether or not any meals are taken away from the home, e.g. at a congregate meal site (Title III, see Chapter 10), a restaurant, or at the home of another person.

*Observation of Actual Diet Consumed.*   Measurement of food ordered, purchased, or prepared does not always give a realistic picture of food consumed. Food may be stored, discarded, shared with family, friends, or pets, or left as plate waste. In order to find out what an elderly person actually eats, records should be made from direct observation of meals prepared for consumption and plate waste. Actual intake can then be assessed by the difference.

*Diet Analyses.*   Cooperative elderly individuals can be instructed to collect a replicate diet. Over 24-hour periods, duplicate samples of *all* foods consumed and beverages ingested are put into plastic jars. It is preferable that beverages are put into separate containers from solid foods. The food and beverage collections are refrigerated. At the end of the 24-hour period, the collection vessels are picked up by the nutritionist. The total diet is homogenized in a gallon blender with distilled water. The total homogenate is weighed, and weighed aliquots of the homogenate are then subjected to nutrient analysis. Samples can be analyzed wet or after freeze-drying. If the quantity of a particular nutrient in the aliquot is determined, then the amount of that nutrient in the total diet can be calculated.

Diet analyses are best combined with 3-day diet records, with the food collections being made on the third day.

## ASSESSMENT OF NUTRIENT INTAKES OF HOUSEBOUND ELDERLY PERSONS

The aims of this method are to utilize records of food purchases by individuals to determine the nutritional quality of diets (Carl, 1980).

The assumption is made that food purchases are only for the elderly person who lives alone, that shopping lists are available for a period of at least 28 days, and that the individual whose food energy and nutrient intake is being examined does not have access to foods which do not appear on the shopping lists.

Food purchases for housebound elderly individuals living alone may be made by relatives, friends, or shopping aides. The cooperation of the person who is responsible for the food shopping must be obtained unless a local agency for the elderly, which supplies shopping aides, keeps the shopping lists in their files.

Purchases of all food items on each shopping list will be determined. Data to be collected by a nutritionist or public health nurse should include food item, weight or liquid measure, and cost. Total food purchases for a 28-day period can then be summed and averaged to yield weekly or daily food available to the person. The nutrient content of the available food can then be computed using USDA Handbook 456 or coded for use with the Ohio State University computerized data base (Adams, 1975; Herzler, 1977).

The RDA for the individual (51+) for calories and the following 16 nutrients is obtained, viz: protein, carbohydrate, fat, calcium, phosphorus, iron, zinc, magnesium*, vitamin A, thiamin, riboflavin, niacin, vitamin C, vitamin $B_6$, vitamin $B_{12}$, and folacin (Recommended Dietary Allowances, 1980). However, for the magnesium, vitamin $B_6$ and folacin content of foods there is a need to utilize data provided by Freeland and Cousins (1976), Murphy et al., (1975), USDA Home Econ. Res. Report (1969) and Perloff and Butrum (1977). (See also Tables 10, 12, and 13 in Appendix.) The percent of the RDA for food energy and these nutrients which are being obtained from the food purchased can be calculated if the food purchases are expressed as nutrients obtained per day.

Simple computations which can also be obtained from shopping list information are the division of purchased foods into food groups and the total number of different foods purchased. The total number of foods purchased in an elderly housebound population has been found to be related to the nutritional quality of the diet. Nutrients consumed per dollar expended can also be determined.

The value of the shopping list method for the determination of the nutritional quality of the diet in elderly housebound people is limited, in that food waste is not measured and information is not obtained on foods that are not eaten during the period of food purchase inventory. Use of this method is being evaluated in circumstances where a food survey of the elderly in a community is being carried out under circumstances in which access to private homes is limited.

The combination of shopping list food surveys with demographic information is important. Information on the age range and income bracket of the target population group can be obtained from housing authorities or from census tract data (Carl, 1979).

## DIETARY ASSESSMENT IN INSTITUTIONS

The goal is to assess the nutritional adequacy of diets provided in institutions including domiciliary care facilities, intermediate care homes, and nursing homes. In order to evaluate the nutritional adequacy of food served, one must calculate the amount of food served, and determine the difference between the

*Food values are omitted from Handbook 456.

amounts of food purchased as of a known date prior to the food inventory, and the amounts of food remaining in the facility on the day of the inventory.

Repeated food inventories are required when the nutritional adequacy of the diet of the institution is to be monitored. The period of the food inventory must be constant. It is recommended that a 28-day inventory be employed because shorter inventories used in computations of the nutritional adequacy of institutional food have been shown to overstate the quality of the food (Davies and Holdsworth, 1979).

The number of patients and residents is then determined and the food energy and nutrients available to the persons in the two groups are calculated. Nutrients for which calculations should be performed include protein, calcium, phosphorous, magnesium, zinc, vitamin A, thiamin, riboflavin, niacin, ascorbic acid, vitamin $B_6$, vitamin $B_{12}$, and folacin.

The Recommended Dietary Allowances of the Food and Nutrition Board of the National Academy of Sciences for men and women over the age of 51 years should be used for these calculations.

To calculate nutrient requirements the RDA for each nutrient per man or woman should be calculated and then multiplied by the number of persons of each sex in the facility. The products are then added together. This figure represents the total RDA for calories and 14 selected nutrients for all residents in the facility for one day.

In order to assess the nutritional adequacy of the food served, the percentage of the RDA's are calculated by dividing the total nutritive quality of all the food served by the RDA for each nutrient, and multiplying by 100.

In order to compute the nutrient composition of the food issued, it is recommended that a computerized data base, such as the Ohio State University program, be employed (USDA Handbook 8.) Limitations of this data base include missing values for several of the key nutrients including magnesium, zinc, folacin, vitamin $B_{12}$, and vitamin $B_6$.

Nutritionists who are computing the nutritional quality of geriatric institutionalized food are advised to keep a file on new and reliable tables of nutrient values and to modify the data base to supply presently missing values by selective additions as new information is published.

## ASSESSMENT OF FEEDING PRACTICES
## IN GERIATRIC CARE FACILITIES

The aims of this type of study are to determine the degree of nutritional risk for the residents, to determine resident satisfaction with the food service, and to assess whether modification in the system would be carried out (Allington et al., 1980).

The questionnaires are prepared for the administrator, the food service manager or dietitian, the cook, and the residents. Questions addressed to the administration pertain to the method of food purchase, food expenditure, staffing pattern and staff responsibilities, and the nutritional assessment of patients and patient care plans. Questions addressed to the food service manager, dietary aide, or dietitian relate to their knowledge of nutrient requirements of the elderly, menus for staff and residents and menu rotation, special diets, standardization of recipes, and arrangements made for feeding or assisted self-feeding of residents, monitoring of plate waste, and food hygiene.

Questions for the cook relate to the use of recipes and cooking methods other than those stipulated by the food service manager, and the use of food preparation methods which cause nutrient destruction.

Questions to the residents relate to satisfaction or dissatisfaction with the food, foods missed, foods enjoyed or disliked, satisfaction with portion size, frequency and times of meals, and whether food suggestions made by residents are heeded.

All questionnaires should ask certain consistent questions pertaining to the food service.

From the completed questionnaires, the nutritionist investigator should be able to assess the quality of the dietary service to the facility. Answers to the following questions should be analyzed using composite information obtained from the four questionnaires:

1. Is the staff (nursing, kitchen, dining room, etc.) adequate in number and qualifications?
2. Are food costs appropriate to patient and staff needs?
3. Do the staff eat different foods than the residents?
4. Do patient care plans specify diet and dietary changes, with reasons?
5. Does the food service manager understand food groups, nutrients supplied by particular foods, and nutrient requirements of elderly persons?
6. Are the patients weighed? How often?
7. Is patient food consumption monitored?
8. What are the methods of food storage?
9. What health screening is required for kitchen staff and others concerned with feeding patients?
10. How are dishes and utensils washed?
11. How are vegetables prepared?
12. Are salads served?
13. How often is milk served?
14. How often is citrus fruit juice served?
15. How often are fortified breakfast cereals served?
16. Is the menu monotonous?
17. Do special diets conform to recommended therapeutic guidelines?
18. Do patients complain that meals are inedible?
19. What foods do patients say they long for?
20. Are patients dissatisfied with menu changes made in response to their suggestions?

21. Is there disagreement in the answers to questions between the administration, the food service manager, the cook, and the residents?

## CLINICAL ASSESSMENT

The aims of the clinical assessment of nutritional status are:

1. To discover whether the person has had symptoms which partially explain or account for a change in nutritional status.
2. To discover whether the person has had medical problems (as described in lay terms by the person) or diagnosed diseases (as told to the patient or recounted by the physician) which could partially explain or account for changes in nutritional status.
3. To determine from physical examination whether the individual has one or more signs which are indicative of nutritional disease.

Symptoms which are related to nutritional disorder or disease are listed in Table 6-1. Physical signs related to nutritional disease are summarized and grouped in Table 6-2.

The clinical assessment of nutritional status presents a special challenge with elderly individuals (Driezen, 1974). Symptoms and signs which may be compatible with nutritional disease may be due to non-nutritional diseases. For example, purpura, particularly when confined to the forearms, may indicate senile purpura due to aging changes in the skin plus mild trauma, but it also could be due to scurvy or vitamin K deficiency due to intake of anticoagulant drugs or liver disease.

If the presenting health complaints, other symptoms, history, and physical signs suggest nutritional disease, then final diagnosis depends on laboratory tests and/or on finding that the condition resolves with specific nutritional intervention (e.g. giving therapeutic doses of the deficient nutrient) or on find-

**TABLE 6-1  Symptoms Which May Be Related to Nutritional Disease**

| | |
|---|---|
| Loss of appetite | Slow healing of wound, sore, or ulcer |
| Loss of taste or smell | Changes in skin color (yellow, brown, grey) |
| Loss of weight | Light sensitivity |
| Gain in weight | Swelling of the legs |
| Pain or discomfort on eating or swallowing, sore lips, tongue, or throat | Hair loss |
| | Thin nails |
| Vomiting | Breathlessness on exertion and/or at rest |
| Regurgitation of food | Burning, pricking, pins and needles, or cramps in the legs |
| Change in bowel habits | |
| Diarrhea | Feeling of walking on cotton |
| Blood in the stools | Loss of balance |
| Bulky, foul stools | Confusion |
| "Rash" (dermatitis) not responding to topical medication | Loss of memory |
| | Depression |
| Bleeding into the skin or easy bruising | |

TABLE 6-2   Physical Signs Which May Be Related
to Nutritional Disease

| | |
|---|---|
| Emaciation | Stomatitis |
| Dependent edema | Pallor (conjunctival) |
| Dermatitis (light exposed areas) | Koilonychia |
| Dry skin with crazy pavement dermatosis | Intertrigo |
| Purpura | Muscle wasting |
| Decubitus ulcer (bed sore) | Paralysis |
| Angular stomatitis | Ataxia |
| Cheilosis | Corneal vascularization |

ing a non-nutritional cause, e.g. cancer, which causes secondary malnutrition (Roe, 1980).

Laboratory tests performed to confirm a clinical diagnosis of malnutrition may lack specificity and/or sensitivity or may not be available. Further, nutritional intervention will not be successful if the cause of malnutrition is not concurrently treated or if the patient has malabsorption and nutrient supplements are given by mouth, or if the patient is unable to utilize nutrients efficiently, as in alcoholic cirrhosis or cancer.

Major problems in the clinical assessment of the elderly patient are loss of memory, failure to complain, acceptance of a medical problem as being due to aging, lack of nutritional specificity of complaints, and multiplicity of disease, only some of which may be nutritional in origin.

Clinical and public health nutritionists as well as therapeutic dietitians need to understand that the medical history which has been obtained by the patient's physician can provide the history necessary to the clinical assessment. Similarly, the physical examination, which includes a review of systems, can provide extensive information on nutritional findings. It is imperative that in hospitals, clinics, and in geriatric institutions, the nutritionists should be able to examine medical records and should have familiarity with medical terms (see Glossary of Medical Terms in Appendix). A complete clinical assessment of the nutritional status includes pertinent information from the physical history and from the physical examination. In most instances, the nutritionist's major responsibilities in clinical assessment are:

1. Analysis of the patient's medical records for
   a. symptoms listed in Table 6-1
   b. physical signs as shown in Table 6-2
   c. medical problems and diagnoses as listed in Table 6-3.
2. Patient interview following the guidelines of a structured questionnaire to obtain information on current health complaints which indicate nutritional disease (Table 6-4).
3. Examination of the patient with the physician to elicit signs of malnutrition.

**TABLE 6-3** Medical Problems and Diagnoses Related to Nutritional Disease

| PATIENT'S DESCRIPTION (OR DESCRIPTION BY RELATIVE) | DIAGNOSIS IN MEDICAL RECORD |
|---|---|
| Loss of flesh | Cachexia (chronic protein-energy malnutrition) |
| Cancer | Neoplastic disease (organ or site and type specified ± metastases) |
| Sore tongue/sore mouth | Glossitis or stomatitis due to ariboflavinosis, pellagra, ill-fitting dentures, candidiasis, radiation therapy, cancer chemotherapy or drug reaction |
| Can't swallow or keep food down | Plummer-Vinson syndrome; systemic sclerosis; carcinoma of the pharynx or esophagus |
| Disease of the bowels ("Food goes right through me," "Blood in my bowel movements," or "stoppage of the bowels") | Gluten-sensitive enteropathy; inflammatory bowel disease; carcinoma of the colon or rectum; diverticular disease; late effects of gastrectomy or intestinal bypass or resection |
| Liver disease | Alcoholic cirrhosis |
| Bleeding problems | Scurvy; vitamin K deficiency due to anti-coagulants |
| Poor (tired) blood | Anemia (nutritional) |
| Skin disease | Exfoliative dermatitis; pemphigus; pemphigoid; pellagra; other nutritional dermatoses |
| Hormone problem, low-thyroid | Obesity; myxedema; thyrotoxicosis |
| Heart disease | Congestive heart failure; alcoholic heart disease; hypertensive heart disease; atherosclerotic heart disease |
| Chest disease | Emphysema; chronic bronchitis; cor pulmonale |
| Stroke/paralysis | Hemiplegia; cranial nerve paralysis; peripheral neuropathy; Parkinson's disease |

## ANTHROPOMETRIC ASSESSMENT

Anthropometric assessment of the elderly should include measurement of weight, height, midarm circumference, and triceps skinfold thickness. Weight is best measured on a beam-type calibrated scale but weight may also be obtained on a bathroom scale which is frequently checked for accuracy of readings. Weighing of patients who cannot stand unaided should be on a scale with a broad base on which a chair of known weight can be placed. For bedridden patients, weighing requires use of a hoist and special weighing device (Figure 6-6).

The patient's height can be measured if the person can stand upright against a wall. The simplest devices for accurate measurement of height are a tape fixed to the wall and a flat board or ruler, which can be placed on the

**TABLE 6-4   Short Form Questionnaire for Use by Nutritionists Interviewing Geriatric Patients**

(Patient's responses are circled. If the patient cannot understand the question, circle "no answer.")

1. How is your appetite?     Very good    Good    Fair    Poor    No Answer

2. Does your food taste as good as usual?    Yes    No    No Answer
   If no, are there certain foods which taste bad?    Yes    No
   If yes, which foods? _____
   _____

3. Do you have difficulty with chewing?    Yes    No    No Answer
   If yes, are there certain foods you can't chew?    Yes    No
   If yes, which foods? _____
   _____

4. Do you have difficulty with swallowing?    Yes    No    No Answer
   If yes, are there certain foods you can't swallow?    Yes    No
   If yes, which foods? _____
   _____

5. Do you have any difficulty in keeping your food down?    Yes    No    No Answer
   If yes, are there certain foods you can't keep down?    Yes    No
   If yes, which foods? _____
   _____

6. Do you get a stomach ache or gas after eating?    Yes    No    No Answer
   If yes, are there certain foods which give you a stomach ache or gas?    Yes    No
   If yes, which foods? _____
   _____

7. Do you have diarrhea (loose bowel movements) after eating?    Yes    No    No Answer
   If yes, is the diarrhea related to certain foods?    Yes    No
   If yes, which foods? _____
   _____

8. Are you frequently constipated?    Yes    No    No Answer
   If yes, are there certain foods you eat to relieve your constipation?    Yes    No
   If yes, which foods? _____
   _____

9. Are you losing weight?    Yes    No    Don't Know    No Answer
   If yes, is this intentional?    Yes    No

10. Are you gaining weight?    Yes    No    Don't Know    No Answer
    If yes, is this intentional?    Yes    No

patient's head. If the patient is confined to bed or is unable to stand, the crown-to-heel length may be substituted for a height measurement (Figure 6-7). Whenever possible, records should be obtained of the person's maximal height and weight at a recent time when he or she was in good health.

Assessment of the person's weight-for-height-for-age should be made using Table 6-5. These measurements and records will indicate whether the patient's weight is within the normal range for height and age, or at or below

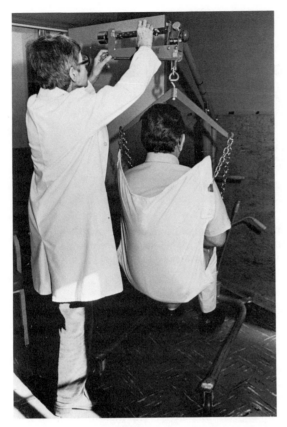

FIGURE 6-6    Patient lifter and beam scale used to weigh elderly patients.

the normative range, whether the person has gained or lost weight, and whether the patient's height has declined (loss of height is most commonly due to osteoporosis of the vertebral column).

Fatness or leanness is assessed by triceps skinfold thickness. Measurement of triceps skinfold thickness should be with calibrated Lange calipers. The midpoint on the arm is determined with a tape measure as halfway between the tip of the acromion process of the shoulder and the olecranium process of the elbow. This point is marked with a pen and the skin and fatfold thickness at this point are measured with the calipers (Figure 6-8).

The midarm circumference is obtained using a nylon tape placed around the arm at the point selected for measurement of skinfold thickness (Figure 6-9). From the combined measurements of triceps skinfold thickness and midarm circumference, the arm muscle area can be computed*. The arm muscle diameter is

$$*\text{Arm muscle area (cm}^2) = \frac{[\text{Arm circumference (mm)} - \pi \times \text{triceps skinfold (mm)}]^2}{400\pi}$$

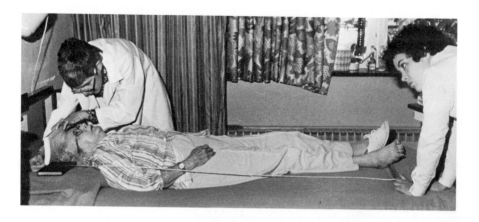

FIGURE 6-7    Crown-to-heel "height" measurement of bedridden patient. (Note that two persons are required to make this "height" measurement—one to place the head against a board and the other to position the feet.)

a measure of lean body mass. Whereas it is usual practice to measure triceps skinfold thickness and midarm circumference using the left arm, choice of arms in the elderly may be determined by neuropathology. Hemiplegia following stroke, which is usually left-sided and associated with wasting of the left arm, will make it necessary to make the anthropometric measurements on the right arm. Other problems which commonly are associated with measurement of triceps skinfold thickness in elderly people are sagging and increased compressibility of the fat folds on the back of the arm and difficulty in measuring triceps skinfold thickness in a recumbent, bedridden patient. It has been recommended that in the elderly and younger person, multiple measurements of skinfold thickness be used to calculate the percent of body fat.

Whether or not it is appropriate or feasible to carry out these more complex measurements depends on the expertise and experience of the nutritionist who is making the anthropometric measurements, as well as on prior establishment that multiple skinfold measurements can, in fact, be obtained with accuracy in particular patients who are being examined.

Serial measurements of triceps skinfold thickness and arm circumference carried out by the same person will provide valuable information on change in fatness and in muscle mass in the elderly. Used together with body weight determinations, it is possible not only to follow increases and decreases in weight, but also to obtain information on whether changes in weight are due to gain or loss in fat or lean body mass.

**TABLE 6-5** Assessment of Weight-for-Height-for Age in Persons 65 Years and Older

| HEIGHT IN INCHES | WEIGHT IN POUNDS |
|---|---|
| MEN | |
| 62 | 148 |
| 63 | 146 |
| 64 | 147 |
| 65 | 155 |
| 66 | 160 |
| 67 | 167 |
| 68 | 169 |
| 69 | 172 |
| 70 | 181 |
| 71 | 188 |
| 72 | 183 |
| 73 | 190[a] |
| 74 | 194[a] |
| WOMEN | |
| 57 | 130 |
| 58 | 133 |
| 59 | 137 |
| 60 | 138 |
| 61 | 144 |
| 62 | 146 |
| 63 | 149 |
| 64 | 152 |
| 65 | 153 |
| 66 | 162 |
| 67 | 173 |
| 68 | 168 |

[a]Estimated values obtained from linear regression equations.
Note: Examined persons were measured without shoes. Clothing weight ranged from 0.20 to 0.62 lb., which was not deducted from weights shown.

Adapted from *Weight by Height by Age for Adults 18-74 Years: U.S., 1971-74,* DHEW Publ. No. (PHS) 79-1656, Sept. 1979.

Arm circumference and arm muscle area for elderly men and women under and over the age of 80 years and of different body weights are shown in Table 6-6. Caution is required in interpreting acute changes in body weight in the elderly. A common cause of sudden weight gain is edema associated with congestive heart failure. Sudden weight loss will occur in edematous patients with congestive heart failure after they receive effective diuretics.

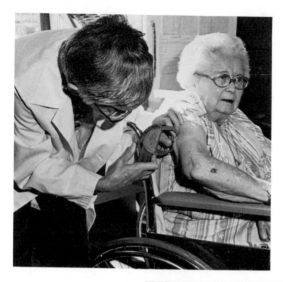

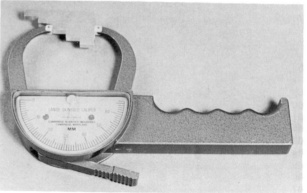

FIGURE 6-8    Measurement of triceps skinfold thickness with Lange skinfold calipers.


## HEMATOLOGICAL ASSESSMENT

In the elderly, as in other age groups, hematological assessment can be used as a means of screening patients for malnutrition. Characteristic changes in the blood count and in the morphology of cells of the red and white cell series occur in response to specific nutritional deficiencies. The extent to which hematological changes and abnormalities can be used in the diagnosis of nutritional deficiency depends on the duration of the deficiency as well as on the supportive evidence of clinical and biochemical findings.

In order to define the presence of anemia, the simplest screening methods are by determination of the hemoglobin level (grams of hemoglobin

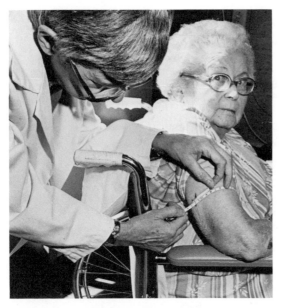

**FIGURE 6-9**    Measurement of mid-arm circumference using a nylon tape.

per 100 ml of blood) and by estimation of the packed cell volume (hematocrit reading as percent of a defined volume of blood). The cyanmethemoglobin method is now the standard method for hemoglobin determination and packed cell volume is estimated using a microhematocrit centrifuge with a scale which can be used to read the percent volume of packed cells in capillary tubes. In anemias, the hemoglobin level and the packed cell volume are reduced (Thompson, 1979).

For definition of nutritional anemias, a complete blood count is required, together with examination of red blood cells on a stained blood film and a differential count of cells of the white cell series. Normal or acceptable values for hemoglobin, hematocrit, red cells (erythrocyte count), total white cells (leukocyte count), and leukocyte differential count are shown in Table 6-7. This table also shows the ranges of acceptable values for the red cell indices. The red cell indices include the mean corpuscular volume (a measure of the average volume of the red cells) as well as the mean corpuscular hemoglobin and the mean corpuscular hemoglobin concentration. Equations for calculations of red cell indices are shown in Table 6-8. Laboratories performing blood counts by automated Coulter counter technique produce reports which include red cell indices. In Table 6-9, changes in these blood parameters in nutritional anemias are indicated.

In chronic iron deficiency anemia, reduction in hemoglobin and hematocrit values are associated with a diminished red cell count. Further, there are characteristic changes in red cell morphology and staining. The red cells appear smaller than normal (microcytic) and they are light in color in the blood

TABLE 6-6    Arm Circumference, Triceps Skinfold Measurements
and Arm Muscle Mass in Elderly Women and Men

| WOMEN | MEAN | ± STANDARD DEVIATION |
|---|---|---|
| Height (cm) | | |
| under 80 years | 153.8 | 7.05 |
| 80 years and over | 151.6* | 6.18 |
| Weight (kg) | | |
| under 80 years | 58.87 | 11.168 |
| 80 years and over | 57.54 | 12.124 |
| Arm circumference (cm) | | |
| under 80 years | 26.8 | 3.88 |
| 80 years and over | 26.1 | 3.70 |
| Arm muscle area (sq cm) | | |
| under 80 years | 36.7 | 10.28 |
| 80 years and over | 36.0 | 10.26 |
| MEN | | |
| Height (cm) | | |
| under 80 years | 166.5 | 6.73 |
| 80 years and over | 164.0* | 6.33 |
| Weight (kg) | | |
| under 80 years | 67.00 | 10.435 |
| 80 years and over | 64.61 | 13.855 |
| Arm circumference (cm) | | |
| under 80 years | 27.2 | 2.91 |
| 80 years and over | 26.4 | 3.88 |
| Arm muscle area (sq cm) | | |
| under 80 years | 46.5 | 10.32 |
| 80 years and over | 44.5 | 11.81 |

*$p < 0.05$. Mean values of subjects 80 years and over were significantly less than the means for those under 80 years of age.

Adapted from *Nutrition and Health in Old Age,* Department of Health and Social Security (London: Her Majesty's Stationery Office, 1979).

films stained with Wright's stain (hypochromic). The mean corpuscular volume is reduced as is the mean corpuscular hemoglobin concentration.

Both folacin and vitamin $B_{12}$ deficiencies cause megaloblastic anemias (Chanarin, 1969). The defect is not, as in iron deficiency, in the production of hemoglobin which requires iron for its biosynthesis, but is a maturational defect in both the red and white cell series. In anemia due to either folacin or vitamin $B_{12}$ deficiency, the red cell count is reduced very early in the development of the disease. As fewer cells are formed, the hematocrit and hemoglobin levels are reduced. The blood film shows red blood cells which are larger than normal (macrocytic), and these cells have an increased mean corpuscular volume. These macrocytic cells tend to be oval when seen on blood films, and

**TABLE 6-7** Acceptable Values for Hemoglobin, Hematocrit, Red Cells and White Cells, and Leukocyte Differential Count

| DIFFERENTIAL COUNT | | NORMAL HEMATOLOGICAL VALUES (M = MALE; F = FEMALE) | | |
|---|---|---|---|---|
| CELL | ADULT (%) | TEST | | NORMALS |
| Neutrophil | 50-60 | WBC | M | 7.8 ± 3 |
| Band | 0-1 | X $10^3$ | F | 7.8 ± 3 |
| Eosinophil | 1-3 | RBC | M | 5.4 ± 0.7 |
| Basophil | 0-1 | X $10^6$ | F | 4.8 ± 0.6 |
| Monocyte | 4-10 | Hgb | M | 16 ± 2 |
| Lymphocyte | 25-40 | g | F | 16 ± 2 |
| | | Hct | M | 47 ± 5 |
| | | % | F | 42 ± 5 |
| | | MCV | M | 87 ± 7 |
| | | $\mu^3$ | F | 90 ± 9 |
| | | MCH | M | 29 ± 2 |
| | | $\mu\mu$g | F | 29 ± 2 |
| | | MCHC | M | 34 ± 2 |
| | | % | F | 34 ± 2 |

**TABLE 6-8** Calculations of Red Cell Indices

$$MCV = \frac{\text{Hematocrit} \times 10}{\text{Red blood count in millions}} \text{ cu}\mu$$

Normal value for the MCV: 80-94 cu$\mu$

$$MCH = \frac{\text{Hemoglobin} \times 10}{\text{Red blood count in millions}} \mu\mu\text{g}$$

Normal value for the MCH: 27-31 $\mu\mu$g

$$MCHC = \frac{\text{Hemoglobin} \times 100}{\text{Hematocrit}} \%$$

Normal value for the MCHC: 32-36%

MCV = Mean corpuscular volume
MCH = Mean corpuscular hemoglobin
MCHC = Mean corpuscular hemoglobin concentration

Taken from B. A. Brown, *Hematology: Principles and Procedures* (Philadelphia: Lea & Febiger, 1973).

they stain deeply (hyperchromic) because they contain more hemoglobin per cell. Macrocytic red cells are also more fragile than normal red cells. When iron deficiency and folacin or vitamin $B_{12}$ deficiency coexist, stained blood films show a mixture of hypochromic microcytic and hyperchromic macrocytic

TABLE 6-9   Criteria for Diagnosis of Nutritional Anemias
from Red Cells Indices

| ANEMIA | MCV | MCH | MCHC |
|---|---|---|---|
| | cu$\mu$ | $\mu\mu$g | % |
| Iron deficiency | <80 | <27 | <32 |
| Folacin or vitamin B$_{12}$ deficiency | >100 | >31 | >35 |

red cells. The white blood cells classified as neutrophils or polymorphonuclear leukocytes show an increased number (hypersegmentation) of lobes.

The bone marrow in folacin and vitamin B$_{12}$ deficiency shows red and white blood cell precursors which are larger than normal (megaloblastic cells).

Elderly men and women can maintain hemoglobin and hematocrit values as well as red blood cell counts within the acceptable ranges for younger adults. However, when comparison is made between the blood picture of older and younger adults, a small but significant reduction in hemoglobin, hematocrit, and red blood cell counts have been shown to occur with advancing years after the age of 65 (Table 6-10). Among independently living elderly persons, anemia has been found to vary with the population group studied (community or institution), with sex, and with age. Anemia is more common in housebound and institutionalized persons, is more common in women than in men, and is also more prevalent in persons over the age of 75 years.

Common causes of iron deficiency in the elderly include low iron intake and excessive iron losses due to gastrointestinal bleeding, high intake of aspirin, diverticular disease, colon cancer, surgical procedures, or hemorrhage associated with anticoagulant drug therapy (Kalchthaler and Tan, 1980).

In the elderly, megaloblastic anemia may be due to pernicious anemia. Folacin deficiency, which can cause megaloblastic anemia in the elderly, is usually due to very low intake of folacin-rich foods such as green leafy vegetables, liver, and fortified breakfast cereals. Other causes include malabsorption syndromes and intake of drugs which impair folacin utilization.

Hematological assessment is important in that when biochemical determination of iron, folacin or vitamin B$_{12}$ deficiency is not available for geriatric patients, the specific nutritional deficiency can be determined by repeated blood counts, estimation of red cell indices, and examination of stained blood films after administration of hematinics. Hematinics include iron, vitamin B$_{12}$, and folic acid. If the initial blood picture shows a microcytic, hypochromic anemia, then administration of an available iron supplement, such as ferrous sulfate, will produce a hematologic response such that there will be an increase in hemoglobin level and in packed cell volume, an increase in mean corpuscular volume towards the normal range, and an increase in the mean corpuscular hemoglobin. Blood films will show the presence of red blood cells of normal size and staining as the anemia responds to iron treatment.

TABLE 6-10  Red Blood Cell Measurements: Population Reference Values as Means + Central 95% Range ($\bar{x}$ ± 1.965)

| SEX & AGE GROUP (yrs.) | RLG (10$^{12}$/L) | HEMOGLOBIN (gm/dl) | HEMATOCRIT (%) | MCV (fl) | MCH (pg) | MCHC (gm/dl) |
|---|---|---|---|---|---|---|
| MALES | | | | | | |
| All ages | 5.40 ± 0.78 | 16.00 ± 1.96 | 47.00 ± 4.90 | 87.00 ± 4.90 | 29.00 ± 1.96 | 34.00 ± 1.96 |
| 65-72 (n=45) | 4.80 ± 0.86* | 14.50 ± 2.53* | 43.67 ± 7.19* | 90.73 ± 15.90 | 30.35 ± 5.45* | 33.36 ± 2.46* |
| 73-80 (n=34) | 4.62 ± 0.94* | 13.66 ± 3.85* | 40.99 ± 10.24* | 88.85 ± 21.10 | 30.00 ± 8.20 | 33.44 ± 3.55* |
| 81-88 (n=21) | 4.55 ± 1.20* | 13.83 ± 3.89* | 40.73 ± 10.20* | 89.38 ± 10.36* | 30.46 ± 4.12 | 33.95 ± 2.85 |
| 89-96 (n=6) | 4.63 ± 1.22* | 14.42 ± 3.63 | 42.82 ± 10.74 | 92.67 ± 12.74 | 31.42 ± 2.47* | 33.92 ± 2.89 |
| All elderly males | 4.68 ± 1.01* | 14.09 ± 3.43* | 42.18 ± 9.50* | 89.97 ± 16.88* | 30.32 ± 6.19* | 33.54 ± 2.98* |
| FEMALES | | | | | | |
| All ages | 4.80 ± 0.59 | 14.00 ± 1.96 | 42.00 ± 4.90 | 87.00 ± 4.90 | 29.00 ± 1.96 | 34.00 ± 1.96 |
| 65-72 (n=64) | 4.54 ± 1.03* | 13.74 ± 3.02 | 41.14 ± 8.95 | 90.77 ± 14.55* | 30.49 ± 4.86* | 33.32 ± 2.20* |
| 73-80 (n=66) | 4.45 ± 1.05* | 13.51 ± 2.80* | 40.30 ± 8.14* | 90.47 ± 16.33 | 30.54 ± 5.18 | 33.64 ± 2.74* |
| 81-88 (n=45) | 4.35 ± 1.19* | 12.74 ± 2.65* | 38.53 ± 7.86* | 88.91 ± 16.09* | 29.68 ± 5.59 | 33.32 ± 2.43* |
| 89-100 (n=11) | 4.31 ± 1.40* | 12.96 ± 4.47 | 39.51 ± 12.71 | 91.55 ± 9.97* | 30.34 ± 3.46* | 32.99 ± 2.17* |
| All elderly females | 4.45 ± 1.12* | 13.37 ± 3.08* | 40.12 ± 8.92* | 90.26 ± 15.44* | 30.35 ± 5.14* | 33.42 ± 2.49* |

*P < 0.05 by Student t test and analysis (differs significantly from laboratory normal values for sex).

Taken from M. S. H. Htoo, R. L. Kofkoff and M. L. Freedman, "Erythrocyte parameters in the elderly: An argument against new geriatric normal values," *J. Amer. Geriatrics Soc.*, 27 (1979), 548.

When the initial blood picture and bone marrow film, if available, shows a megaloblastic anemia, it is essential that the initial hematinic be vitamin $B_{12}$, which has to be administered by intramuscular injection. The rationale for initial administration of vitamin $B_{12}$ is that if folic acid is given prior to vitamin $B_{12}$ in pernicious anemia, there will be a hematologic response which will mislead the physician to accept a diagnosis of folacin deficiency. The correct diagnosis of pernicious anemia may be overlooked which imposes a risk that the patient will develop neurological signs of pernicious anemia which do not respond to administration of folic acid.

When vitamin $B_{12}$ injections are given in the appropriate dosages to treat pernicious anemia, early hematological responses include normalization of the megaloblastic bone marrow and the appearance in the blood of reticulocytes. Reticulocytes are late precursors of red blood cells. The presence of reticulocytes in the blood can be demonstrated by special staining techniques. An increase in the red cell count and in the packed cell volume will also follow; the mean corpuscular volume will decrease towards the normal range and the blood film will then show the appearance of normocytic (normal sized) red blood cells and the disappearance of hypersegmented polymorphonuclear leukocytes (neutrophils).

When a megaloblastic anemia does not respond to therapeutic doses of parenteral vitamin $B_{12}$, then folic acid should be administered orally unless it has already been demonstrated that severe malabsorption is present when the folic acid may be administered by injection. Hematologic response to folic acid in folacin deficiency follows a similar sequence to that of pernicious anemia treated by injection of vitamin $B_{12}$.

Hematological assessment can be used as an indicator of vitamin $B_6$ deficiency. This deficiency is rarely due to dietary insufficiency in elderly persons. Causes in the elderly include use of drugs which are vitamin $B_6$ antagonists and chronic alcohol abuse (Lindenbaum, 1980).

The anemia associated with vitamin $B_6$ is a hypochromic anemia due to impairment in heme synthesis. Iron can be demonstrated in granules, bone marrow red cell precursors, and in red cells in the peripheral blood cells containing these iron granules, called sideroblasts. The presence of sideroblasts in the bone marrow and in the blood of patients with vitamin $B_6$ deficiency is a reflection of malutilization of iron in the formation of hemoglobin. Since vitamin $B_6$ deficiency is usually due to use of drugs which are vitamin $B_6$ antagonists or to toxic effects of alcohol on the bone marrow, administration of vitamin $B_6$ will not produce amelioration in the anemia or, at best, will produce an inadequate hematologic response unless the responsible drug or alcohol intake is discontinued.

The total lymphocyte count can be used as a means of screening for adequacy of cellular immune function (Bistrian et al., 1975). Reduction in the total lymphocyte count is indicative of a depression of cellular immune function which can develop rapidly when food is withheld prior to or after surgery or in cachetic patients who are also severely anorectic. Normative values for lymphocyte counts and values in acute and chronic protein-energy malnutrition are shown in Table 6-11.

**TABLE 6-11** Malnutrition and Immune Competency

| | TOTAL LYMPHOCYTE COUNT/MM$^3$ | SKIN TEST MM REACTION |
|---|---|---|
| Normal | ⩾1500 | ⩾10 |
| Moderate | 800-1200 | 5-10 |
| Severe malnutrition (Kwashiorkor-like) | <800 | <5 |

Taken from G. L. Blackburn and P. A. Thornton, "Nutritional assessment of the hospitalized patient," *Med. Clin. North America,* 63: 1111, 1979. © W. B. Saunders Co. Reprinted by permission.

## BIOCHEMICAL ASSESSMENT

The biochemical assessment of nutritional status can be employed to determine the level of recent intake of specific nutrients, to estimate nutrient stores in body fluids (serum or plasma) or tissues (red or white blood cells), to obtain functional measures of nutritional adequacy or deficiency, and to determine nutritional risk (Sauberlich et al., 1974). In the development of nutritional deficiencies, biochemical changes precede clinical signs of deficiency. Biochemical assessment is used to confirm or refute nutritional diagnoses which are based on clinical, anthropometric, or hematological assessment. Biochemical tests used to screen geriatric patients for nutritional disease are shown in Table 6-12. Limitations in conducting biochemical assessment of the vitamin, mineral, or absorptive function status of the elderly are:

1. Ignorance of normative values for older age groups.
2. Inadequate laboratory facilities and expertise.
3. Problems in collecting samples, e.g. 24-hour urine samples from incontinent, noncatheterized patients.
4. Impaired absorptive function for test substance (as in xylose tolerance test).
5. Decreased renal function leading to slowed clearance of test substance.

Examples of plasma or serum levels of nutrients usually reflect intake but may also reflect nutritional status. Quantitative biochemical tests for the assessment of levels of recent intake of specific nutrients include plasma (or serum) folacin and plasma ascorbic acid.

**TABLE 6-12** Biochemical Tests and Test Values for Assessment of Normative Nutritional Status in the Elderly

| TEST | VALUES FOR PERSONS ≥ 60 BY RACE AND SEX | | | |
|------|-------|-------|-------|-------|
| | BLACK | | WHITE | |
| | MALE | FEMALE | MALE | FEMALE |
| Total proteins g/dl | 7.22± 0.17 | 7.31± 0.45 | 7.10± 0.22 | 7.01± 0.37 |
| Serum albumin g/dl | 4.13± 0.09 | 4.14± 0.07 | 4.17± 0.10 | 4.29± 0.11 |
| Hemoglobin g/dl | 15.09± 1.08 | 13.55± 1.99 | 16.43± 1.41 | 15.09± 1.08 |
| Serum iron mg/dl | 0.076± 0.025 | 0.059± 0.025 | 0.093± 0.386 | 0.085± 0.269 |
| Serum glucose mg/dl | 95.1± 24.0 | 115.3± 78.2 | 92.1± 11.9 | 91.2± 12.3 |
| Serum cholesterol mg/dl | 193.4± 66.4 | 246.9± 106.1 | 206.2± 53.8 | 212.4± 42.3 |
| Vitamin C | 0.64± 0.40 | 0.74± 0.38 | 0.99± 0.39 | 0.93± 0.34 |

Taken from E. T. Koh, M. S. Chi, and F. W. Lowenstein, "Comparison of selected blood components by race, sex, and age," *Amer. J. Clin. Nutr.* 33 (1980), 1828-35.

Linear relationships have been demonstrated between the intake of available dietary folacin and plasma (serum) folacin levels and between intake of vitamins and leukocyte ascorbic acid levels.

Plasma or serum carotene levels may reflect recent intake of food sources of carotenes, but low plasma carotene levels also occur with malabsorption.

Plasma or serum retinol levels are generally accepted as a measure of vitamin A status.

Nutrient stores can be estimated by a determination of levels of specific nutrients in red or white blood cells. Examples of biochemical tests for the determination of nutrient "stores" include red cell folacin determination and leukocyte ascorbate levels. It is assumed that levels of these nutrients in cells of the peripheral blood reflect body stores of the vitamins. However, it must be emphasized that it is presently unclear whether in elderly people levels of these nutrients in blood cells are in precisely the same normative range of values accepted for younger persons.

Functional tests of vitamin status include the erythrocyte glutathione reductase assay for riboflavin status, the erythrocyte transketolase test for measurement of thiamin status, and the plasma pyridoxal phosphate level for estimation of vitamin $B_6$ status. Acceptable low and deficient values for key vitamin levels or assay values are shown in Table 6-13.

A mineral profile of geriatric patients should be obtained at regular intervals, preferably monthly, if intake of specific minerals is precarious, if patients are receiving drugs which cause mineral depletion, or if they have medical problems which are associated with excessive mineral losses or mineral retention. Biochemical tests of mineral status available at most hospital laboratories are plasma (serum), sodium, potassium, and calcium and phosphorus. Acceptable, deficient, and excessively high levels for these minerals are shown in Table 6-14. A low product of calcium and phosphorus (CaXP in mg/dl)<40 is indicative of osteomalacia in an elderly patient.

Patients with liver disease (especially those with alcoholic cirrhosis), patients with congestive heart failure, and persons receiving diuretics may become magnesium and zinc deficient. Plasma magnesium and zinc levels are not precise measures of magnesium and zinc status, but can be used, if the tests are available, to monitor patient progress and response to treatment. Acceptable and deficient levels for serum magnesium and zinc are shown in Table 6-15.

**TABLE 6-13** Biochemical Assessment of Vitamin Status in the Elderly (Assay Values)

|  | ACCEPTABLE | LOW | DEFICIENT |
|---|---|---|---|
| Plasma retinol ($\mu$g/100 ml) | > 20.0 | 10-20.0 | < 10.0 |
| Serum folate (ng/ml) | > 6.0 | 3-6.0 | < 3.0 |
| Red cell folate (ng/ml) | > 150 | 100-150 | < 100 |
| Serum vitamin $B_{12}$ (pg/ml) | > 200 | 100-200 | < 100 |
| Serum vitamin $B_6$ (ng/ml) | > 4.0 | 3-4.0 | < 3.0 |
| Red cell vitamin $B_6$ (ng/ml) | > 14.0 | 12-14.0 | < 12.0 |
| Serum ascorbic acid (mg/100 ml) | > 0.30 | 0.20-0.29 | < 0.20 |
| Leukocyte ascorbic acid (mg/100 ml) | > 15 | 8-15 | < 8 |
| Red cell transketolase TPPE % | < 15 | 16-20 | > 20 |
| Red cell glutathione reductase AC | > 1.2 | 1.2-1.4 | > 1.4 |

**TABLE 6-14    Reference Values for Plasma or Serum Electrolytes in SI and Conventional Units**

| PLASMA OR SERUM CONSTITUENT | SI UNITS* (mmol/liter) | CONVENTIONAL UNITS |
|---|---|---|
| Calcium | 2.12-2.62 | 8.5-10.5 mg/100 ml |
| Chloride | 100-107 | 100-107 meq/l |
| Phosphate (fasting) | 0.8-1.4 | 2.5-4.5 mg/100 ml |
| Potassium | 3.8-5.2 | 3.8-5.2 meq/l |
| Sodium | 136-149 | 136-149 meq/l |

*SI Units = Systeme International d'Unites

Adapted from L. G. Whitby, I. W. Percy-Robb, and A. F. Smith, *Lecture Notes on Clinical Chemistry*, 3rd Printing (Oxford, London: Blackwell Sci. Publ., 1978).

**TABLE 6-15    Acceptable and Deficient Values for Serum Magnesium and Zinc**

| CONSTITUENT | ACCEPTABLE | DEFICIENT |
|---|---|---|
| | (VALUES IN USUAL UNITS) | |
| Magnesium | 0.7-1.0 mmol/l | < 0.7 mmol/l |
| Zinc* | >80 µg/dl | ≤70 µg/dl |

*Serum zinc values between 70 and 80 µg/dl are low.

## QUESTIONS

1. What are the appropriate conditions for use of specific dietary assessment methods in the elderly? Pair methods and conditions correctly:

|  | Method |  | Conditions |  |  |
|---|---|---|---|---|---|
|  | House | (H) | Cooperative | (C) | R.D. |
|  | M.D. Office | (O) | Semicooperative | (SC) | M.D. |
|  | Nursing Home | (N) | Noncooperative | (NC) | P.P.* |

a) Food frequency        i.    H        C        R.D.
b) Food service
   questionnaire         ii.    O        NC       M.D.
c) Food inventory       iii.    N        NC       R.D.
d) Shopping lists        iv.    O        C        M.D.
e) Diet record            v.    H        SC       P.P.

*P.P. = Health Paraprofessionals

2. Distinguish between the following *symptoms* and *signs* of malnutrition.

   a) feeling of walking on cotton    f ) koilonychia
   b) loss of appetite    g) diarrhea
   c) dependent edema    h) ataxia
   d) glossitis    i ) loss of memory
   e) pain on swallowing    j ) pallor (conjunctival)

3. The following instruments and methods are used in nutritional assessment. Indicate appropriate applications:
   a) Lange calipers
   b) cyanmethemoglobin method
   c) Coulter counter
   d) erythrocyte glutathione reductase assay
   e) total lymphocyte count

4. Iron deficiency can be determined by use of which two of the following tests?
   a) plasma retinol
   b) plasma ferritin
   c) red cell folacin
   d) red cell protoporphyria
   e) serum iron

5. Which of the following statements is correct?
   a) The blood picture in folacin and vitamin $B_{12}$ deficiency is similar.
   b) The blood picture in folacin and vitamin $B_{12}$ deficiency is entirely different.

## REFERENCES

ADAMS, C.F., "Nutritive value of American foods in common units," *Agric. Handbook No. 456*, USDA, Washington, D.C., 1975.

ALLINGTON, J.K., M.E. MATTHEWS, V.K. JOHNSON, and N.E. JOHNSON, "A short method to ensure nutritional adequacy of food served in nursing homes. 1. Identification of need; 2. Development of a model food plan." *J. Amer. Dietet. Assoc.*, 76 (1980), 458–70.

BISTRIAN, B.R., G.L. BLACKBURN, N.S. SCRIMSHAW, and J.P. FLATT, "Cellular immunity in semi-starved states in hospitalized adults," *Amer. J. Clin. Nutr.*, 28 (1975), 1148.

BLACKBURN, G.L., B.R. BISTRIAN, B.S. MAINI, H.T. SCHLAMM, and M.F. SMITH, "Nutritional and metabolic assessment of the hospitalized patient," *J. Parenteral and Enteral Nutr.*, 1 (1977), 11–22.

BURKE, B.S., "The dietary history as a tool in research," *J. Amer. Dietet. Assoc.*, 23 (1947), 1041–46.

CHANARIN, I., *The Megaloblastic Anemias*. Oxford and Edinburgh: Blackwell Scientific Publ., 1969, pp. 389–91.

CAIRD, F.I., "Problems of interpretation of laboratory findings in the old," *Brit. Med. J.*, 4 (1973), 348–51.

CARL, J.W., "Food purchases of housebound elderly," M.N.S. Degree Thesis, Cornell University, 1980.

DAVIES, L., and M.D. HOLDSWORTH, "A technique for assessing nutritional 'at risk' factors in residential homes for the elderly," *J. Human Nutr.*, 33 (1979), 165–69.

DRIEZEN, S., "Clinical manifestations of malnutrition," *Geriatrics*, 29 (1974), 97–103.

FREELAND, J.H., and R.J. COURSIN, "Zinc content of selected foods," *J. Amer. Dietet. Assoc.*, 68 (1976).

HERZLER, A.A., and L.M. HAEVER, "Development of food tables and uses with computers," *J. Amer. Dietet. Assoc.*, 70 (1977), 20.

KALCHTHALER, T., and M.E.R. TAN, "Anemia in institutionalized elderly patients," *J. Amer. Geriat. Soc.*, 28 (1980), 108–13.

LINDENBAUM, J., "Nutritional anemia in alcoholism," *Amer. J. Clin. Nutr.*, 33 (1980), 2727–35.

MURPHY, E.W., B.W. WILLIS, and B.K. WATT, "Provisional tables on the zinc content of food," *J. Amer. Dietet. Assoc.*, 66 (1975).

"Pantothenic acid, vitamin $B_6$ and vitamin $B_{12}$ in foods," *USDA Home Econ. Res. Rept.*, No. 36, 1969.

PERLOFF, B.P., and R.R. BUTRUM, "Folacin in selected foods," *J. Amer. Dietet. Assoc.*, 70 (1977).

ROE, D.A., *Clinical Nutrition for the Health Scientist.* Boca Raton, FL: CRC Press. Inc., 1980.

SAUBERLICH, H.E., J.H. SKALA, and R.P. DOWDY, *Laboratory Tests for the Assessment of Nutritional Status.* Cleveland, OH: CRC Press, Inc., 1974.

THOMPSON, R.B., *A Short Textbook of Hematology*, 5th Ed. Turnbridge Wells, Kent, England: Pitman Medical Publ. Co., Ltd., 1979.

WATT, B.K., and A.L. MERRILL, "Composition of foods — raw, processed, prepared," *Rev. USDA Agric. Handbook No. 8*, Washington, D.C., 1963.

# CHAPTER SEVEN
# Nutritional Deficiencies

Nutritional deficiencies in the elderly can result from short-term or long-term ingestion of a diet which is inadequate in food energy or lacking in one or more specific nutrients. Under physiological conditions, a diet is deficient if it does not meet the needs of most healthy individuals of a particular age group. Since the nutritional needs of most elderly people differ from the needs of younger people (including the middle-aged) for which the Recommended Dietary Allowances are set, and since the elderly differ one from another in their food energy and nutrient requirements, dietary adequacy for the elderly is better defined as a diet which, for a given individual, prevents malnutrition, and cannot be improved by additions and/or modifications in the levels of food-energy nutrients supplied.

Diets which lead to development of nutritional deficiency are a) monotonous, b) low in food energy, c) restrictive, and d) low in nutrient-calorie ratio.

Variety or dietary diversity will increase the quality of the diet, as will calorie adequacy. Conversely, the fewer the number of foods eaten, the greater the risk that sources of essential nutrients will be excluded or will be inadequate. Diets high in sweets or which include heavy daily intake of alcoholic beverages satisfy the hunger needs of the elderly without providing needed nutrients.

An example of a nutritionally adequate meal is shown in Figure 7-1. Examples of daily food intake patterns which if eaten on a usual or regular basis will induce nutritional deficiency are shown in Figures 7-2 through 7-5.

In the U.S., diets of the elderly are often deficient in folacin. Diets low in food energy are also low in iron. Elderly persons not consuming milk will have inadequate intakes of calcium, vitamin D, and riboflavin.

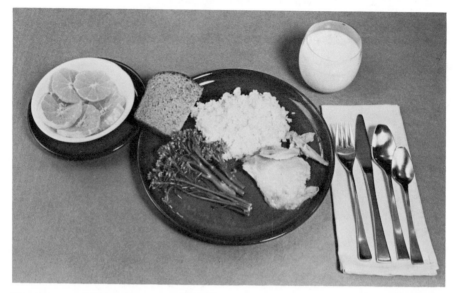

FIGURE 7-1    Well-balanced main meal: Foods of high nutrient-to-calorie ratio including roast chicken, enriched steamed rice, broccoli, whole wheat enriched bread, orange slices and milk.

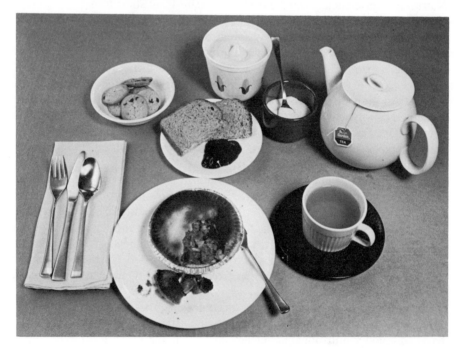

FIGURE 7-2    Monotonous diet with few different foods: Breakfast and lunch include tea, bread and jelly, and supper consists of a beef pot pie.

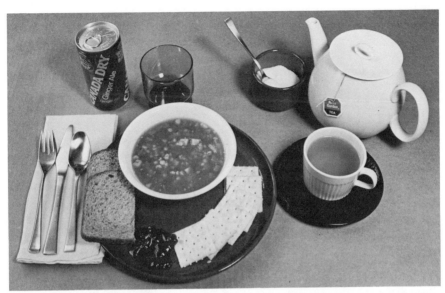

FIGURE 7-3   Low calorie, low nutrient, high sodium menu: Includes lunch of bread, jelly and tea and supper of soup, salted crackers and ginger ale.

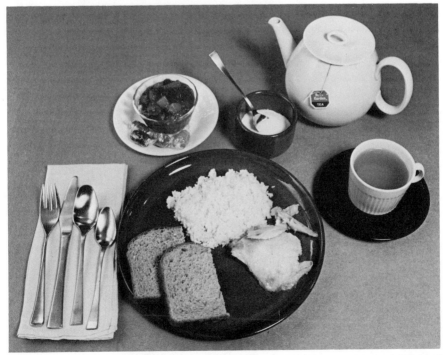

FIGURE 7-4   Sodium-restricted diet low in nutrients: Includes tea, sugar, Jello, hard candy, chicken, bread, and rice.

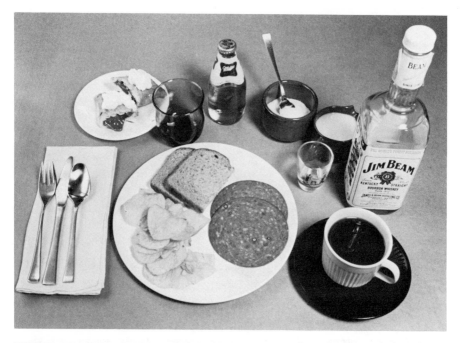

FIGURE 7-5    High calorie, low nutrient diet of an elderly alcoholic: Includes bread, salami, potato chips, pastry with whipped cream, coffee with non-dairy creamer, beer, and whiskey.

## DISEASES

Acute and chronic diseases are likely to reduce food intakes, because of associated loss of appetite (Exton-Smith, 1979; Hodkinson, 1980). Acute diseases and injuries which convey a nutritional risk are shown in Table 7-1. In the presence of acute disease, intake of food is likely to be markedly reduced, or to cease altogether. At the same time, catabolic effects of disease increase nutrient requirements. Nutritional needs for wound healing after injury or surgery can magnify nutrient deficits. In elderly surgical patients, protein-energy malnutrition is frequently found both in the pre- and postoperative periods. Pre- and postoperative causes of malnutrition in the elderly are shown in Table 7-2.

Chronic diseases which are associated with malnutrition in the elderly are listed in Table 7-3. Types of nutritional deficiency commonly associated with these diseases are indicated, together with etiological factors. Chronic disease processes lead to malnutrition by impairment of food intake or retention, by causing maldigestion and malabsorption, by increasing renal losses of nutrients, and by decreasing the efficiency of nutrient utilization.

TABLE 7-1   Acute Diseases and Injuries of the
Elderly Associated with Anorexia

Acute bronchitis
Pneumonia (viral or bacterial)
Other bacterial infections
Other viral infections
Oral candidiasis (yeast infections of the mouth)
Generalized dermatitis or other dermatoses with severe itching
Acute confusional psychoses
Acute cholecystitis
Burns
Fractures
Intestinal obstruction

TABLE 7-2  Pre- and Postoperative Causes of Malnutrition

| PREOPERATIVE | POSTOPERATIVE |
|---|---|
| Pain | Intravenous fluids |
| Vomiting | No food allowed by mouth |
| No food allowed by mouth | Catabolic effects of surgery |
| Alcoholic binge prior to hospitalization | Lack of nutritional support |
| Intravenous fluids | Deficiencies of formula feeds (enteral or parenteral) |
| Burn losses | Short bowel syndrome |
| | Postgastrectomy syndromes |

TABLE 7-3  Chronic Diseases Associated with Malnutrition in the Elderly

| | |
|---|---|
| Congestive heart failure | Arthritis |
| Cancer | Organic brain syndromes |
| Chronic neurological diseases with paralysis | Psychotic depression |
| | End stage renal disease |
| Alcoholic cirrhosis | Maldigestion/malabsorption syndromes, |
| Chronic bronchitis and emphysema | e.g. chronic pancreatitis, radiation enteritis |

## DRUGS

Drug groups and individual drugs which cause malnutrition are shown in Table 7-4. The drugs listed are all in common use by geriatric patients living at home or in hospitals or extended care facilities. Several drugs which can lead to malnutrition may be taken by patients on multiple drug regimens (Roe, 1979; 1981). It is also significant that drugs used for different pharmacological purposes can have additive effects in producing nutrient depletion. Thus, whereas laxatives and most diuretics increase potassium depletion, taken together they can induce a potassium deficiency if the potassium intake is insufficient to meet drug-imposed as well as physiological requirements.

Nutritional deficiencies caused by common drugs are shown in Table 7-5.

**TABLE 7-4    Common Drugs Which Cause Malnutrition in the Elderly**

| DRUG USE | DRUG |
|---|---|
| Cardiac disease | Digitalis |
| Hypertension | Thiazides (e.g. hydrochlorothiazide) Furosemide Ethacrynic acid Mercurial diuretics Triamterene |
| Arthritis | Aspirin |
| Gout | Indomethacin Colchicine |
| Indigestion (Antacids) | Magnesium and aluminum hydroxide |
| Constipation (Laxatives) | Mineral oil, phenolphthalein |
| Insomnia/anxiety (Sedatives) | Barbiturates |

**TABLE 7-5    Nutritional Deficiencies Caused by Common Drugs Taken by the Elderly**

| DRUG AND DRUG GROUP | DEFICIENCY | |
|---|---|---|
| 1. Cardiac glycosides Digitalis | Anorexia → protein energy malnutrition Zinc and magnesium deficiency | |
| 2. Diuretics | Thiazides → Furosemide Ethacrynic acid | Potassium, zinc, and magnesium depletion |
| | Triamterene → Hg. diuretics | Folacin deficiency Protein deficiency |
| 3. Antiinflammatory drugs Aspirin Indomethacin Colchicine | GI Blood loss → iron deficiency Malabsorption of fat soluble and water soluble vitamins | |
| 4. Antacids (antacid abuse) | Phosphate depletion; ostemalacia | |
| 5. Laxatives (laxative abuse) | Mineral oil → Deficiency of vitamins A, D, and K Phenolphthalein (Potassium deficiency) Multiple nutrient deficiencies due to malabsorption Folacin and vitamin D deficiency | |

## MULTIFACTORIAL CAUSES

Whereas it can be generalized that in the elderly, malnutrition is due to the combined effects of poor diet, disease, and drugs, in practice, if malnutrition is subdivided into the categories of protein-energy malnutrition, avitaminosis, and mineral deficiencies, causative factors can be seen to have differing importance. Thus, protein-energy malnutrition is most likely to be due to acute and chronic disease, avitaminoses are usually due to a deficient diet, and mineral deficiencies are due mainly to the effects of drugs. In each of these types of malnutrition, multiple causation is frequent but the relative importance of any one etiological factor is different.

## PROTEIN-ENERGY MALNUTRITION

Protein-energy malnutrition in the elderly as in younger persons may be acute or chronic.

### Acute protein-energy malnutrition (PEM)

Acute protein-energy malnutrition develops in previously well-nourished or obese people when they are on a starvation regimen while undergoing the catabolic stress of infection, injury, or surgery (Butterworth and Weinsier, 1980). Acute PEM occurs in hospitalized patients whose previous nutritional status may have been satisfactory, but who are denied access to food. Alternatively, acute PEM can develop in patients who cannot eat due to disease-related causes. Signs of acute PEM are apathy, weakness, edema, delayed wound healing, intolerance of anesthesia, susceptibility to adverse drug reactions, and impaired cellular immune function. Diagnosis is by history, by clinical examination and identification of edema, including wound edema, by hematological studies showing lymphocytopenia, by biochemical determinants including the finding of hypoalbuminemia, and by skin tests showing a lack of allergic responses to standard antigens including candida and mumps antigens.

### Chronic protein-energy malnutrition

Chronic PEM is synonymous with *cachexia*. Cachexia usually results from low food intake, secondary to anorexia. In the elderly, common causes of cachexia are cancer (particularly disseminated neoplastic disease), chronic neurological disease associated with paralysis, end-stage hepatic or renal disease, and high dosage digitalis therapy. While cachexia is mainly due to reduced energy and protein intake, additional causal factors are catabolic effects of disease and excessive losses of nutrients by malabsorption or through protein-losing enteropathy.

Signs of cachexia are emaciation, loss of subcutaneous fat, loss of lean body mass, brittleness of the hair, ridged or banded nails, and crazy-pavement dermatosis of the lower legs. Acute protein-energy malnutrition may be superimposed on cachexia.

## Protein malnutrition

Severe protein malnutrition is the result of excessive protein losses as produced by extensive burns, bullous (blistering) dermatoses (pemphigoid or pemphigus), by protein-losing enteropathy which may occur with cancer, or in renal disease with massive albuminuria. The latter may develop in the elderly with inorganic mercury intoxication secondary to administration of mercurial diuretics. Severe protein malnutrition causes edema, hypoalbuminemia, and failure of wound healing. The clinical appearance of an elderly patient with chronic protein energy malnutrition and exfoliative dermatitis is shown in Figure 7-6.

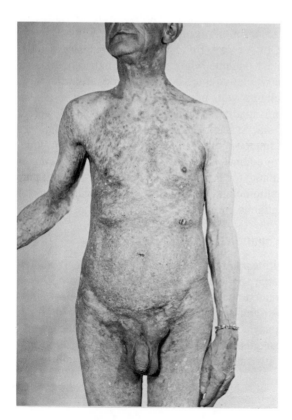

**FIGURE 7-6**   **Elderly man with chronic exfoliative dermatitis and protein energy malnutrition due to inorganic mercury toxicity.**

## Fat Soluble Vitamin Deficiencies

*Vitamin D Deficiency.*    In the elderly, the disease osteomalacia, which is due to a vitamin D deficiency, develops in people who are housebound or institutionalized and not exposed to sunlight (Lawson et al., 1979). Etiological factors which frequently coexist are low dietary intake of vitamin D and chronic intake of drugs such as barbiturates and diphenylhydantoin which interfere with the hydroxylation of vitamin D in the liver. Causes of vitamin D deficiency in the elderly are summarized in Table 7-6.

**TABLE 7-6   Causes of Vitamin D Deficiency in the Elderly**

1. Environmental
   a. Lack of exposure to sunlight
   b. Wearing of heavy clothing and/or use of light barriers

2. Dietary
   a. Lack of intake of milk or other dietary sources of vitamin D

3. Malabsorption
   a. Gluten-sensitive enteropathy—senile type
   b. Postgastrectomy
   c. Resection of small intestine
   d. Pancreatic insufficiency
   e. Drugs causing malabsorption
      i. Laxative abuse—mineral oil, phenolphthalein
      ii. Cholestyramine
   f. Geriatric intestinal mucosal atrophy
   g. Biliary obstruction
      i. Intrahepatic
      ii. Extrahepatic
   h. Radiation enteritis—chronic

4. Impaired hepatic 25-hydroxylation of vitamin D
   a. Cirrhosis
   b. Geriatric effect

5. Increased catabolism of vitamin D due to drugs
   a. Diphenylhydantoin (Dilantin)
   b. Phenobarbital
   c. Glutethimide

6. Impaired 1-hydroxylation of vitamin D metabolites in the kidney
   a. Chronic renal failure
   b. Geriatric effect
   c. Diphosphonates

7. Phosphate depletion
   a. Antacid abuse (phosphate binding)
   b. Malabsorption syndromes
   c. Hyperparathyroidism
   d. Hemodialysis
   e. Total parenteral alimentation
   f. Metabolic acidosis
   g. Fanconi syndrome—adult type

Symptoms and signs of osteomalacia in the elderly are:

1. Pain related to the back, chest, and limbs; worsened by sudden movement, muscle strain, weight-bearing, and pressure.
2. Bone tenderness elicited by pressure.
3. Skeletal deformities including loss of height, kyphosis, scoliosis, pigeon chest, and bowing of long bones.
4. Muscle weakness involving proximal limb muscles.
5. Waddling gait secondary to muscle weakness.
6. Paresthesias, muscle cramps, and tetany secondary to severe hypocalcemia.

Diagnostic tests for osteomalacia are:

1. Radiological examination. Findings are a) decreased skeletal radiodensity indicative of demineralization and b) pseudofractures (Looser's zones, which are symmetrical radiolucent bands at the ends of long bones, in the ribs, pubic bones, and scapulae). Osteoporosis frequently coexists with osteomalacia.
2. Bone biopsy. Findings are osteoid seams and undermineralization.
3. Biochemical tests. In geriatric patients, there is hypophosphatemia with or without hypocalcemia. Alkaline phosphatase is usually increased. Total urinary hydroxyproline is elevated. Serum parathyroid hormone (PTH) may be elevated in the early stages of the disease. Serum 25-hydroxycholecalciferol may be lowered. Biochemical findings alone are not diagnostic but biochemical tests may corroborate diagnosis and indicate causal mechanisms.
4. Therapeutic intervention. Administration of vitamin D or a vitamin D-metabolite, or exposure to ultraviolet light will relieve symptoms, heal radiological changes, and reverse abnormal biochemical findings. Cure may require treatment of causal pathology on discontinuation of drugs.

*Vitamin A Deficiency.*   Overt vitamin A deficiency is uncommon in the elderly in the U.S. Subgroups of the elderly population may be at risk. These include elderly alcoholics and elderly persons with malabsorption syndromes. Alcohol metabolism and vitamin A metabolism are competitive. Vitamin A absorption is impaired by certain drugs, including mineral oil and cholestyramine.

Mild to moderate vitamin A deficiency is usually symptom free. Patients may complain of difficulty in finding their way about at night or difficulty in adapting to the light in darkened rooms. Night blindness can be identified by dark adaptation tests. Improvement in dark adaptation follows administration of vitamin A. Night blindness in elderly alcoholics is due to vitamin A and/or zinc deficiency.

Diagnostic tests for vitamin A deficiency include a) measurement of plasma retinol, b) performance of dark adaptations tests, and c) administration of vitamin A in therapeutic doses (Garry, 1981).

*Vitamin K Deficiency.*   Vitamin K deficiency in the elderly can be caused by drugs or disease (Roe, 1976).

Drugs causing vitamin K deficiency are:

1. Coumarin anticoagulants (vitamin K antagonists)
2. Broad spectrum antibiotics (tetracycline)
3. Cholestyramine

Diseases causing vitamin K deficiency are:

1. Alcoholic cirrhosis
2. Other severe liver disease

Low dietary intake of vitamin K per se will not cause a vitamin K deficiency because vitamin $K_2$ is synthesized by bacteria in the large intestine. Massive intake of vitamin E can precipitate vitamin K deficiency in patients on coumarin anticoagulant drugs. Patients who are on anticoagulant drugs and barbiturates may become vitamin K deficient when the barbiturates are discontinued. This is because the stimulation by barbiturates of the anticoagulant drug metabolism is removed and anticoagulant drug effects are prolonged. Vitamin K deficiency may also develop in patients on anticoagulant drugs whose vitamin K intake is low and who, at the same time, are given oral broad-spectrum antibiotics which inhibit vitamin $K_2$ synthesis.

Vitamin K deficiency is manifested by hemorrhage. Hemorrhage into the skin is called purpura. Purpura is common in vitamin K deficiency, but in the elderly may be due to changes in the skin. Oozing hemorrhage may occur from wound sites, from hemorrhoids, into the gastrointestinal tract, or from other sites of trauma.

Diagnostic tests for vitamin K deficiency are:

1. Measurement of prothrombin time and related indices. Prothrombin times are prolonged in vitamin K deficiency.
2. Discontinuation of anticoagulant drugs.
3. Administration of vitamin K by oral or parenteral routes.


## Water Soluble Vitamin Deficiencies

*Vitamin $B_{12}$ Deficiency.* In the elderly, a vitamin $B_{12}$ deficiency is commonly due to lack of gastric intrinsic factor (IF), which causes vitamin $B_{12}$ malabsorption. Gastric intrinsic factor is lacking in pernicious anemia (Addison's anemia). A late effect of partial or total gastrectomy is inadequate production of IF, and this also causes vitamin $B_{12}$ deficiency. Table 7-7 offers a classification of causes of vitamin $B_{12}$ deficiency. Other frequent causes of vitamin $B_{12}$ deficiency in the elderly are vitamin $B_{12}$ malabsorption due to ileal disease or ileal resection (Hoffbrand, 1971).

Symptoms of vitamin $B_{12}$ deficiency can be divided according to etiology. Symptoms associated with anemia are:

1. Weakness
2. Dyspnea

**TABLE 7-7   Causes of Vitamin B$_{12}$ Deficiency in the Elderly**

1. Malabsorption
   a. due to lack of gastric intrinsic factor
      i. Addison's disease (pernicious anemia)
      ii. Partial gastrectomy
      iii. Total gastrectomy
   b. due to loss of ileal absorption site
      i. Regional enteritis
      ii. Radiation enteritis
      iii. Ileal resection
   c. due to drugs
      i. Paraaminosalicylic acid
      ii. Colchicine
      iii. Neomycin
2. Diet
   Vegan diet (rare cause)

## Gastrointestinal symptoms are:

1. Sore tongue or mouth
2. Anorexia
3. Nausea
4. Gastric discomfort
5. Flatulence
6. Abdominal pain
7. Episodic diarrhea

## Neurological symptoms are:

1. Burning pains in limbs
2. Tingling of fingers and toes
3. Numbness, cold, or tightness of skin
4. Difficulty in walking
5. Unsteadiness
6. Incontinence

## Physical signs are:

1. Pallor
2. Lemon-yellow color of skin
3. Tachycardia
4. Hypotension
5. Systolic murmur
6. Loss of position and vibration sense, particularly in lower limbs
7. Ataxia (worse when eyes are closed)
8. Depression

9. Memory impairment
10. Visual impairment
11. Abnormal tendon reflexes (Babinski sign + )

Diagnostic tests are:

1. By history, symptoms, and physical signs.
2. By presence of megaloblastic anemia with megaloblasts in the bone marrow and peripheral blood.
3. Serum vitamin $B_{12}$ levels in deficient range.
4. Schilling test results indicative of vitamin $B_{12}$ malabsorption.
5. Resolution of anemia and of all symptoms including neurological symptoms following injection of vitamin $B_{12}$.

*Folacin Deficiency.* Folacin deficiency is reported as the most common nutritional deficiency in the elderly (Hurdle, 1966; Chanarin, 1973). Causes include low intake due to avoidance of rich food sources of the vitamin such as liver, green leafy vegetables, and breakfast cereals which are fortified with folic acid. Folacin deficiency is prevalent in elderly alcoholics due to grossly inadequate diets, malabsorption, loss of folacin into the stomach (Menetrier's disease), and impaired metabolism or storage of folacin coenzymes in the liver. Drugs taken by the elderly which cause folacin deficiency include diphenylhydantoin (Dilantin), phenobarbital, glutethimide (Doriden), cholestyramine, salicylazosulfapyridine, and methotrexate (Roe, 1982). Folacin deficiency may be due to disease-associated malabsorption syndromes. A full list of causes of folacin deficiency in the elderly is shown in Table 7-8.

Clinical features of folacin deficiency include megaloblastic anemia,

**TABLE 7-8  Causes of Folacin Deficiency in the Elderly**

*Malabsorption of Folacin*
   Gluten-sensitive enteropathy (senile type)
   Tropical sprue
   Radiation enteritis
   Alcoholic enteritis
   Inflammatory bowel disease
   Cholestyramine
   Salicylazosulfapyridine

*Hyperexcretion and Malutilization of Folacin*
   Cirrhosis
   Congestive heart failure
   Menetriers disease (loss of folacin into the stomach)

   Methotrexate ⎫
   Triamterene  ⎬   Folacin antagonists
   Trimethoprim ⎭

   Diphenylhydantoin
   Phenobarbital
   Glutethimide

which always occurs in severe folacin deficiency. This megaloblastic anemia is identical with that found in vitamin $B_{12}$ deficiency. An organic brain syndrome may also occur and is characterized by mental confusion and loss of memory. The organic brain syndrome associated with folacin deficiency is different from the neurological manifestations of vitamin $B_{12}$ deficiency.

Diagnostic tests for folacin deficiency are:

1. Complete blood count including red cell indices.
2. Examination of stained blood films.
3. Determination of plasma and red cell folacin.
4. Hemopoietic response to folacin supplementation.

Differentiation of folacin deficiency from vitamin $B_{12}$ deficiency is essential because therapeutic doses of folic acid will not prevent progression of the neurological signs of vitamin $B_{12}$ deficiency, which can only be halted or resolved by vitamin $B_{12}$ injections. It is therefore important to exclude the diagnosis of vitamin $B_{12}$ deficiency before administering therapeutic doses of folic acid to patients with megaloblastic anemia.

*Riboflavin Deficiency.* The causes of riboflavin deficiency are low intake and malabsorption, particularly in patients with laxative abuse or disease-induced chronic diarrhea with malabsorption. Impaired synthesis or liver storage of flavin coenzymes occurs in elderly alcoholics with liver disease (Nichoalds, 1981).

Clinical features of riboflavin deficiency include 1) angular stomatitis, 2) glossitis (purplish or beefy tongue which may be sore or burning), and 3) dermatitis, localized to the face, particularly the nose, nasolabial folds and skin in front of the ears; also dermatitis of the scrotum. In both sexes the dermatitis may be generalized with a tendency to localization in skinfolds. Skin changes are particularly widespread in elderly persons with ariboflavinosis. In the elderly, the most common causes of angular stomatitis (cracks at the corners of the mouth) are an edentulous condition or ill-fitting dentures and not riboflavin deficiency.

Diagnosis is by erythrocyte glutathione reductase assay. Measurement of riboflavin excretion in the urine as a diagnostic test is not recommended in the elderly. Whereas in younger persons riboflavin excretion is related to riboflavin intake, in the elderly, daily riboflavin excretion in the urine may be difficult to measure because 24-hour urine samples cannot be obtained. Further, riboflavin excretion may be high in riboflavin-deficient elderly patients due to potentiation of urinary losses of this vitamin by catabolic disease, infection, ingestion of broad spectrum antibiotics, or accidental boric acid ingestion. Corroboration of the diagnosis is by administration of riboflavin, which will clear the dermatitis and mucosal changes.

*Thiamin Deficiency.* In geriatric patients, the major cause of thiamin deficiency is alcohol abuse. Classical beri beri is rare and the usual manifestation of thiamin deficiency in elderly alcoholics is the Wernicke-Korsakoff syndrome. Whether or not the Wernicke-Korsakoff syndrome will occur in alcoholics is determined by genetic predisposition. Genetic predisposition occurs in those who have abnormal (mutant) transketolase enzyme. Thiamin deficiency has been reported in elderly patients with gastric carcinoma and in hemodialysis patients.

The Wernicke-Korsakoff syndrome occurs in longstanding alcoholics who have been on prolonged drinking sprees and are not eating (Roe, 1979). Onset is rather abrupt. In the acute phases of the disease (Wernicke's encephalopathy), ocular signs occur with drooping of the eyelids (ptosis), small pupils (miosis), paralysis or partial paralysis of muscles controlling upward gaze, and nystagmus. Ataxia and muscle weakness are common. Since the disease is usually first recognized following sudden discontinuation of alcohol ingestion, symptoms associated with alcohol withdrawal may confuse the clinical picture. Apathy, listlessness, indifference, disorientation, drowsiness, and a semicomatose state are usually present. Korsakoff's psychosis, the late stage of the disease, is associated with confabulation (making up of events to fit memory gaps), severe memory loss, loss of perceptual function, and an inability to perform simple tasks without supervision (Victor et al., 1971). Beri beri presents with signs of peripheral neuritis or congestive heart failure. Heart disease in elderly alcoholics is more likely to be due to the toxic effects of alcohol than to beri beri (Douglas Talbott, 1975).

The diagnosis of thiamin deficiency is made by history of alcohol abuse, determination of erythrocyte transketolase, and by administration of thiamin. Wernicke's encephalopathy is reversible by megadosages of thiamin, recommended dosages of 100–200 mg thiamin given i.v. followed by oral dosages of 50–100 mg orally. Signs of Korsakoff's psychosis tend to improve with administration of high dosages of thiamin, but reversal of clinical signs is incomplete (Riggs and Boles, 1944-45).

*Vitamin B$_6$ Deficiency.* Vitamin B$_6$ deficiency can be due to drugs which are vitamin B$_6$ antagonists. In the elderly, chronic intake of isoniazid (isonicotinic acid hydrazide, INH), cycloserine, L-dopa, or penicillamine can cause vitamin B$_6$ deficiency both because complexes of the vitamin with the drug are excreted in the urine and because these drugs may inhibit activity of pyridoxal kinase which converts vitamin B$_6$ to its active form, pyridoxal phosphate (Roe, 1976).

Alcohol abuse can lead to a functional vitamin B$_6$ deficiency due to ethanolic inhibition of pyridoxal kinase (Lumeng and Li, 1974).

Dietary deficiency of vitamin B$_6$ sufficient to cause symptoms is rare. However, calculation of vitamin B$_6$ intakes of hospitalized aged suggests that dietary intakes of vitamin B$_6$ by many older persons are deficient (Vir and Love, 1977).

Signs of vitamin $B_6$ deficiency include dermatitis which may be generalized, peripheral neuritis, depression, and sideroblastic anemia. Sideroblastic anemia indicates a condition in which iron is not utilized optimally for heme synthesis and instead is deposited within red cell precursor cells.

Diagnosis is 1) by history and clinical findings, 2) by determination of erythrocyte glutamic pyruvic transaminase before and after *in vitro* stimulation with pyridoxal phosphate, and 3) determination of serum vitamin $B_6$ and pyridoxal phosphate (Hampton et al., 1977). In drug-induced vitamin $B_6$ deficiency or alcohol-induced vitamin $B_6$ deficiency, normalization of laboratory tests as well as resolution of clinical signs may require high doses of vitamin $B_6$.

*Vitamin C (Ascorbic Acid) Deficiency.* The major cause of ascorbic acid deficiency in the elderly is an inadequate dietary intake of the vitamin. Dietary deficiency of ascorbic acid occurs with exclusively milk diets or with diets lacking fruit, green vegetables, and potatoes (Hodges et al., 1969).

High doses of salicylates (aspirin) may cause vitamin C depletion (Coffey and Wilson, 1975).

Signs of vitamin C deficiency may be rather nonspecific in elderly people. For example, mental confusion can occur with vitamin C deficiency or from other causes. Similarly, vitamin C deficiency may present with lassitude and fatigue. Signs of scurvy include purpura, subperiosteal hemorrhages, bleeding from the gums, and delayed wound healing, which are common complaints in the elderly and do not offer diagnostic clues. Healing of bed sores is also slowed. Skin changes other than purpura may occur including follicular hyperkeratosis.

Diagnosis is by history, by physical examination, and by determination of serum, leukocyte and platelet ascorbate. Diagnosis is confirmed by cure with administration of ascorbic acid in therapeutic dosages (Vir and Love, 1978).

## Deficiencies of Major Minerals and Trace Elements

*Phosphate Depletion.* Phosphate depletion may occur in geriatric patients receiving antacids as self-prescribed treatment for flatulence, indigestion, or other symptoms referrable to the gastrointestinal tract, or when phosphate binding antacids are prescribed in end-stage renal disease, or when such antacids are used as prophylaxis against steroid-induced peptic ulcer. Further, phosphate depletion is particularly liable to occur in patients with steroid-related or alcohol-related ulcer disease (Lotz et al., 1968).

Symptoms of phosphate depletion are those suggestive of myopathy with severe muscle weakness. Muscle weakness is usually of proximal muscles.

Fatigue, malaise, and bone pain due to osteomalacia may be present. Diagnostic tests are biochemical with demonstration of hypophosphatemia, hypophosphaturia, hypercalciuria, and normocalcemia (Fitzgerald, 1978). Symptoms are relieved by stopping antacids and by administration of phosphate.

*Potassium deficiency.*   Potassium deficiency is common in the elderly. Causes are dietary, disease- and drug-related (Judge et al., 1974).

Low potassium intakes in the elderly are due to reliance on carbohydrate foods and avoidance of food sources rich in potassium, particularly vegetables, fruits, and milk.

Major causes of potassium deficiency include prolonged vomiting or diarrhea, and diabetic acidosis. In hospital patients, potassium deficiency may occur with starvation or with intravenous alimentation if care is not taken to maintain electrolyte balance.

Potassium deficiency in the elderly is often drug-induced. Excessive losses of potassium into the urine occur with use of diuretics including thiazide diuretics, furosemide, and ethacrynic acid. Abuse of laxatives and cathartics can also cause potassium depletion. Prolonged or high dosage intake of corticosteroid hormones also causes potassium deficiency and hypokalemia (Roe, 1981). Table 7-9 summarizes causes of hypokalemia (low serum potassium).

It is important to note that patients on reduced potassium intakes may be the same patients who are taking potassium depleting drugs or who have diseases which contribute to potassium depletion. Hypokalemia is a cause of digitalis-related arythmias.

Symptoms of potassium deficiency are weakness, anorexia, nausea, vomiting, listlessness, apprehension, sometimes diffuse pain, drowsiness, stupor, and irrationality. However, hypokalemia can exist without any abnormal clinical findings. When symptoms of hypokalemia are present, the most common finding is profound muscle weakness. Electrocardiographic changes are also characteristic (Nardone et al., 1978).

Diagnosis is from determination of serum or red cell potassium levels and electrocardiogram. Symptoms are relieved by administration of potassium

TABLE 7-9   Causes of Hypokalemia

1. Deficient diet
2. Gastrointestinal potassium wasting
3. Renal potassium wasting due to disease
4. Drug-induced potassium wasting
   a. diuretics including organomercurial thiazides, ferrosemides, and ethacrynic acid
   b. antibiotics including carbenicillin and penicillin
   c. liquorice and extracts of liquorice
   d. laxatives
   e. corticosteroids
   f. nephrotoxic drugs, e.g. outdated tetracycline

salts. It is to be noted, however, that potassium toxicity can occur from ingestion of concentrated potassium chloride solution, which can induce small bowel ulceration. No toxicity is associated with increasing the level of potassium in the diet.

*Magnesium Deficiency.* Magnesium deficiency is most frequently seen in elderly patients with gastrointestinal diseases leading to malabsorption in patients with hyperparathyroidism, bone cancer, hyperaldosteronism, diabetes mellitus, and thyrotoxicosis. Alcoholics may become magnesium depleted because of high renal losses and low intake (Rude and Singer, 1981). (See Appendix, Table 13.)

Drugs which may induce magnesium depletion include digitalis and oral diuretics.

Diet per se is not a cause of magnesium deficiency but intake may be reduced to zero when patients are not allowed any food and are maintained on intravenous dextrose-saline.

Clinical signs of magnesium deficiency are neuromuscular in type, including generalized seizures, vertigo, muscle weakness, tremors, depression, irritability, and psychotic behavior.

Diagnosis is by measurement of serum magnesium and by response of patients to magnesium salt supplementation.

*Zinc Deficiency.* Zinc deficiency in the elderly is due to combined effects of diet, disease, alcohol, and therapeutic drugs. Diet-related factors include low intake of zinc-rich foods and high intake of foods that reduce zinc availability including high phytate-containing cereals such as oatmeal and high fiber foods such as bran cereals. When elderly surgical patients are on prolonged intravenous feeding or are maintained on chemically defined diets, zinc intake is negligible unless zinc salts have been added to the formula (Underwood , 1977; Pulmissaro, 1974; Greger and Sciscoe, 1979).

Disease states leading to zinc deficiency include all catabolic disorders associated with muscle wasting as well as hepatic and renal disease. Alcohol abuse may be associated with zinc deficiency because of low zinc intake, malabsorption, and hyperexcretion of zinc in the urine. Acute zinc deficiency in the alcoholic is likely to occur when malnourished patients who have been on drinking sprees are admitted to hospital for surgical procedures and are given intravenous dextrose-saline only.

Drugs which cause zinc deficiency in the elderly are diuretics and digitalis glycosides, which increase renal losses of zinc.

Signs of zinc deficiency include symmetrical dermatitis, which begins on the hands and spreads over the arms and to the lower limbs before appearing on the trunk. The skin lesions are crusted and fissured. Loss of taste is characteristic of zinc deficiency. However, loss of taste in the aged may be due to other causes including the aging process itself. Wound healing is delayed after injury or surgery. Depression occurs in some zinc-deficient patients (Jacob, 1981).

Diagnosis is by measurement of zinc in hair and serum and by resolution of the signs of deficiency when zinc supplements are administered.

*Iron Deficiency.* Iron deficiency is common in the elderly. A major cause is blood loss (Bowering et al., 1976). Blood loss is due to hemorrhage from malignant tumors in the gastrointestinal tract, bleeding esophageal varices in portal hypertension with cirrhosis, bleeding peptic ulcer or hemorrhage outside the gastrointestinal tract. High intake of aspirin or indomethacin, as antiinflammatory analgesics for relief of arthritic pain, can induce capillary bleeding in the stomach or intestine, which, over time, can lead to severe iron deficiency anemia (Leonards and Levy, 1973; Boardman and Hart, 1967).

A low total intake of iron is correlated with a low intake of food energy (average iron intake equals 6 mg/1000 Kcal). An inadequate intake of heme iron is associated with low animal protein consumption. High intake of tea impairs iron absorption as does deficient intake of vitamin C.

Signs of iron deficiency include nonspecific signs of anemia such as pallor, weakness, and breathlessness. In the Plummer-Vinson syndrome (Patterson-Kelly syndrome) iron deficiency is associated with dysphagia (painful swallowing). The painful swallowing in this condition is related to a precancerous condition of the pharynx which may be associated with very prolonged iron deficiency. Patients with this condition may develop pharyngeal or esophageal cancer.

Screening tests for anemia include hemoglobin and hematocrit determination. Diagnosis of iron deficiency is from complete blood counts including red cell indices, examination of stained blood films and bone marrow, serum iron, erythrocyte protoporphyrin, and serum ferritin values. The anemia will respond to iron supplements, e.g. ferrous sulfate, when iron absorption is normal and when the primary disease or drug cause of the anemia is removed (Sayers, 1981).

Causes and signs of less common nutritional deficiencies to be found occasionally in elderly persons are shown in Table 7-10.

**TABLE 7-10 Infrequent Nutritional Deficiencies in the Elderly**

| NUTRITIONAL DEFICIENCY | CLINICAL SIGNS |
| --- | --- |
| Niacin | Pellagra (light sensitivity, diarrhea, depression, mental confusion) |
| Essential fatty acid | Scaly dermatitis |

## QUESTIONS

1. Diets associated with the development of nutritional deficiencies in the elderly have one or more of the following characteristics. Circle all correct answers:
   a) low cholesterol
   b) low fiber
   c) low in nutrient-calorie ratio
   d) high alcohol
   e) low number of foods

2. Circle the one chronic disease not associated with malnutrition:
   a) glaucoma
   b) end-stage renal disease
   c) chronic pancreatitis
   d) alcoholic cirrhosis
   e) cancer

3. Deficiency diseases in the elderly are usually multifactorial but one causative factor predominates. Pair the following types of malnutrition with the predominant cause.

   a) avitaminoses          i.   drugs
   b) mineral deficiencies   ii.  diseases
   c) protein-energy         iii. diet
      malnutrition

4. Protein–energy malnutrition can be acute or chronic. Which of the following are signs of acute, which of chronic malnutriton?

   a) wound edema            f) crazy pavement dermatosis
   b) emaciation             g) lymphocytopenia
   c) apathy                 h) impaired cellular immune function
   d) ridged nails           i) loss of subcutaneous fat
   e) delayed wound healing  j) hair brittleness

5. Following are the medical terms denoting specific vitamin deficiencies. Identify the vitamin deficiency producing each of the diseases listed below.
   a) Wernicke-Korsakoff psychosis
   b) scurvy
   c) osteomalacia
   d) pellagra
   e) pernicious anemia

## REFERENCES

BOARDMAN, P.L., and E.D. HART, "Side effects of indomethacin," *Ann. Rheum. Dis.*, 26 (1967), 127.

BOWERING, J., A.M. SANCHEZ, and M.I. IRWIN, "A conspectus of research on iron requirements of man," *J. Nutr.*, 106 (1976), 987–1074.

BUTTERWORTH, C.E. JR., and R.L. WEINSIER, "Malnutrition in hospitalized patients: assessment and treatment," in *Modern Nutrition in Health and Disease*, 6th Ed., eds. R.S. Goodhart and M.E. Shils. Philadelphia: Lea & Febiger, 1980, pp. 667–84.

CHANARIN, I., "Dietary deficiency of vitamin $B_{12}$ and folic acid," in *Nutritional Deficiencies in Modern Society*, eds. A.N. Howard and I. McLean Baird. Newman Books Ltd., 1973, pp. 17–26.

COFFEY, G., and C.W.M. WILSON, "Ascorbic acid deficiency and aspirin induced haematemesis," *Brit. Med. J.*, 1 (1975), 208.

DOUGLAS TALBOTT, G., "Primary alcoholic heart disease in medical consequences of alcoholism," *Ann. N.Y. Acad. Sci.*, 252 (1975), 237–42.

DRIEZEN, S., "Clinical manifestations of malnutrition," *Gerontology*, 29 (1974), 97–103.

EXTON-SMITH, A.N., "Nutritional deficiencies in the elderly," in *Nutritional Deficiencies in Modern Society*, eds. A.N. Howard and I. McLean Baird. London: Newman Books, 1973.

EXTON-SMITH, A.N., and P.W. OVERSTALL, *Geriatrics*. Lancaster, England: MTP Press Ltd., Internat. Med. Publ., 1979.

FITZGERALD, F., "Clinical hypophosphatemia," *Ann. Rev. Med.*, 29 (1978), 177–89.

GARRY, P.T., "Vitamin A," *Clinics in Lab Med.*, 1 (1981), 699–711.

GREGER, J.L., and B.S. SCISCOE, "Zinc nutriture of elderly participants in an urban feeding program," *Amer. J. Clin. Nutr.*, 32 (1979), 1859.

HAMPTON, D.J., B.M. CHRISLEY, and J.A. DRISKELL, "Vitamin $B_6$ status of the elderly in Montgomery County, VA," *Nutr. Rep. Internat.*, 16 (1977), 743–50.

HODGES, R.E. et al., "Experimental scurvy in man," *Amer. J. Clin. Nutr.*, 22 (1969), 535–48.

HODKINSON, H.M., *Common Symptoms of Disease in the Elderly*, 2nd Ed. Oxford, London, Edinburgh, Melbourne: Blackwell Scientific Publ., 1980.

HOFFBRAND, A.V., "The Megaloblastic Anaemias," in *Recent Advances in Hematology*, eds. A. Goldberg and M.C. Brain. Edinburgh: Churchill Livingstone, 1971, pp. 1–76.

HURDLE, A.D.F., AND P. WILLIAMS, "Folic acid deficiency in elderly patients admitted to hospital," *Brit. Med. J.*, 2 (1966), 202–5.

JACOB, R.A., "Zinc and copper," *Clinics in Lab. Med.*, 1 (1981), 743–66.

JUDGE, T.G., F.I. CAIRD, R.G.S. LEASK, and C.C. MACLEOD, "Dietary intake and urinary excretion of potassium in the elderly," *Age and Aging*, 3 (1974), 167–73.

LAWSON, D.E.M., A.A. PAUL, A.E. BLACK, et al., "Relative contributions of diet and sunlight to vitamin D state in the elderly," *Brit. Med. J.*, 2 (1979), 303–5.

LEONARDS, J.R., and G. LEVY, "Gastrointestinal blood loss during prolonged aspirin administration," *New Eng. J. Med.*, 289 (1973), 1020.

LOTZ, M., E. ZISMAN, and F.C. BARTTER, "Evidence for a phosphorus depletion syndrome in man," *New Eng. J. Med.*, 278 (1968), 409–15.

LUMENG, L. and T-K. LI, "Vitamin $B_6$ metabolism in chronic alcohol abuse. Pyridoxal phosphate levels in plasma, and the effects of acetaldehyde on pyridoxal phosphate synthesis and degradation in human erythrocytes," *J. Clin. Invest.*, 53 (1974), 693–704.

NARDONE, D.A., W.J. MCDONALD, and D.E. GIRARD, "Mechanisms of hypokalemia: clinical correlation," *Medicine*, 57 (1978), 435–46.

NICHOALDS, G.A., "Riboflavin," *Clinics in Lab Med.*, 1 (1981), 685–98.

PULMISSARO, D.J., "Nutrient deficiencies after intensive parenteral alimentation," *New Eng. J. Med.*, 291 (1974), 188.

RIGGS, H.E., and R.S. BOLES, "Wernicke's disease. A clinical and pathological study of 42 cases," *Quart. J. Stud. Alc.*, 5 (1944–45), 361–370.

ROE, D.A.,  *Alcohol and the Diet*. Westport, CT: AVI Publ. Co., 1979.

ROE, D.A.,  *Clinical Nutrition for the Health Scientist*. Boca Raton, FL: CRC Press, Inc., 1979, pp. 71–84.

ROE, D.A.,  *Drug-Induced Nutritional Deficiencies*. Westport, CT: AVI Publ. Co., 1976, pp. 36–38.

ROE, D.A.,  "Drug interference with the assessment of nutritional status," *Clin. Lab. Med.*, 1 (1981), 647–64.

ROE, D.A.,  "Drug-nutrient interrelationships," *Newer Knowledge Practical Gastroenterol.*, 6 (1982), 32–38.

ROE, D.A.,  "Interactions between drugs and nutrients," *Med. Clin. N. Amer.*, 63 (1979), 985–1007.

RUDE, R.K., and F.R. SINGER,  "Magnesium deficiency and excess," *Ann. Rev. Med.*, 32 (1981), 245–59.

SAYERS, M.A.,  "Iron," *Clinics in Lab. Med.*, 1 (1981), 729–41.

UNDERWOOD, E.J.,  *Trace elements in animal and human nutrition*, 4th Ed. New York: Academic Press, 1977, p. 545.

VICTOR, M., R.D. ADAMS, and G.H. COLLINS,  *The Wernicke-Korsakoff syndrome. A clinical and pathological study of 245 patients, 82 with post mortem examination*. Philadelphia: F.A. Davis Co., 1971.

VIR, S.C., and A.H.G. LOVE,  "Vitamin $B_6$ status of institutionalized and non-institutionalized aged," *Internat. J. Vit. Nutr. Res.*, 47 (1977), 364–72.

VIR, S.C., and A.H.G LOVE,  "Vitamin C status of institutionalized and non-institutionalized aged," *Internat. J. Vit. Nutr. Res.*, 48 (1978), 274–80.

# CHAPTER EIGHT
# Diseases Which Respond
# To Diet Modification

## OBESITY

Obesity is common in persons 65 years or older. Common causes are failure to reduce food-energy intake in response to diminished energy expenditure in physical activity, overeating due to boredom, large meals and snacks, and institutional provision of and intake of drugs which increase appetite.

A diet higher in calories than is required for energy needs leads to energy storage and fat deposition. Excess calories (food energy) from fat, carbohydrate, and protein foods leads to obesity. Intake of calories from alcoholic beverages, consumed in addition to a diet providing sufficient food-energy to meet caloric needs, can also lead to obesity, though alcohol calories are not utilized by the body as efficiently as food calories. In the elderly, drugs which promote appetite (hyperphagic drugs) lead to obesity because of increased food intake. These drugs include tranquilizers and lithium carbonate, used in the treatment of mental disease.

The efficiency with which dietary energy sources are utilized to maintain body weight varies from person to person and is influenced by age, sex, exercise, disease, and drugs. Moderately overweight individuals require slightly excessive calories to maintain their body weight, while massively obese persons have to keep up a very large intake of food to maintain their body weight constant, but require maintenance of low to semistarvation diets over a long period of time in order to reduce their body weight to reach the normal range. Reduction in body weight in massively or morbidly obese persons is commonly retarded or impeded by disinclination for exercise. Exercise may also be restricted because of secondary effects of obesity leading to physical disabilities. Variables related to obesity in the elderly are shown in Table 8-1.

Obesity is the most common nutritional problem of public health concern in the United States. While gross obesity is uncommon in the very old, because persons who are morbidly obese are more likely to die earlier of complications of their obesity, obesity is still a serious disability in the elderly.

Medical disabilities of obesity are associated with the complication of obesity. Causal relationships have been identified between obesity and the development of maturity-onset diabetes, as well as essential hypertension and hypertensive heart disease. Obesity is also associated with the development of abdominal hernia. Gall bladder disease and gout are more common in obese

**TABLE 8-1   Demographic and Medical Variables Related to Obesity in Elderly Persons**

| VARIABLE | RISK FACTOR |
|---|---|
| Age | Less than 75 years |
| Sex | Females > males |
| Socioeconomic status (SES) | Low SES > high SES in females<br>High SES > low SES in males |
| Education | Less than 12th grade |
| History | Past obesity<br>Past repeated attempts to diet<br>Lack of physical exercise |
| Diseases | Maturity-onset diabetes<br>Hypertension<br>Osteoarthritis (with symptoms related to weight-bearing joints)<br>Abdominal hernia<br>Varicose veins ± stasis dermatitis and ulcers<br>Gall bladder disease<br>Gout<br>Psychiatric, neurological, musculo-skeletal and other diseases causing confinement to wheelchair or bed* |

Drugs: Hyperphagic agents, including phenothiazine and benzodiazepine tranquilizers and lithium carbonate as well as sedatives such as barbiturates.

Drugs used in the treatment of obesity: including amphetamines, thyroid hormones.

Drugs used in the treatment of diseases complicating obesity: including oral hypoglycemic agents, diuretics, other antihypertensive drugs, and non-narcotic analgesics used to treat diabetes, hypertension, osteoarthritis and gout, respectively.

*Obese wheelchair or bedfast elderly patients are those who maintain food energy intake in excess of their needs and do not have diseases which cause energy wastage.

people, though causal relationships are not adequately identified. Most importantly in the elderly, obesity is associated with increased symptoms of degenerative osteoarthritis (osteoarthrosis). Complications of varicose veins including stasis dermatitis and stasis ulcers are more frequent in the obese. Morbid (massive) obesity is associated with bacterial and yeast infections between fat folds and under the breasts. The Pickwickian Syndrome, characterized by somnolence and respiratory failure, is a life-threatening complication of morbid obesity. Obese elderly patients are poor operative risks.

Massive obesity is a hindrance to independent living in the elderly. Such persons become breathless on mild exertion, and therefore are unable to cope with stairs, with housework, and with the exertion required in getting to food markets. Physically disabled patients are the most difficult to care for and nurse both at home and in institutions. Problems include difficulties in lifting and bathing. Obesity also makes physical examinations difficult, and abnormal physical findings (more particularly abdominal traumas and infections), may be missed by the attending physicians (Van Itallie, 1979).

Measures for the control of obesity in the elderly have not met with outstanding success. Approaches include diet restriction (particularly prescribed restriction in food-energy intake), exercise, behavior modification, and drugs. The most effective programs utilize combinations of diet and exercise with a personalized behavior modification program. Behavior modification is difficult to achieve. In the elderly, requirements for modification of eating practices differ according to living circumstances. Independently living elderly persons must understand and interpret instructions, be motivated to lose weight, keep food records, and preferably eat away from the kitchen-refrigerator area and the TV set.

When behavior modification is proposed in a situation where the elderly person is living with a spouse, other family member, or companion, this person can be most supportive and undertake the responsibility of acting as a guide to the patient to promote compliance with the recommended changes in eating activities. We assume that the obese, independently living elderly person would be advised to eat only when hungry, to eat in a constant place (which should be the dining area), to eat at similar times every day, and not to eat except when he or she has full awareness of the amount eaten. Snacking in front of the TV set would therefore be forbidden.

Successful modification of eating behavior in the elderly is more likely in those persons who have full preservation of mental functions and also a strong motivation to lose weight. Newly diagnosed elderly diabetics and cardiac patients with potentially life-threatening disease will often follow behavior modification programs. Compliance is facilitated by the presence of an eating partner who will follow the same regime, by responsibility for cooking being in the hands of someone other than the patient, and by a living situation which includes a defined dining area. Specific types of behavior modification can be used in domiciliary care facilities for the elderly, in intermediate care homes, and in skilled nursing homes. When cooperation of the patient is possible, social activities at which no food is provided can be provided between scheduled meal times. Visitors can be discouraged from bringing in snack foods. Snack carts and refrigerators in the institution to which patients have access can be stocked only with fruits or fruit juices. Obese patients can also be given nonfood token rewards for dietary compliance and weight loss (Stuart, 1974).

The use of anorectic drugs, including unsubstituted and substituted amphetamines, is never justified in the elderly, because hunger does not dictate excessive food consumption in the obese, and also because the side effects of these drugs, including insomnia and excitement, are serious contraindications to their use. There is also no justification for giving elderly persons thyroid hormones for the purpose of weight reduction, because these drugs may cause cardiac arythmias and otherwise adversely affect cardiac function. Diuretics will only produce weight loss when edema is present and should never be used in the treatment of obesity (Roe, 1979).

The food intake of patients receiving tranquilizers, sedative drugs, and lithium carbonate as well as their body weight should be monitored. If their food intakes and body weights are clearly increasing, caloric restriction is necessary. In many patients, however, weight can be controlled by decreasing intake of the prescribed hyperphagic drug.

## CARDIOVASCULAR DISEASE

Common forms of cardiovascular disease in the elderly are congestive heart failure, atherosclerotic heart disease, hypertensive heart disease, and peripheral vascular disease due to diabetes and/or atherosclerosis.

### Salt Restriction

Indications for sodium restriction in the elderly are a) prevention and treatment of congestive heart failure, and b) management of essential hypertension (Wintrobe et al., 1970).

High intake of sodium chloride and other sodium sources in the diet (including sodium nitrate and nitrite and monosodium glutamate) and in drugs such as sodium bicarbonate, as well as other sodium compounds, mitigates against control of congestive heart failure and hypertension. Hypertension in the elderly is multifactorial and never solely attributable to high sodium intake. Reduction in sodium intake does, however, reduce blood pressure. Weight reduction in obese, elderly patients promotes a drop in blood pressure but the effect of weight reduction on blood pressure in these patients is enhanced by concurrent sodium restriction.

Mild, moderate, and severe hypertension should be treated by prescription of antihypertensive drugs as well as by sodium restriction and weight reduction if the patient is obese.

Commonly prescribed antihypertensive drugs are listed in Table 8-2, which also shows the indication for each antihypertensive drug or drug combination. Diuretics which are used in the drug management of hypertension may cause potassium, calcium, magnesium, and zinc depletion (Nickerson and Ruedy, 1975). For reference to diuretics which can cause mineral depletion, see Table 7-5.

Dietary sodium restriction has to be tailored to the needs of individual patients. Mild sodium restriction requires that the patient lower his or her intake of high sodium foods, and high sodium drugs should be discontinued. Moderate sodium restriction requires also that no salt be added to foods in the kitchen or at the table. Severe sodium restriction requires the use of low sodium foods. Patients who must adhere to a very low sodium diet should have their drinking water tested for sodium content, which should not exceed 20 mg per liter (Safe Drinking Water Committee, 1980). On the assumption that the average daily intake of water is two liters per day, the goal is to maintain an intake of sodium from drinking water and beverages made from this water at less than 50 mg per day. With a low to moderate intake of sodium from drinking water, it is possible for elderly patients with congestive heart failure to adhere to a strict low sodium diet (500 mg/day). When, for any reason, the sodium content of the domestic water supply is high, patients on a severely restricted sodium diet should be advised to drink from an alternate water source, for example bottled spring water.

Dietary guidelines to be followed by elderly patients who are on sodium restricted diets are given in Table 8-3. Patients on moderate to strict low

**TABLE 8-2  Commonly Prescribed Antihypertensive Drugs with Indications for Their Specific Usage***

| DRUG | INDICATION |
| --- | --- |
| Thiazide diuretics, e.g. hydrochlorothiazide triamterene reserpine | Mild hypertension |
| Propranolol | Moderate hypertension |
| Methyldopa | Severe hypertension |
| Hydralazine | |
| Captopril | |
| Diazoxide | Hypertensive emer- |
| Clonidine | gencies |

*Combination therapy is used in moderate to severe hypertension.

**TABLE 8-3   Dietary Guidelines for Elderly Patients on Sodium Restricted Diets**

1. Patients (or responsible household member) should be given instructions on the total amount of sodium intake permitted daily.

2. Use of Table 6 in the *Appendix* to determine the sodium content of foods is recommended to plan a mildly restricted, moderately restricted, or severely restricted low sodium diet.

3. Potassium values are also given in these tables to enable patients on diuretics to choose low sodium, high potassium foods which will offset the potassium losing effects of the diuretics.

4. Severely restricted sodium diets must be carefully planned to ensure that the diet is nutritionally adequate, i.e. meets RDA 1980. (See *Appendix,* Table 3)

5. Patients on severely restricted, low sodium diets should be told which nondietary sodium sources to avoid, including high sodium over-the-counter and prescription drugs and water treated with domestic water softeners.

sodium diets should be encouraged to use exchange lists of low sodium foods which will provide the Recommended Dietary Allowances for essential nutrients.

### Lipid Restriction

Epidemiological associations have been demonstrated between high intake of dietary fats, high serum cholesterol, and coronary heart disease (CHD) incidence (Glueck, 1979). The risk factors in this multifactorial disease include a high cholesterol diet, high intake of saturated fat, hyper-cholesterolemia, high serum/low density lipoproteins, hypertension, and cigarette smoking (Dwyer and Hetzel, 1980). A decrease in CHD mortality in European countries in the immediate post-World War II period was associated with diminished intake of total calories, fewer total calories from fat (mostly saturated fat), and a reduction in dietary cholesterol. Dietary restriction of total fat, saturated fat, and cholesterol have not, however, been shown to influence CHD mortality in older adults. This could be because athero-sclerosis, causing the CHD, has been so advanced that it is irreversible by the time that the lipid restricted diet has been instituted. Regression of disease has been demonstrated in patients with atherosclerosis of the femoral arteries, but only when a lipid restricted diet has been combined with hypolipidemic drugs (Leren, 1966; Barndt, 1977).

Elderly individuals who have adhered to a prudent diet over a lifetime or for most of their lives, with food-energy intakes in keeping with their needs and a low intake of dietary fat and cholesterol, may have a lower risk of dying from CHD, especially if they are nonsmokers. While restriction of total fat as well as of total food intake is most advisable in the elderly in order to avoid obesity and the complications of obesity, we do not presently advocate sudden, stringent restriction of cholesterol in the diet of the elderly for the express purpose of reducing the risk of mortality from CHD. Cessation of smoking is highly recommended. As previously mentioned, restricted cholesterol intake is also advisable in the management of diabetes in the elderly.

### Alcohol Consumption

Moderate consumption of alcoholic beverages has been shown to have a protective influence against CHD mortality (Spritz, 1979). When alcohol is consumed, serum levels of high density lipoproteins are increased, which lowers CHD risk. While elderly people who are used to drinking a glass of wine a day should not be discouraged from doing so, both because the drink may provide a sense of well-being and because of the protective effect against CHD, we would caution against encouragement of higher alcohol intakes by the elderly. Risks of heavy drinking in the elderly include not only alcoholic liver disease but also alcoholic bone disease, psychosis (Korsakoff's psychosis), alcoholic heart disease, and falls resulting in injury (Roe, 1979).

## DIABETES

Diabetes in the elderly is most commonly of the maturity-onset type. Etiological factors in the development of maturity-onset diabetes include obesity and declining glucose tolerance associated with aging (Ireland et al., 1980). Most patients with maturity-onset diabetes do not require insulin. Indeed, pancreatic insulin production is high in the early phases of the disease and may remain high throughout. In these patients, diabetes is related to peripheral insulin resistance. Maturity-onset diabetes may convert to the insulin-requiring type late in the disease due to "exhaustion" of pancreatic endocrine functions, whereby insulin is no longer produced in sufficient amounts to meet body needs. Maturity-onset diabetes may be associated with Type IV hyperlipoproteinemia.

Elderly insulin-requiring diabetics, however, can be juvenile diabetics who have grown older. Nutritional and dietary management of diabetes in the elderly requires full appreciation by the nutritionist that goals may be a) weight reduction in order to improve glucose tolerance, b) control of hyperlipemia in insulin-requiring diabetics, and c) maintenance of blood sugar within an appropriate range to avert both hyperglycemia and hypoglycemia. It has been shown that persistent hyperglycemia is associated with the development of serious complications of diabetes including renal, retinal, and degenerative vascular disease (Nutall, 1980).

Most maturity-onset elderly diabetics can be controlled by diet only. Oral hypoglycemic drugs may be prescribed particularly for elderly patients for whom dietary compliance is a major problem. However, it must be understood that in the elderly, unwanted outcomes of oral hypoglycemic drug therapy include increased mortality from cardiovascular disease and adverse drug reactions, usually due to interaction of oral hypoglycemic agents with other drugs (Diabetes, 1970).

In the dietary treatment of maturity-onset diabetes the primary objective is weight reduction, and, through weight reduction, improvement in glucose tolerance. Dietary modifications which are presently advocated to produce overall energy restriction include:

1. *Reduced intake of simple carbohydrates* with exclusion of sucrose and sucrose-containing foods as well as exclusion of foods containing lactose, glucose, and fructose as intentional food additives. The aim is to reduce body weight to the average weight for the height and age of that individual. When reduced intake of simple sugars is inadequate to meet this goal, further advice on dietary restriction includes defined intake of fat and of animal protein foods. The desirable distribution of food-energy would have carbohydrate supplying 42 percent, protein, 20 percent, and fat, 38 percent. The approach is didactic. Complicated protein exchange lists are not discussed. While patients are encouraged to eat vegetables with main meals, no specific instructions are given on intake of dietary fiber. Levels of complex carbohydrate are defined for each patient to meet the food-energy distribution between carbohydrates, protein, and fat.

   This simple dietary approach has been advocated in the United Kingdom as a means of meeting therapeutic goals in patients with maturity-onset diabetes who have ingrained dietary habits and who may have difficulty in understanding more complicated dietary instructions (Wilson et al., 1980).

2. *Reduced intake of simple carbohydrates and fats.* Guidelines to be followed are close to the U.S. Dietary Goals, except that intake of refined sugar is minimized to avoid postprandial increases in blood glucose. Total carbohydrate provides 55–60 percent of energy intake. Fat consumption is reduced, or held at not more than 30 percent of energy intake. Fats should include 10 percent saturated fat, 10 percent polyunsaturated fat, and 10 percent monosaturated fat. Cholesterol intake is reduced to 250 mg per day. These general dietary guidelines are best adopted by the mildly obese diabetic. Caloric restriction is essential. Sample menus should be provided. Foods to be included in the diet to achieve nutritional adequacy (to meet the RDA) must be discussed with the patient. Dietary compliance is usually best achieved by use of the exchange system (See Appendix, Table 1).

Dietitians, clinical nutritionists, and physicians must be cautious in advising persons of advanced age to markedly change dietary patterns established over a lifetime, because it is unlikely that the new diet will be followed, and also because if the changes are made, the patients may be worried and unhappy.

Improved glucose tolerance and better long-term control of the diabetic state may also be achieved by changing the carbohydrate content of the diet with or without energy restriction as follows:

1. *A high carbohydrate/high fiber diet may be prescribed.* Complex carbohydrates from commercially available and acceptable cereal foods and tuberous vegetables should account for about 60 percent of the total daily energy requirements. Simple sugars are restricted.

   It has been suggested that the higher carbohydrate content of the diet decreases fasting blood glucose concentrations and that diets high in fiber reduce postprandial blood glucose concentrations, and follow-up of patients treated by this diet have demonstrated a drop in glycosylated hemoglobin which indicates a long-term improvement in diabetes control (Anderson and Ward, 1978). Whereas this diet has been successfully used in highly motivated elderly patients with maturity-onset diabetes, doubt has been cast on any special role for the fiber content of this diet which is derived both from cereal grains and from vegetable sources. An alternate explanation of the good effects of the high carbohydrate-high fiber diet is that benefits accrue from the restriction in sugar intake. This is a modified fat diet in that the rate of polyunsaturated fatty acids to saturated fatty acid is 1:1.

The high carbohydrate-high fiber-modified fat diet has also been advocated for use in the management of insulin-requiring diabetics (Simpson et al., 1979). In these patients, diabetic control requires completion of prescribed meals. A problem, however, which is not inconsiderable in elderly patients is that with a change from a low carbohydrate to a high carbohydrate-high fiber diet, the bulkier characteristics of the foods make total consumption difficult. It is our experience that dietary adherence in those of advanced age is poor, and that any advantage to be gained from the high carbohydrate-high fiber diet through small reduction in insulin requirements may be outweighed by the discomfort imposed on the patient.

2.  *Guar gum* has been used to treat patients with maturity-onset diabetes and patients with minimal insulin requirement (Jenkins et al., 1978). Certain unabsorbable plant polysaccharides such as guar gum, a galactomannan from the cluster bean, reduces postprandial hyperglycemia. The gum is used by the food industry as a thickener and emulsion stabilizer. It has been suggested that the guar gum, by increasing the viscosity of gastrointestinal contents, slows gastric emptying and thereby slows absorption of dietary sugar. No malabsorption of carbohydrate has been reported, but stool losses of fat are increased. We would caution nutritionists concerning use of guar gum in any form for the treatment of elderly diabetics in whom the risk of malabsorption of micronutrients may be greater than the advantages to be gained by this unusual pharmacological approach to the treatment of diabetes.

We emphasize that the dietary management of elderly diabetics has to be tailored to the needs, the understanding, and the situation of the individual. Management requires that:

1.  All elderly obese diabetics be given a calorically restricted diet.
2.  Elderly diabetics, irrespective of body weight, be advised to reduce intake of fat and cholesterol.
3.  Elderly diabetics be told that there is no need to restrict intake of carbohydrate foods, provided these consist in whole grain cereals (not sweetened breakfast cereals) and vegetables.
4.  All elderly diabetics be given diets which, after food selection, will meet their nutrient requirements.
5.  Elderly diabetics who require insulin must have dietary carbohydrate spread out through the day, such as to avoid hypoglycemia or hyperglycemic periods.

Diabetic exchange lists are provided in the Appendix, Table 1, which also indicates how these lists should be used in diet prescription. Comparison of diet essentials for diabetics not requiring insulin and for insulin-requiring diabetics is given in Tables 8-4 and 8-5. For further information on the dietary management of elderly diabetics, readers are advised to consult a handbook on diabetes (Ireland et al., 1980) as well as recent position papers on diabetes management.

TABLE 8-4    Guidelines on Diets for Elderly Diabetic
             Patients Not Requiring Insulin

Caloric restriction (use diabetic exchange list)
Total fat restriction
Cholesterol restriction
Dietary fiber increase

TABLE 8-5    Guidelines on Diets for Insulin-Requiring
             Elderly Diabetics

Caloric restriction (use diabetic exchange list)
Increased frequency of feeding
Consistent intake of carbohydrate, fat, and protein
Meals at the same time every day
Use food or sugar to prevent early signs of hypoglycemia
Restrict total fat and cholesterol intake

## CONSTIPATION

In the elderly, constipation is complex in etiology (Bouchier, 1977). Contributing causes are:

1.  *Low fiber diet*. The intestinal transit time is prolonged in persons habitually consuming a diet low in dietary fiber which contributes to fecal bulk. When low fiber diets are eaten, stool weight and volume are reduced. The water content of the stool is diminished, and the frequency of defecation is usually reduced. Diet-related constipation can occur when dietary fiber consists of lignin (e.g. in tomato pips or fruit seeds) which does not contribute significantly to stool bulk.

2.  *Irregular bowel habits*. The urge to defecate is promoted by physiological stimuli which cause mass movement of the large intestine. The gastrocolic reflex which occurs in response to food or fluid intake initiates mass movement of colon contents. When the urge to defecate is neglected or ignored, or when food or warm drinks are not taken regularly as a stimulus to the gastrocolic reflex, simple constipation results. Neglect of the urge to defecate is most likely when defecation induces pain, e.g. with hemorrhoids or anal fissure, or when the patient is confused.

3.  *Debility*. Weakness and poor abdominal musculature make defecation difficult in the elderly. It is particularly difficult and may be painful for an elderly debilitated person to expel small, hard stools which occur when a low fiber diet is consumed.

4.  *Constipating drugs*. Narcotic analgesics, notably opioids such as morphine, are constipating. These drugs increase tone in the colon and churning activity is induced in the large intestine, which together cause resistance to luminal transit. Opioids are administered to elderly patients for relief of severe pain such as may occur in cancer.

5.  *Obstruction*. Change in bowel habit in the elderly with sudden or relatively rapid development of constipation should cause suspicion that there is an obstruction to the passage of bowel contents. Obstructive constipation in the elderly is most commonly due to cancer of the colon or rectum.

Treatment of constipation in the elderly must be preceded by identification of the cause or causes. The physician must exclude obstruction as the cause of constipation before any dietary or drug measures are adopted. Obstructive constipation usually requires surgical intervention. Constipation occurring in patients who are receiving opioids can seldom be ameliorated by dietary management alone. Laxatives are usually also required. Debility in the elderly may be relieved by treatment of underlying disease, by nutritional rehabilitation, and by mild exercise according to the causal mechanism. When total food intake is increased and dietary quality is improved, the effect may be twofold in that stool size is increased and abdominal muscles may be stronger so that it is easier for the person to defecate.

Regularity of bowel movements in the elderly may be achieved when a hot breakfast or a hot morning beverage is supplied at the same time each morning and a visit to the toilet is encouraged soon thereafter.

Increase in dietary fiber should be achieved by inclusion of whole grain cereal breads or muffins, and by giving a bowl of bran-containing breakfast cereal each morning. Other measures for increasing intake of dietary fiber include increasing the frequency of intake of vegetables, which may be cooked or raw (Mendeloff, 1976). Usually the former are preferred by the elderly.

It should be stressed that sudden increases in the fiber content of the diet of elderly people are not easily tolerated. Patients may complain of gas pain, abdominal bloating, and loose bowel movements. Further, if the ''new'' high fiber diet is bulky, the elderly individual may not be able to consume that amount of food.

A moderately high fiber diet suitable for management of constipation of dietary origin in the elderly is given in Table 4 in the Appendix.

## DIVERTICULAR DISEASE

Diverticulosis and diverticulitis are disorders of later life (Bouchier, 1977). Diverticulosis denotes a condition in which pouches arise in the wall of the colon. Diverticulitis is a complication of diverticulosis in which a pouch becomes inflamed. Diverticulitis requires active treatment with hospitalization. When a diverticulum is inflamed, hemorrhage and/or perforation of the diverticulum may ensue. Elderly patients with diverticulosis should be given moderately high fiber diets from which lignin sources are excluded. With this diet, conditions causing symptomatic diverticular disease are avoided, including constipation, diarrhea, and irregular defecation.

## GLUTEN-SENSITIVE ENTEROPATHY

Gluten-sensitive enteropathy (celiac-sprue syndrome) may present for the first time in the elderly (Hovdenak, 1980). Younger ''celiacs'' who developed the disease in middle-life may now have lived on to become elderly, since the life-saving, gluten-free diet has been in use for more than 30 years.

Among persons who develop gluten-sensitive enteropathy in later years, most are women. Typical symptoms are loss of weight, diarrhea, steatorrhea, and evidence of multiple nutritional deficiencies. However, often the presenting clinical features are atypical. Symptoms and signs may include gurgling abdominal noises, flatulence, abdominal pain, diarrhea or constipation, aphthous stomatitis, anemia, skeletal pain (due to osteomalacia and/or osteoporosis), and confusional psychosis. Patients may present with intensely pruritic (itching), blistering, symmetrical skin lesions which, on biopsy, are shown to be dermatitis herpetiforms. Low whole-blood folacin and low fasting serum calcium levels are common.

Patients show remarkable improvement with a relief of symptoms when they are kept on a gluten-free diet. Elderly patients must be carefully instructed on cereal foods to be avoided. No foods or beverages containing wheat, oats, or rye should be taken and patients should be told particularly to avoid high gluten health breads and gluten-enriched pasta. During the period when the disease is active, lactose intolerance may be severe and patients may be unable to take milk or other lactose-containing foods without developing fermentative diarrhea. As recovery proceeds with the patient in the gluten-free diet, tolerance for lactose gradually returns to normal.

Nutritional rehabilitation must be undertaken in accordance with findings of nutritional deficiencies. Most commonly, patients are folacin and vitamin D deficient.

### QUESTIONS

*Circle the correct answers to the following questions.*

1. Causes of constipation in the elderly are:
   a) debility
   b) opioids (narcotic analgesics)
   c) cheese
   d) low-fiber diet
   e) rectal cancer

2. In the dietary management of maturity-onset diabetes, which of the following guidelines should be followed:
   a) restriction of food-energy intake
   b) restriction of total carbohydrate to less than 40 percent food-energy
   c) restriction of soluble carbohydrate
   d) maintenance of dietary carbohydrate as 50–60 percent of food-energy
   e) restriction of dietary fat and cholesterol

3. Complications of obesity are:
   a) hypertension
   b) cirrhosis
   c) intertrigo
   d) Pickwickian syndrome
   e) diabetes

4. Justification for sodium restriction of the elderly is based on which of the following statements:
   a) High sodium intake precipitates congestive heart failure.
   b) Sodium restrictions in the elderly can prevent development of hypertension.
   c) Sodium restriction is important in the management of hypertension.
   d) Sodium restriction may induce weight reduction when edema is present.
   e) Sodium restriction will induce weight reduction when edema is absent.

5. Whole wheat bread should be avoided in patients with which of the following health problem(s):
   a) diabetes
   b) diverticulosis
   c) gluten-sensitive enteropathy
   d) coronary heart disease
   e) obesity

## REFERENCES

ANDERSON, J.W., and K. WARD, "Long term effects of high carbohydrate, high fiber diets on glucose and lipid metabolism. A preliminary report on patients with diabetes," *Diabetes Care*, 1 (1978), 77–82.

BARNDT, R. JR., D.H. BLANKENHORN, D.W. CRAWFORD, and S.H. BROOKS, "Regression and progression of early femoral atherosclerosis in treated hyperlipoproteinemia patients," *Ann. Intern. Med.*, 86 (1977), 139.

BOUCHIER, I.A.D., *Gastroenterology*, 2nd Ed. London: Bailliere Tindall, 1977, pp. 192–93.

Diabetes. The University Group Diabetes Program. "A study of hypoglycemic agents on vascular complications in patients with adult-onset diabetes, II." *Diabetes*, 19 (Suppl. 2) (1970), 789–830.

DWYER, T., and B.S. HETZEL, "A comparison of trends of coronary heart disease mortality in Australia, USA and England and Wales with reference to three major risk factors—hypertension, cigarette smoking and diet," *Internat. J. Epidemiol.*, 9 (1980), 65–71.

GLUECK, C.J., "Dietary fat and atherosclerosis," *Amer. J. Clin. Nutr.*, 32 (1979), 2703–11.

HOVDENAK, N., "Prevalence and clinical picture of adult gluten induced enteropathy in a Norwegian population," *Scand. J. Gastroenterol.*, 15 (1980), 401–4.

IRELAND, J.T., W.S.T. THOMSON, and J. WILLIAMSON, *Diabetes Today. A Handbook for the Clinical Team*. Aylesbury, Buckinghamshire, England: HM & M Publishers, 1980.

JENKINS, D.J.A., T.M.S. WOLEVER, and R. NINEHAM, "Guar crispbread in the diabetic diet," *Brit. Med. J.*, 2 (1978), 1744–46.

LEREN, P., "The effect of plasma cholesterol lowering diet in male survivors of myocardial infarction: a controlled trial," *Acta Med. Scand.* (Suppl.) 5, 1966.

MENDELOFF, A.I., "Dietary fiber," in *Present Knowledge in Nutrition*, 4th Ed. New York: Nutrition Foundation, Inc., 1976.

NICKERSON, M., and O. RUEDY, "Antihypertensive agents and the drug therapy of hypertension," in *The Pharmacological Basis of Therapeutics*, 5th Ed., eds. L.S. Goodman and A. Gilman. New York: Macmillan Publ. Co., Inc., 1975, pp. 705–14.

NUTTALL, F.Q., "Dietary recommendations for individuals with diabetes mellitus, summary of report from the Food and Nutrition Committee of the American Diabetes Association," *Amer. J. Clin. Nutr.*, 33 (1980), 1311–12.

ROE, D.A., *Alcohol and the Diet*. Westport, CT: AVI Publ. Co., 1979.

ROE, D.A., "Interactions between drugs and nutrients," *Med. Clin N. Amer.*, 63 (1979), 985–1007.

Safe Drinking Water Committee, *The Contribution of Drinking Water to Mineral Nutrition in Humans*, vol. 3. Washington, D.C.: Safe Drinking Water Committee, Nat. Acad. Press, 1980, pp. 283–293.

SIMPSON, R.W., J.I. MANN, and J. EATON, "High carbohydrate diets and insulin-dependent diabetics," *Brit. Med. J.*, 2 (1979), 523–25.

SIMPSON, R.W., J.I. MANN, J. EATON, R.A. MOORE, R. CARTER, and T.D.R. HOCKADAY, "Improved glucose control in maturity onset diabetes treated with high carbohydrate-modified fat diet," *Brit. Med. J.*, 1 (1979), 1753–56.

SPRITZ, N., "Appraisal of alcohol consumption as a causative factor in liver disease and atherosclerosis," *Amer. J. Clin. Nutr.*, 32 (1979), 2654–58.

STUART, R.B., "Behavioral control of overeating," in *Obesity in Perspective*, ed. G.A. Bray. DHEW Publ. No. (NIH) 75-708, 1974, pp. 367–85.

VAN ITALLIE, T.B., "Obesity: Adverse effects on health and longevity," *Amer. J. Clin. Nutr.*, 32 (1979), 2723–33.

WILSON, E.A., D.R. HADDEN, J.D. MERRETT, D.A.D. MONTGOMERY, and J.A. WEAVER, "Dietary management of maturity-onset diabetes," *Brit. Med. J.*, 1 (1980), 1367–69.

WINTROBE, M.M., G.W. THORN, R.D. ADAMS, I.L. BENNETT, E. BRAUNWALD, K.J. ISSELBACHER, and R.G. PETERSDORF, eds., *Harrison's Principles of Internal Medicine*. New York: McGraw-Hill Book Co., 1970, p. 2016.

# CHAPTER NINE
## Drugs and Nutrition
## In the Elderly

### DRUG USE AND ABUSE

Although people 65 years and over make up only about 10 percent of the population in the United States, they consume 25 percent of the country's prescription drugs (U.S. Task Force on Prescription Drugs, 1968). Chronic diseases, for which single or multiple drug therapies are commonly prescribed, are more common in the elderly. Management by physicians of hypertension, ischemic heart disease, congestive heart failure, peripheral vascular disease, chronic bronchitis and emphysema, Parkinson's disease, dementias and cerebrovascular disease, diabetes, arthritis, and cancer is by prescription of drugs which confer the risk of nutritional or diet-related side effects. In any one patient, one or more drugs may be prescribed which can affect nutritional status.

The elderly also take prescription and nonprescription drugs for relief of health complaints such as weakness, headache, nervousness, forgetfulness, vertigo (dizziness), flatulence, constipation and diarrhea, and pain. They are also easily persuaded to take nutrient supplements and tonics to improve appetite, to gain in strength and well-being, and to prevent acute infections.

Excessive use or misuse of medications is common (Guttman, 1977; Hulka et al., 1975; Raffoul et al., 1981). Reasons for this include:

1. Prescriptions from several physicians.
2. Belief that if a low drug dose is ineffective in relieving symptoms, a higher dose will produce the desired effect.
3. Hypochondriasis.

4. Health-related obsessions (e.g. preoccupation with bowel function leading to laxative abuse).
5. Inadequate review of patient care plans.
6. Failure to relate drugs in use to actual health problems present.
7. Inappropriate use of drugs, including sedatives and tranquilizers, to make the patient ''more manageable.''
8. Forgetfulness or mismanagement, leading to increased frequency of drug intake or overdose.
9. Difficulty in following medication regimens.
10. Use of drugs prescribed for others (spouse, other household member, or friend).
11. Drug dose unrelated to current body weight.
12. Advice from the mass media.

## AGING AND DRUG DISPOSITION

### Drug Absorption

With aging, physiological changes occur in the gastrointestinal tract which could affect drug absorption. The pH of the stomach is increased, reflecting a decrease in production of hydrochloric acid in the stomach. Splanchnic (GI) blood flow is decreased. Intestinal motility is decreased. There is a decrease in the number of cells lining the intestine which are capable of absorption of nutrients and drugs. Although there are these several aging changes in the structure and function of the gastrointestinal tract which could diminish the rate or quantity of drug absorbed, no significant reduction in drug absorption attributable to aging has been identified. It is presumed that the very large capacity of the gastrointestine for absorption of small molecular weight compounds, such as drugs, outweighs aging effects which could reduce absorption (Vestal, 1980).

### Drug Distribution

Several changes in body composition occur with aging which can affect the distribution of drugs (Novak, 1972). There is a reduction in lean body mass and a reduction in body water. Body fat is increased; plasma albumin concentrations are decreased, even in the absence of protein malnutrition. Due to these physiological changes, the volume of distribution of drugs is reduced. Fat-soluble drugs may be retained to a greater extent because of deposition in body fat stores. Protein binding of drugs (binding to plasma albumin) is decreased. With less plasma protein binding of drugs, more free drug is available to diffuse to receptor sites which can potentiate drug action.

## Drug Metabolism

Rates of drug metabolism have been shown to be slower in the old than in the young (O'Malley et al., 1971). Change in the rate of drug metabolism may be related to aging, to change in nutritional status and/or diet which may occur in the elderly, and to a decline in liver function due to alcohol consumption or hepatic diseases. Evaluation of observed changes in the rate of metabolism in the elderly are further complicated by the interactive effects of smoking. In younger people, smoking increases the rate of drug metabolism while in the elderly, the effect of smoking on drug metabolism is diminished (Vestal et al., 1979).

## Drug Elimination

Major routes of drug elimination are via the biliary system and via the renal tract into the urine. Decreased liver size and decreased hepatic blood flow occur with aging and could contribute to less efficient hepatobiliary excretion of drugs. However, no definitive evidence has been obtained that slowed elimination of drugs by the elderly is due to these causes.

Glomerular filtration rate declines with age. Slowed elimination of certain drugs in the elderly may be due to age-related decline in renal function even in the absence of renal disease. The renal excretion of digitalis glycosides (e.g. Digoxin), lithium carbonate, and aminoglycoside antibodies is reduced with decreased renal function.

## Drug Disposition and Geriatric Disease

In many geriatric patients, disposition of drugs is impaired by the presence of chronic disease including malabsorption syndromes, hepatic dysfunction associated with alcoholic cirrhosis, congestive heart failure, and chronic renal disease. Multiple organ dysfunctions may occur in one patient. Adverse outcomes include less efficient drug absorption, metabolism, and elimination of drugs (Ouslander, 1981).

## Drug Dispostion in Malnourished Patients

Malnutrition also affects the transport, metabolism, and elimination of drugs (Hurwitz, 1969). Protein malnutrition leads to reduction in plasma albumin so that the protein binding of drugs is reduced. As previously stated, reduction in protein binding allows more of a drug to diffuse out of the vascular compartment (through capillaries) and across interstitial spaces and tissues to reach the drug receptor sites. Protein malnutrition also impairs drug metabolism in the liver. Other nutritional deficiency states which may impair drug metabolism include ascorbic acid, niacin, and riboflavin deficiency. Starvation or semistarvation also slows drug metabolism. Renal excretion of drugs is diminished by the presence of edema which may be associated with both protein malnutrition and congestive heart failure.

## DEFINITION OF ADVERSE DRUG REACTIONS

Adverse drug reactions include a) lack of desired therapeutic effects, and b) toxic side effects (Caranasas, 1974). The elderly are at high risk for the development of adverse drug reactions due to:

1.   The chronicity of their disease processes and the multiplicity of their diseases, which increase the chances that they will take drugs over a long period of time and will take a number of drugs.
2.   Drug misuse due to:
     a.   sensory impairment (drug instructions are not heard or read)
     b.   lack of instruction (the M.D., nurse, or pharmacist does not explain how the drug(s) should be taken or the label is unclear)
     c.   mental confusion
     d.   misplaced lay advice
     e.   personal decision
     f.   economic problem (it is cheaper to take old medications than to see a new physician).
3.   Delayed drug metabolism and elimination.
4.   Hazards of over-the-counter drugs.
5.   Taking medication intended for others.
6.   Alcohol intake while on drugs.
7.   Drug-food incompatibilities.
8.   Drug-nutrient interactions.
9.   Use of folk medicines.
10.  Circumstances which impose risks of adverse drug reactions not recognized by the M.D.

## EFFECT OF DIET ON THERAPEUTIC EFFICACY

Food components affect drug absorption and bioavailability (Toothaker and Welling, 1980). Absorption of drugs may be increased or decreased by physiological changes which occur in the gastrointestinal tract in the fed versus the fasting state. Nutrients in foods can promote drug absorption. Non-nutrient components of the diet, including specific forms of dietary fiber, may adsorb drugs, producing a transient or net reduction in drug absorption. Delayed absorption of common drugs can occur when the drug is taken at the same time as food or within 1–2 hours after food has been eaten. When drug absorption is delayed by food this does not mean that less drug is totally absorbed, but rather that the time for a drug to reach peak blood levels after a single dose is lengthened. Delaying effects of food on drug absorption may be due to specific food components, e.g. pectin, or to physiological changes in the gastrointestinal tract and its blood supply associated with food intake. Splanchnic blood flow increases after food is consumed. Stomach emptying time influences the rate of drug absorption. In the fasting state or when there is little food in the stomach, the drug leaves the stomach rapidly, so that it will very soon reach the small intestine where drugs are optimally absorbed. However, if the drug formulation is such that disintegration of drug particles, as well as dissolution of the drugs, in stomach fluid must precede absorption, then rapid stomach emptying mitigates against efficient drug absorption. Drug tablets, particularly those containing certain fillers, require more prolonged residence in the stomach for their disintegration and dissolution.

Drugs that can be absorbed from the stomach, which are either lipid-soluble or non-ionized at the acid pH of the gastric environment, are more slowly absorbed when the stomach is full. Slower diffusion of the drug increases the time it takes for the drug to reach the mucosal lining of the stomach where absorption takes place.

Slower gastric emptying times may, however, promote absorption of drugs. Reasons are either that delayed stomach emptying will permit more drug to be dissolved in the stomach before it passes into the small intestine to be absorbed or more drug may be absorbed when it reaches the absorption site of the small intestine slowly (Welling 1977). Slow stomach emptying occurs particularly after heavy meals or meals containing fat and, to a lesser extent, with intake of foods which are mainly sources of carbohydrate. It is now known that different dietary components may leave the stomach at different rates. Retention of dietary fiber sources in the stomach is longer than retention of fluid or semifluid components. The rate at which a drug leaves the stomach depends on whether it is adsorbed to dietary fiber or suspended or dissolved in the fluid contents of the stomach. Dietary and gastrointestinal physiological factors influence the speed and efficiency of absorption of drugs which are formulated for sustained release.

The volume of beverage taken with a drug and the characteristics of the beverage also influence drug absorption. Drugs are more efficiently absorbed when they are in dilute solution and hence when the drug is taken with water or other liquids which have no specific pharmacological function (Borowitz et al., 1971).

When drugs are taken with food or beverages containing caffeine or theobromine, such as coffee, tea, chocolate and cola drinks, metabolism of the related drug theophylline may be slowed. Abstention from methylxanthines promotes clearance of theophylline and related drugs (Monks et al., 1979).

Absorption of L-dopa is diminished when this drug is taken with a high protein meal or with an amino acid mixture. Competitive inhibition of L-dopa absorption occurs when other amino acids, absorbed from the same intestinal absorptive site, are present (Goldin and Goldman, 1973). Similarly, a high protein meal taken with methyl dopa may diminish absorption of the drug because absorption of amino acids derived from protein foods in the meal is competitive with the drug, which, like L-dopa, is an amino acid (Sved et al., 1980).

Tables 9-1 and 9-2 show the effects of food on drug absorption. Table 9-3 shows dietary factors which influence drug metabolism.

Important diet-related factors which promote drug metabolism include:

1. The protein content of the diet. A high protein diet increases the rate of drug metabolism. Low protein-high carbohydrate diets slow drug metabolism. Change in the rate of drug metabolism may be due to change in the protein content of the diet, which is likely to occur with hospitalization or on discharge of a patient from hospital.
2. Eating of vegetables of the Brassica family, including cabbage and brussels sprouts.
3. Eating charcoal-broiled steak.

Changes in the diet which increase the rate of drug metabolism will shorten or modify the duration of effective blood levels. Higher blood levels

**TABLE 9-1   Drugs Whose Absorption May Be Reduced or Delayed by Food**

| DRUG | DOSAGE FORM | FOOD | EFFECT |
|------|-------------|------|--------|
| Penicillin V | Suspension | Milk, liquid formula | Reduced absorption |
| Penicillin G | Suspension | Milk, liquid formula | Reduced absorption |
| Cephalexin | Suspension | Milk, liquid formula | Reduced absorption |
| Nafcillin | Tablets | Breakfast? | Reduced absorption |
| Tetracycline | Capsule | Milk | Reduced absorption |
| Erythromycin stearate | Film coated tablets | Carbohydrate, fat, and protein meals | Reduced absorption |
| Erythromycin stearate | Film coated tablets | Standard breakfast | Reduced absorption |
| ASA | Tablets | Carbohydrate, fat, and protein meals | Reduced absorption |
| ASA | Enteric coated tablets | Standard breakfast | Reduced absorption |
| Sotalol | Tablets | Breakfast, milk | Reduced absorption |
| Cephalexin | Capsules | Standard hospital meal? | Delayed absorption |
| Cephalexin | Suspension | Standard hospital meal? | Delayed absorption |
| Cefaclor | Capsules | Standard breakfast | Delayed absorption |
| Metronidazole | Tablets | Standard breakfast | Delayed absorption |
| ASA | Tablets | Standard breakfast | Delayed absorption |
| Alclofenac | Suspension | Standard breakfast | Delayed absorption |
| Ibuprofen | Capsules | Standard breakfast | Delayed absorption |
| Digoxin | Tablets | Standard breakfast | Delayed absorption |
| Cimetidine | — | Standard breakfast | Delayed absorption |

Adapted from Toothaker and Welling, *Ann. Rev. Pharmacol. Toxicol.*, 1980. © 1980 by Annual Reviews, Inc. Reprinted by permission.

**TABLE 9-2  Drugs Whose Absorption May Be Promoted by Food**

| DRUG | DOSAGE FORM | FOOD |
|---|---|---|
| Erythromycin ethylsuccinate | Suspension | Milk, children's formula |
| Erythromycin estolate[a] | Capsules | Standard breakfast |
| Erythromycin stearate[a] | Film coated tablets | Breakfast? |
| Nitrofurantoin | Tablets | Standard low lipid meal |
| Diftalone | Capsules | "Standard Italian lunch" |
| 8-Methoxsalen | Coated tablets | Standard breakfast |
| Propranolol | — | Standard breakfast |
| Metoprolol | — | Standard breakfast |
| Dicoumarol | Tablets | Standard breakfast |
| Diazepam | Tablets | Standard breakfast |
| Hydrochlorothiazide | Tablets | Standard breakfast |

[a]Single and repeated dose study.

Adapted from Toothaker and Welling, *Ann. Rev. Pharmacol. Toxicol.,* 1980. © 1980 by Annual Reviews, Inc. Reprinted by permission.

of drugs will be sustained longer when the diet is changed so that drug metabolism is retarded (Anderson et al., 1979). There is a critical need to monitor blood levels of drugs with change in diet to improve drug efficacy and prevent toxicity, which can occur when the drug is retained at high levels in the body for an excessive time. Particular consideration must be given to the frequency of drug administration, which must be related to the rate of metabolism and clearance of drugs.

**TABLE 9-3  Dietary Factors Which Influence Drug Metabolism**

Protein level
Alcohol content
Charcoal broiling
Vegetables eaten
  (cabbage, brussels sprouts)
Coffee, tea, cocoa
  (methylxanthine-containing foods)
Dietary fiber
  (or other factors influencing intestinal microflora)
Eating times (in relation to drug intake)

Adapted from A. H. Conney, E. J. Pantuck, C. B. Pantuck, J. G. Forbner, A. P. Alvares, K. E. Anderson, and A. Kappas, "Variability in human drug metabolism," in *Proc. First World Conf. Clin. Pharmacol. Therap.* London, U.K., Aug. 3-9, 1980 (London and Basingstoke: Macmillan Publishers, 1980).

## NUTRITIONAL PROBLEMS RELATED TO SELF-MEDICATION

### Laxative Use and Abuse

Laxative use increases with age. Surveys have shown that approximately 50 percent of people in the United States who are 60 years or older take occasional or regular doses of laxatives. It is reported that only a quarter of these people consider themselves constipated (Fingl and Freston, 1979).

Reasons for laxative use and abuse are:

1. Simple constipation due to low fiber diet.
2. Medical disorders mitigating against easy defecation or defecation unattended by physical distress.
3. Long-term use of laxatives.
4. Intake of drugs which are constipating.
5. Bowel obsessions.

Laxatives are classified into six groups as follows:

1. *Bulk-forming agents.* These include natural and semisynthetic disaccharides or polysaccharides. Laxative properties are related to the hydrophilic, bulk-forming properties of these compounds. An additional laxative effect is due to intestinal bacterial fermentation of these compounds with release of osmotically active substances. Bulk-forming agents include methyl cellulose, food fiber sources (particularly cereal brans), psyllium seeds, and lactulose. Lactulose is a semisynthetic disaccharide which is not hydrolyzed by intestinal enzymes. Its laxative properties are similar to those of lactose in people with lactase deficiency. This unabsorbed disaccharide is metabolized by intestinal bacteria with formation of acetic, lactic and other organic seeds. The pH in the colon is reduced by this fermentation. Water and electrolytes are kept in the intestinal lumen by the intact disaccharide. The organic acid derivatives increase gastrointestinal motility. Large doses of lactulose can induce fermentative diarrhea.

2. *Osmotic agents.* Magnesium and sodium sulfate are osmotic, saline laxatives. After administration these salts are incompletely absorbed. By osmosis, more fluid is drawn into the intestine. The stool passed is admixed with liquid. Osmotic diarrhea occurs when larger doses of osmotic or saline laxatives are taken. It has been suggested that both magnesium and sodium sulfate may release intestinal hormones, including cholecystokinin which can increase both secretion and motility in the small intestine.

3. *Agents that alter electrolyte transport.* Surface active agents which are used as laxatives include bile salts which normally contribute to "bowel evacuation" and dioctylsulfosuccinate.

4. *Agents that alter intestinal motility.* Intestinal motility may be increased by dietary fiber. Fiber sources which increase intestinal motility include hemicellulose from cereal brans, and fruits and vegetables containing pectin and lignin. Lignin from fruit and vegetable seeds is not employed as a laxative because of its irritant effect on the intestine. While natural fiber sources affect intestinal motility and may also act as bulk-forming agents, other substances that promote intestinal motility also alter transport of electrolytes in the intestine.

5. *Agents that alter both electrolyte transport and intestinal motility.* Examples of laxatives which have these dual effects are castor oil, anthraquinone drugs including senna and cascara, and diphenylmethane derivatives including phenolphthalein and bisacodyl. These drugs induce net intestinal losses of sodium and water. Glucose and amino acid absorption may be inhibited. Mucosal permeability may be increased, particularly with high and prolonged intake of these drugs. Ricinoleic acid, the active metabolite of castor oil, not only inhibits absorption of sodium and glucose but also increases the intestinal permeability to macromolecules. Plasma protein losses into the intestine may thereby be increased. Dietary fiber sources which have some effect on intestinal transport do not exert significant effects on intestinal absorption except by adsorption of micronutrients such as trace elements in the intestinal lumen (Reinhold et al., 1976).

6. *Stool softeners.* Drugs function as stool softeners if they increase stool bulk, or if they prevent absorption of water from the feces in the large intestine by providing a physical barrier to water loss. Mineral oil provides an inert physical barrier to water loss from the feces in the large intestine. It also lubricates the stool, thereby facilitating defecation.

## Side Effects of Laxatives

In the elderly, bulk-forming agents taken before food can reduce appetite because the individual feels full. While intake of bulk-forming laxatives seldom has a major anorectic effect, it may be a contributing cause of early satiety. Animal studies, presently unconfirmed in elderly people, indicate that bulk-forming laxatives such as psyllium seed reduce absorption of dietary minerals including calcium, magnesium, and zinc (Smith et al., 1980).

Laxative abuse can cause potassium deficiency (Schwartz et al., 1953). Hypokalemia with or without clinical evidence of potassium deficiency is most likely to develop in elderly people taking laxatives to excess who are also on a marginal potassium intake and take potassium-losing diuretics (Roe, 1979). Types of laxatives most commonly associated with potassium deficiency are agents that affect electrolyte transport.

Malabsorption with steatorrhea can occur in laxative abusers when the laxative taken has a primary effect on the small as well as on the large intestine. Severe malabsorption has been reported in abusers of phenolphthalein and bisacodyl with steatorrhea and decreased calcium absorption. Decreased calcium absorption is a contributory cause of osteomalacia which may develop in elderly laxative abusers. Protein-losing enteropathy with massive plasma protein loss via the gastrointestinal tract is another complication of laxative abuse, which occurs in persons taking phenolphthalein, bisacodyl, or castor oil. Protein-losing enteropathy causes hypoalbuminemia and edema (Levine et al., 1981; Heizer et al., 1968).

Mineral oil, if taken at mealtimes or in the postprandial absorptive period, will prevent or reduce absorption of beta carotene and the fat soluble vitamins. The most common vitamin deficiency reported in elderly mineral oil abusers is osteomalacia. Osteomalacia in these patients is usually multifactorial, being determined not only by intake of mineral oil but also by very low consumption of vitamin D and little or no exposure to sunlight so that vitamin D synthesis in the skin is minimized (Curtis and Ballmer, 1939; Fitzgerald, 1978).

## Antacid Abuse

Antacid abuse is of frequent occurrence in elderly people for the following reasons:

1. Upper gastrointestinal tract symptoms including flatulence and belching are common complaints.
2. Antacids may be taken to counteract gastric side effects of other drugs, viz. corticosteroids and non-narcotic analgesics such as aspirin and indomethacin.
3. Antacids may be taken to relieve acute alcoholic gastritis.
4. Antacids are taken to relieve pain or acute indigestion associated with organic disease of the stomach, e.g. cancer of the stomach.
5. Media advertising strongly suggests that antacids have a positive effect on health.
6. Antacids are taken by cardiac patients with angina or with postprandial dyspnea.

Antacids may contain aluminum or magnesium hydroxide or mixtures of these substances. A phosphate depletion syndrome is known to occur in elderly people on heavy doses of these antacids. Dietary phosphate combines with aluminum and magnesium hydroxide to form insoluble aluminum and magnesium phosphates which are excreted by the gastrointestinal tract. The risk of phosphate depletion is greatest when there is an interactive effect with a low phosphate diet. Symptoms of phosphate depletion are profound muscle weakness which may be limited to proximal limb muscles, malaise, paresthesias (pins and needles), anorexia, and convulsions. In some patients phosphate depletion leads to low phosphate osteomalacia or hemolytic anemia.

Sodium overload with development of congestive heart failure can result from intake of antacids containing sodium bicarbonate (Yokel, 1977).

## Analgesic Abuse

Elderly people commonly have arthritis or other painful musculoskeletal disorders for which they take aspirin or other over-the-counter non-narcotic analgesics. Long-term use of high doses of aspirin causes erosion of the gastrointestinal mucosal, leading to multiple small hemorrhages and chronic blood loss via the gastrointestinal tract. Aspirin overuse is a prominent cause of iron deficiency anemia in the elderly. It should be pointed out that although aspirin has the potential for causing these nutritional side effects, it is a most useful drug and is a safer drug than other analgesics. However, if iron deficiency anemia is discovered in an elderly person, questions should be asked about aspirin usage, and dosage should be modified to avoid gastrointestinal bleeding. Indomethacin, commonly used to treat degenerative arthritis in the elderly, can also cause gastrointestinal bleeding and iron deficiency anemia.

Aspirin overuse is also a contributory cause of folacin deficiency, though the causal mechanism is not well identified (Weiss, 1974). The risk of folacin deficiency leading to macrocytic anemia in aspirin users is greatest in those whose folacin intake is low (Gough, 1964).

Another non-narcotic analgesic which can cause toxicity, having nutritional implications, is acetaminophen. Acetaminophen is the active ingredient of Tylenol and is also present in over-the-counter sedatives and cold mixtures. High doses cause hepatic and renal damage. Massive doses of acetaminophen cause liver necrosis which can be prevented or diminished by administration of sulfur-containing amino acids and related compounds, such as methionine or cysteamine. The nephrotoxic effects of acetaminophen develop with prolonged intake. Manifestations include a progressive loss of renal function and hypoalbuminemia (Rumack and Peterson, 1980)

### Abuse of Alcohol-Containing Mixtures

Numerous over-the-counter drugs in liquid formulation contain alcohol. The alcohol may be present in up to 25 percent of the total volume. Over-the-counter drugs which contain alcohol include cough syrups (elixirs), cold medicines, geriatric tonics, and sleep medicines (Roe, 1979).

Reasons why elderly people take alcohol-containing mixtures are as follows:

1. Alcohol has a sedative effect.
2. Elderly alcoholics want a socially acceptable form of alcohol.
3. Alcohol-containing mixtures are promoted as palliative treatment for common health problems which disable the elderly, e.g. coughs, insomnia, poor appetite, and loss of memory. Certain geriatric tonics which contain nicotinic acid (niacin) in an alcohol-containing vehicle are claimed to induce dilatation of cerebral blood vessels and thus improve memory. There is no scientific basis for these claims. Vitamin mixtures in an alcohol base are to be avoided, both because of the risks of alcohol intake in the elderly, e.g. risk of falls because of alcohol-related confusion, and because the vitamins present in these mixtures, e.g. thiamin, may not be stable or optimally available for absorption.

Alcohol-based tonics may contain methionine. Methionine supplements taken by elderly alcoholics with liver disease can precipitate liver failure (hepatic encephalopathy).

### Abuse of Nutrient Supplements—Vitamins

Hypervitaminoses in the elderly are likely to result from self-medication. Elderly people should be warned against self-medication with potent vitamin preparations. Whereas in the U.S., availability of the fat-soluble vitamins A and D has been reduced by legislation which controls over-the-counter sale of individual capsules or tablets containing high doses of these vitamins, it is still possible for elderly people to obtain an unlimited supply of these vitamins by buying more of the lower dose tablets or capsules. Elderly people may be encouraged to take vitamin A to improve their eyesight and vitamin D to prevent or control fragile bones. Hypervitaminoses A causes bone pain, headache, alopecia, and may also cause jaundice. Hypervitaminoses D causes hypercalcemia and hypertension and progressive renal failure (Roe, 1966).

Other vitamins commonly taken to excess by the elderly are vitamins E, C, and niacin (Herbert, 1979). High doses of vitamin E can be dangerous in patients receiving anticoagulants, because the vitamin E enhances the antivitamin K effects of the drug. Megadoses of vitamin C are not dangerous but can cause gastrointestinal disturbances including ''gas'' and diarrhea. Claims that megadoses of vitamin C prevent or cure colds or prevent or cure cancer are unfounded. High doses of nicotinic acid may produce unpleasant flushes and may also cause impairment of liver function.

### Abuse of Mineral Supplements

Claims have been made that elderly people have special mineral needs which are not supplied in the diet. Calcium, particularly calcium from ''natural'' sources such as bone meal, is advocated for persons with osteoporosis to harden bones. Zinc is advised to promote healing of ulcers and to improve taste sensation. Iodine, especially from kelp, is supposed to be health-giving and to improve thyroid function. Risks are that bone meal may contain lead, and therefore cause lead poisoning, that high intake of zinc causes zinc toxicity, and that kelp, because of the high iodine content, can cause iodide goiter and, in people with pre-existing thyroid enlargement, hypo or hyperthyroidism, depending on previous thyroid status and cancer of the thyroid. Cancer of the thyroid is a rare complication of prolonged iodide overdose. Life-threatening hypersensitivity reactions can occur when iodide is taken in cough medicines by elderly people who are allergic to iodine (Roe, 1979).

### Other Nutrient Supplements

Elderly people may be persuaded that massive intake of fructose or of amino acids such as lysine confers protection against metabolic or infectious disease. There is no scientific basis for these claims.

Elderly people with health complaints are advised to seek advice, diagnosis, and treatment from their physicians and not to self-medicate. Pharmacists can provide guidance to the elderly on the advisability of taking over-the-counter drugs.

## ADVERSE NUTRITIONAL EFFECTS OF DRUGS

The two principal adverse effects of drugs on the elderly's nutritional health are obesity and malnutrition (Roe, 1979; 1980). Drugs which enhance the risk of obesity are hyperphagic drugs or drugs which increase appetite. Psychotropic drugs including phenothiazine and benzodiazepine tranquilizers, antidepressant drugs including the monamine oxidase inhibitors and tricyclics, as well as lithium carbonate may cause marked increases in appetite which, if food is available, lead to excessively large food intake and development of obesity. Change in appetite with this drug is related to relief from anxiety, depression, and phobias. Conversely, when phenothiazine or benzodiazepine tranquilizers are given to elderly, underweight, bedridden patients, they may eat less because the tranquilizing and sedative effects of these drugs detract from interest in food. Because drug metabolism and elimination is slowed in the elderly, "sleep time" after sedative or tranquilizing drugs may be prolonged so that patients may not be awake at meal times.

Drugs which induce protein-energy malnutrition are most commonly those which induce nausea, vomiting, or other adverse reactions to food. Cancer chemotherapeutic drugs commonly cause nausea and vomiting immediately after drug administration but with certain cancer chemotherapy regimens, nausea is prolonged after the drugs are given (Carter, 1981). Combined chemotherapy and radiation therapy produce profound anorexia and, unless nutritional support is given, severe weight loss will follow. Elderly patients who have repeated courses of cancer chemotherapeutic drugs may develop aversion to foods which are offered in the immediate postdrug period and subsequently they may refuse to eat these foods.

Digoxin in high dosages (high dose for body weight) causes serious anorexia with or without nausea and vomiting. "Digitalis cachexia" is a severe type of chronic protein-energy malnutrition which may simulate cancer cachexia. Loss of weight in elderly people on digitalis glycosides may also be due to loss of edema fluid, and therefore may be desirable (Banks and Nayab, 1974).

Protein-energy malnutrition may occur in the elderly, as in younger people, as a consequence of drug-induced maldigestion or malabsorption. Drugs causing maldigestion and malabsorption are listed in Table 9-4, which also shows fecal nutrient losses.

Vitamin deficiencies may be due to inadequate intake because of drug-induced anorexia, maldigestion, malabsorption, hyperexcretion, or impaired vitamin utilization.

Acute vitamin deficiencies occur when vitamin antagonists are administered. Vitamin antagonists commonly used in the elderly are coumarin anticoagulants (vitamin K antagonists) and methotrexate, a folacin antagonist

**TABLE 9-4  Drug-Induced Malabsorption**

| DRUG | USAGE | NUTRIENTS LOST | MECHANISM |
|---|---|---|---|
| Mineral oil | Laxative | Fat soluble vitamins | Physical barrier to absorption; nutrient dissolved ($\beta$ carotene); micelle formation ↓ |
| Phenolphthalein | Laxative | Calcium; fat | Intestinal hurry; K depletion; loss of structural integrity |
| Neomycin | Antibiotic | Fat; nitrogen; K; Fe; calcium; lactose; vit. $B_{12}$ | Mucosal "injury" Pancreatic lipase ↓ Maldigestion |
| Cholestyramine | Hypocholesterolemic agent | | Binding of bile acids and absorption of nutrients (e.g. folacin) |
| Colestipol | Hypocholesterolemic agent | Fat soluble vitamins; folacin | " " |
| Colchicine | Anti-inflammatory agent in gout | | Mitotic arrest; structural defect in intestinal mucosa |
| Methyldopa | Antihypertensive agent | | Autoimmune mechanism? |
| Cimetidine | $H_2$ receptor antagonist (used in peptic ulcer patients) | Vit. $B_{12}$ | Hypochlorhydria |
| Methotrexate | Cancer chemotherapeutic agent | Calcium | Acute folacin deficiency |

used in the treatment of cancer (Carter, 1981). Although the desired pharmacologic effects of these drugs are related to their antivitamin properties, high drug doses can cause life-threatening situations, e.g. hemorrhage with the anticoagulant drugs due to inability to use vitamin K and failure of hemopoiesis when methotrexate is given due to inability of the body to form folacin coenzymes because of methotrexate induced enzyme block (block of the dihydrofolate reductase enzyme). The antidote for methotrexate toxicity is folinic acid. Table 9-5 lists vitamin antagonist drugs and their usage.

Mineral depletion is often caused by drugs in the elderly. As described earlier, severe forms of mineral depletion may result from abuse of over-the-counter drugs. Other drugs causing mineral depletion are oral diuretics (Morgan, 1980). However, although a fall in serum potassium levels is a

**TABLE 9-5  Vitamin Antagonists**

|  | DRUG | USAGE |
|---|---|---|
| Folacin antagonists | Methotrexate | Cancer chemotherapy |
|  | Pyrimethamine | Antimalarial |
|  | Triamterene | Diuretic |
|  | Trimethoprim | Antibacterial |
| Vitamin $B_6$ antagonists | Isoniazid | Antituberculosis agent |
|  | Hydralazine | Antihypertensive agent |
|  | Cycloserine | Antituberculosis agent |
|  | Levodopa | Anti-Parkinsonism agent |
| Vitamin K antagonists | Warfarin | Anticoagulants |

Taken from D. A. Roe, "Interactions between drugs and nutrients," *Med. Clin. N. Amer.,* 63 (5): 1001, 1979. © W. B. Saunders Co. Reprinted by permission.

well-known effect of the thiazide and "loop" diuretics (furosemide and ethacrynic acid), chronic intake of these diuretics does not commonly result in severe hypokalemia in patients taking these drugs for hypertension or congestive heart failure unless intake of potassium from the diet is marginal or patients are laxative abusers. Drugs causing mineral depletion are shown in Table 9-6.

Other folacin (folate) antagonists commonly taken by the elderly are the antibacterial drug trimethoprim and the potassium-sparing diuretic triamterene. These two drugs are mild folacin antagonists.

**TABLE 9-6  Mineral Depletion Induced by Drugs**

| | |
|---|---|
| Diuretics | Calcium (not thiazides) |
| | Potassium |
| | Magnesium |
| | Zinc |
| Laxatives (Laxative abuse) | Potassium |
| | Calcium |
| Glucocorticoids | Calcium |
| | Potassium |
| Chelating agents (penicillamine) | Zinc |
| | Copper |
| Ethanol | Potassium |
| | Magnesium |
| | Zinc |
| Antacids | Phosphates |
| Non-narcotic analgesics (aspirin, indomethacin) | Iron (by GI blood loss) |

Taken from D. A. Roe, "Interactions between drugs and nutrients," *Med. Clin. N. Amer.,* 63 (5): 998, 1979. © W. B. Saunders Co. Reprinted by permission.

## DRUG-FOOD AND DRUG-NUTRIENT INCOMPATIBILITIES

Adverse reactions to drugs can be precipitated by intake with certain foods or alcoholic beverages. Reactions vary greatly in intensity, some being sufficiently unpleasant to make the person want to avoid going through the experience again, while other reactions are life-threatening (Roe, 1979). The major types of drug-food and drug-alcohol incompatibilities are summarized in Table 9-7.

Major risk factors related to adverse nutritional effects of drugs and drug-food incompatibilities occur when:

**TABLE 9-7   Drug-Food and Drug-Alcohol Incompatibilities**

| CLASSIFICATION | REACTANTS | | EFFECT |
|---|---|---|---|
| | 1 | 2 | |
| 1. Tyramine reactions | *MAO Inhibitors* | *High tyramine/ dopamine foods* | |
| | Antidepressants, e.g., phenelzine | Cheese | Flushing |
| | Procarbazine | Red wines | Hypertension |
| | Isoniazid (INH, Isonicotinic acid hydrazide) | Chicken liver Broad beans Yeast extracts | Cerebrovascular accidents |
| 2. Disulfiram reactions | *Aldehyde dehydrogenase inhibitors* | *Ethanol* | |
| | Disulfiram (Antabuse) | Beer | Flushing, headache |
| | Calcium carbimide | Wine | Nausea, vomiting |
| | Metronidazole | Liquor | Chest and |
| | Nitrofurantoin | Foods containing | abdominal pain |
| | C. atramentarius* Sulfonylureas | alcohol | |
| 3. Hypoglycemic reactions | *Insulin releasers* | *Ethanol* | |
| | Oral hypoglycemic agents | | Weakness |
| | Sugar (as in sweet mixes) | | Mental confusion |
| | | | Irrational behavior |
| | | | Loss of consciousness |
| 4. Flush reactions | *Miscellaneous* Chlorpropamide [+ diabetes] | *Ethanol* | Flush Dyspnea |
| | Griseofulvin Tetrachlorethylene | | Headache |

*Coprinus atramentarius = Inky cap mushroom.

Taken from D. A. Roe, "Interactions between drugs and nutrients," *Med. Clin. N. Amer.*, 63 (5): 985, 1979. © W. B. Saunders Co. Reprinted by permission.

1. The drug is an antinutrient.
2. The drug, which has adverse nutritional effects, is taken for a long time.
3. The patient is on a multidrug regimen.
4. The diet is nutritionally inadequate.
5. There is excessive drug use or abuse of prescription or over-the-counter drugs.
6. Disease-related malabsorption is present.
7. The patient is malnourished.
8. The patient is not given special diet instructions.
9. Physicians and nutritionists are unaware of the risks.

## QUESTIONS

*Circle all correct answers.*

1. Over-the-counter drug abuse in the elderly is due to:
   a) chronic allergies
   b) chronic constipation
   c) chronic aches and pains
   d) promotional advertising
   e) alcohol content of drug mixtures

2. Potassium deficiency is associated with:
   a) high sodium intake
   b) low cholesterol diet
   c) intake of oral diuretics
   d) heavy use of laxatives
   e) diet of bread, cold cuts and sodas

3. Tranquilizing drugs may lead to gain in weight. Reasons are:
   a) increased appetite and food intake
   b) fluid retention
   c) decreased physical activity
   d) gain in muscle mass
   e) gain in bone mass

4. Adverse drug reactions occur more frequently in the elderly because:
   a) more drugs are taken
   b) patients do not understand medication instructions
   c) drug metabolism is slowed with aging
   d) over-the-counter drugs are abused
   e) drugs are taken which are intended for others

5. Acute adverse reactions (drug-food and drug-beverage incompatibilities) occur under one or more of the following circumstances:
   a) aspirin is taken with eggs
   b) milk is taken with antihistamines
   c) aged cheese is taken with antidepressants (MAOI)
   d) alcohol is taken with metronidazole (Flagyl)
   e) cookies are taken with propranolol (Inderol)

## REFERENCES

ANDERSON, K.E., A.H. CONNEY, and A. KAPPAS, "Nutrition and oxidative drug metabolism in man: relative influence of dietary lipids, carbohydrate and protein," *Clin. Pharmacol. Therap.*, 26 (1979), 493–501.

BANKS, T., and A. NAYAB, "Letter. Digitalis cachexia." *New Eng. J. Med.*, 290 (1974), 746.

BOROWITZ, J.L., P.F. MOORE, G.K.W. YIM, and T.S. MIYA, "Mechanisms of enhanced drug effects produced by dilution of the oral dose," *Toxicol. Appl. Pharmacol.*, 19 (1971), 164–68.

CARANASOS, C.J., R.B. STEWART, and L.E. CLUFF, "Drug-induced illness leading to hospitalization," *J. Am. Med. Assoc.*, 228 (1974), 713–17.

CARTER, S.K., "Nutritional problems associated with cancer chemotherapy," in *Nutrition and Cancer. Etiology and Treatment*, eds. G.R. Newell and N.M. Ellison. New York: Raven Press, 1981, pp. 303–17.

CURTIS, A.C., and R.S. BALLMER, "The prevention of carotene absorption by liquid petrolatum," *J. Am. Med. Assoc.*, 113 (1939), 1785–88.

FINGL, E., and J.W. FRESTON, "Antidiarrhoeal agents and laxatives: changing concepts," *Clin. Gastroenterol.*, 8 (1979), 161–86.

FITZGERALD, F., "Clinical hypophosphatemia," *Ann. Rev. Med.*, 29 (1978), 177–89.

GOLDIN, B.R., and P. GOLDMAN, "The metabolism of L-dopa. The role of the intestinal microflora," *Fed. Proc.*, 32 (1973), 798.

GOUGH, K.R. et al., "Folic acid deficiency in rheumatoid arthritis," *Brit. Med. J.*, 1 (1964), 212–17.

GUTTMAN, D.V., "A study of legal drug use by older Americans," *Services Research Report* (NIDA), 1977.

HEIZER, W.D., A.L. WARSHAW, T.A. WALDMAN, and L. LASTER, "Protein losing gastroenteropathy and malabsorption associated with factitious diarrhea," *Ann. Intern. Med.*, 68 (1968), 839–52.

HERBERT, V.D., "Megavitamin therapy," in *Contemporary Nutrition Controversies*, eds. T.P. Labuza and E.A. Sloan. St. Paul, New York, Los Angeles, San Francisco: West Publ., 1979, pp. 223–27.

HULKA, B.S., L.L. KUPPER, J.C. CASSEL, R.L. EFIRD, and J.A. BURDETTE, "Medication use and misuse: Physician-patient discrepancies," *J. Chronic Dis.*, 28 (1975), 7–21.

HURWITZ, N., "Predisposing factors in adverse reactions to drugs," *Brit. Med. J.*, 1 (1969), 536–39.

LEVINE, D., A.W. GOODE, and D.L. WINGATE, "Purgative abuse associated with reversible cachexia hypogamma globulinaemia and finger clubbing," *Lancet*, 1 (1981), 919–20.

MONKS, T.J., J. CALDWELL, and R.L. SMITH, "Influence of methylxanthine-containing foods on theophylline metabolism and kinetics," *Clin. Pharmacol. Ther.*, 26 (1979), 513–24.

MORGAN, D.B., and C. DAVIDSON, "Hypokalaemia and diuretics: an analysis of publications," *Brit. Med. J.*, 1 (1980), 905–8.

NOVAK, L.P. "Aging, total body potassium, fat-free mass and cell mass in males and females between ages 18 and 85 years," *J. Gerontol.*, 27 (1972), 438–43.

O'MALLEY, K., J. CROOKS, E. DUKE, and I.H. STEVENSON, "Effect of age and sex on human drug metabolism," *Brit. Med. J.*, 3 (1971), 607–9.

OUSLANDER, J.G., "Drug therapy in the elderly," *Ann. Intern. Med.*, 95 (1981), 711–22.

RAFFOUL, P.R., J.K. COPPER, and D.W. LOVE,   "Drug misuse in older people," *Gerontologist*, 21 (1981), 146–50.

REINHOLD, J.G., B. FARADJI, P. ABADI, and F. ISMAEL-BEIGI,   "Decreased absorption of calcium, magnesium, zinc and phosphorus by humans due to increased fiber and phosphorus consumption as wheat bread," *J. Nutr.*, 106 (1976), 493–503.

ROE, D.A.   *Alcohol and the Diet.* Westport, CT: AVI Publ. Co., 1979.

ROE, D.A.,   "Interaction between drugs and nutrients," *Med. Clin. N. Amer.*, 63 (1979), 985–1007.

ROE, D.A.,   "Nutrient toxicity with excessive intake. 1. Vitamins," *New York State J. Med.*, 66 (1966), 869–71.

ROE, D.A.,   "Nutrition and chronic drug administration: Effects on the geriatric patient," *American Pharmacy*, NS20 (1980), 33–35.

ROE, D.A.,   *Nutrition and the Health Scientist.* Boca Raton, FL: CRC Press, Inc., 1979, pp. 67–69.

RUMACK, B.H., and R.G. PETERSON,   "Clinical toxicology," in *Casarett and Dou-ll's Toxicology. The Basic Science of Poisons*, 2nd Ed., eds. J. Dou-ll, C.D. Klaassen, and M.O. Amdur. New York: Macmillan Publ. Co., Inc., 1980, pp. 682–83.

SCHWARTZ, W.B., and A.S. RELMAN,   "Metabolic and renal studies in chronic potassium depletion resulting from overuse of laxatives," *J. Clin. Invest.*, 32 (1953), 258–71.

SMITH, R.G., M.J. ROWE, A.N. SMITH, M.A. EASTWOOD, E. DRUMMOND, and W.G. BRYDON,   "A study of bulking agents in elderly patients," *Age and Ageing*, 9 (1980), 267–71.

SVED, A.F., I.M. GOLDBERG, and J.D. FERNSHAM,   "Dietary protein intake influences the antihypertensive potency of methyl dopa in spontaneously hypertensive rats," *J. Pharm. Exp. Therapeut.*, 214 (1980), 147–51.

U.S. Task Force on Prescription Drugs: "The Drug Users." Washington, D.C.: USDHEW, 1968, pp. 126–29.

VESTAL, R.E.,   "Methodological problems associated with studies of drug metabolism in the elderly," ed. P. Turner. First World Conf. on Clin. Pharmacol. and Therapeut., London, Aug. 3-9, 1980. London: Macmillan, 1980, pp. 110–16.

VESTAL, R.E., A.J.J. WOOD, R.A. BRANCH, D.J. SHAND, and G.R. WILKINSON,   "Effects of age and cigarette smoking on propranolol disposition," *Clin. Pharmac. Therap.*, 26 (1979), 8–15.

WEISS, H.J.,   "Aspirin—a dangerous drug?" *J. Am. Med. Assoc.*, 229 (1974), 1221–22.

WELLING, P.G.,   "Influence of food and diet on gastrointestinal absorption: A review," *J. Pharmacokinet. Biopharmaceut.*, 5 (1977), 291–331.

YOKEL, R.A.,   "Sodium and potassium levels in antacids," *Am. J. Hosp. Pharm.*, 34 (1977), 200–202.

# CHAPTER TEN
# Nutrition Services

## NUTRITIONAL COUNSELLING FOR THE ELDERLY

In recent years, target groups for nutrition education have included the elderly. The overall aim has been to influence older people to consume an adequate diet (Wurtman, 1979; Smith, 1978; Harper, 1978). Recognition that certain elderly people need nutrition counselling is due in part to a growing awareness of the difficulties these people may have in buying and preparing food and more especially in choosing and obtaining foods required for special diets (Clarke and Wakefield, 1975). Other special needs of the elderly, coming under the umbrella of nutrition education, include strategies to modify eating times and content of meals to avoid symptoms generated by food and adverse drug reactions, combatting nutrition misinformation, and instruction on the risks of food and alcohol abuse (Roe, 1979; 1980). Nutrition counselling for the elderly may be direct education in a classroom or a community setting but more commonly is by counselling of elderly individuals or groups or by giving information to those with responsibility for the direct care of the elderly.

Goals of nutritional counselling are:

1. To explain personal food-energy and nutrient needs.
2. To show how nutritional requirements can be met using available foods.
3. To offer simple and feasible menu and exercise plans for weight control or reduction.
4. To develop skills in food procurement and preparation which are related to situational factors and disabilities which are present.

5. To give information on locally available nutrition support services, food delivery services, and congregate meal centers.
6. To interpret prescribed diets intended for the control of chronic disease and to ensure that restrictive diets are nutritionally adequate.
7. To give practical advice on foods which are desirable to prevent gastrointestinal complaints including flatulence and constipation.
8. To establish eating times which allow optimal absorption, utilization, and tolerance of prescribed medications.
9. To combat use of fad diets.
10. To encourage socialization at meal times.
11. To obtain information on alcohol abuse, to make referrals on alcoholism counselling, and to counsel alcoholics on dietary needs.
12. To promote the best use of a limited food budget.

### Who receives counselling?

1. The elderly individual if he or she is living independently and is responsible for food procurement and preparation.
2. The homemaker who purchases and/or prepares food for the elderly person.
3. The food service manager at a domiciliary care facility or nursing home.
4. The nurse or personal care attendant who is responsible for feeding and assisting in feeding the individual.

## Guidelines on Implementation of Counselling Goals

*Meeting Energy and Nutrient Needs.* The food-energy needs of the individual should be explained with emphasis on adjustment of calorie intake downwards in accordance with age, lower metabolic rate, decreased muscle mass and, most importantly, physical exercise. It should be emphasized that if the person's weight is within the desirable range for his or her height, his usual food-energy intake is meeting his requirements.

Using oral presentation and charts as shown in Figure 10-1, food sources of key nutrients should be explained. Special emphasis should be placed on food sources rich in calcium, vitamin D, riboflavin, and folacin, which are frequently deficient in the diets of the elderly. It should also be stressed that if a variety of foods rich in essential nutrients are consumed, this will markedly increase the chance that the diet will be nutritionally adequate.

*Weight Reduction.* When weight reduction is required, it is necessary to determine the person's current and/or usual food-energy intake. For an individual who is living independently, this requires repeated 24-hour dietary recalls (a minimum of three so that the average daily intake can be calculated) or a diet record. It is seldom feasible to obtain a diet record for more than three days, one of which should be a weekend day. Instruction should be given either to the elderly individual or to a responsible spouse, home companion, or

| Food/beverage | Nutrient |
|---|---|
| Enriched bread, pasta, and flour | Carbohydrate<br>B vitamins |
| Milk | Protein<br>Vitamin A<br>Vitamin D<br>Calcium |
| Margarine | Fat<br>Vitamin A |
| Fruit juices (citrus) | Vitamin C<br>Potassium |
| Fortified breakfast cereals | Carbohydrate<br>Vitamin A<br>Vitamin D<br>Vitamin C<br>B vitamins<br>Iron |
| Green leafy vegetable | Folic acid<br>Potassium |

**FIGURE 10-1    Food sources of key nutrients (to be consumed daily).**

domestic worker, on how the diet record should be kept. It is very important that the 24-hour recalls or diet records indicate eating times, all foods and beverages consumed, and portion sizes. Then the individual's weight and height should be measured. An ideal body weight for a man or woman of that height can be determined using Table 10-1. By subtracting the ideal weight from the patient's weight, a desirable weight loss can be calculated. It is only justifiable, however, to calculate the desired weight loss by this means if edema and ascites are absent. When a diuretic is prescribed to treat edema but has not yet been taken, then measurement of body weight and calculation of desirable weight loss should be delayed until a ''dry'' weight can be obtained, that is, the patient should be weighed again when the edema fluid has been lost. When the patient has ascites, prescription of weight-reducing diets is seldom justifiable.

The feasibility of attaining the desired weight loss has to be evaluated by the nutritionist in consultation with the patient's physician and preferably also following discussion with another family member or a close companion of the patient, who can assess motivation and ability of the patient to change or modify his or her eating habits.

TABLE 10-1  Suggested Desirable Weights for Heights and Ranges for Adult Males and Females

| HEIGHT[a] | | WEIGHT[b] | | | | | | | |
| --- | --- | --- | --- | --- | --- | --- | --- | --- | --- |
| | | MEN | | | | WOMEN | | | |
| in. | cm | lb | | kg | | lb | | kg | |
| 58 | 147 | — | | — | | 102 | (92-119) | 46 | (42-54) |
| 60 | 152 | — | | — | | 107 | (96-125) | 49 | (44-57) |
| 62 | 158 | 123 | (112-141) | 56 | (51-64) | 113 | (102-131) | 51 | (46-59) |
| 64 | 163 | 130 | (118-148) | 59 | (54-67) | 120 | (108-138) | 55 | (49-63) |
| 66 | 168 | 136 | (124-156) | 62 | (56-71) | 128 | (114-146) | 58 | (52-66) |
| 68 | 173 | 145 | (132-166) | 66 | (60-75) | 136 | (122-154) | 62 | (55-70) |
| 70 | 178 | 154 | (140-174) | 70 | (64-79) | 144 | (130-163) | 65 | (59-74) |
| 72 | 183 | 162 | (148-184) | 74 | (67-84) | 152 | (138-173) | 69 | (63-79) |
| 74 | 188 | 171 | (156-194) | 78 | (71-88) | — | | — | |
| 76 | 193 | 181 | (164-204) | 82 | (74-93) | — | | — | |

[a]Without shoes.
[b]Without clothes. Average weight ranges in parentheses.

The food-energy content of the weight-reducing diet has to be selected. Severe food restriction and semifasting regimens are inappropriate in elderly persons.

Predicted rate of weight loss of elderly, sedentary people on diets of defined caloric content can be calculated using the information shown in Table 10-2.

Simple menus for use in weight reduction which are planned to provide an adequate intake of nutrients are illustrated in Figures 10-2 and 10-3. By using exchange lists, these menus can be varied (see Tables 1 and 2 in the Appendix).

Further increase in the rate of weight loss could be obtained by increasing energy expenditure through exercise. Appropriate forms of physical activity in a person over 65, who does not have severe cardiac or respiratory disease or other severe physical handicaps, are walking, bicycling, gardening, golf, bowling, and daily exercises. Gradual acclimation to increased physical activity is essential. Individuals using a walker can exercise under supervision.

Individuals who are confined to a wheelchair may also be able to increase their energy expenditure by performing simple exercises which involve arm and head movements. However, the extent to which such exercise can contribute to weight loss in a wheelchair patient is very limited. Exercise plans for the disabled elderly person need to be worked out by a physiatrist or physical therapist who has extensive experience in working with geriatric patients.

**TABLE 10-2    Defining Goal of Weight Loss, Rate of Weight Loss, and Kilocalorie Level of Diets for Sedentary Obese Elderly**

1. Obtain measurements of weight and height of patient.

2. Determine, by use of Table 10-1, the "ideal" weight for a person of the individual's sex, height, and age. We will assume the goal of weight reduction is attainment of "ideal" weight.

3. Obtain a 3-day diet record and, from this record, determine the person's current food-energy intake in kcal.

4. Estimate on the basis of the individual's medical needs and food-related behavior whether it is better to recommend loss of 1 or 2 lbs per week.

5. a.  To lose 1 lb per week, subtract 500 kcal daily from current intake in kcal.*
   b.  To lose 2 lbs per week, subtract 1000 kcal daily from current intake in kcal.

6. Explain to individual or responsible household member or health professional how long it will take for the individual to reach the "ideal" weight without change in activity pattern.

*Estimation of kcal reduction is from the following calculation:

1 lb of body fat = 454 gm

1 gm of body fat yields 7.7 kcal

454 gm of body fat yields 454 X 7.7 = 3,496 kcal/lb body fat (3500 kcal)

If 3500 kcal is divided into 7 days, then to reduce 1 lb in body fat per week requires reduction of $\frac{3500}{7}$ = 500 kcal/day.

**FIGURE 10-2    Simple menu for weight reduction (1000 kcal).**

*Breakfast*
   Prune juice, 1/4 cup
   Cereal, fortified, 3/4 cup
   Skim milk, 8 oz.
   Tea

*Lunch*
   Lean roast beef, 3 oz.
   Carrots, 1/2 cup
   Rice, 1/2 cup
   Fruit (fresh orange), 1 small
   Margarine, 1 tsp.
   Coffee

*Dinner*
   Cottage cheese, 1/2 cup
   Tomato
   Lettuce
   Whole wheat enriched bread, 1 slice
   Margarine, 1 tsp.

*Snack*
   Cantaloupe, 1/4 medium
   Skim milk, 8 oz.

For 1200 kcal, add 1 meat, 1 bread, and 1 fat.

**FIGURE 10-3    Alternate menu for weight reduction (1000 kcal).**

*Breakfast*
>  Orange juice, 1/2 cup
>  Cereal, fortified, 3/4 cup
>  Skim milk, 8 oz.
>  Coffee

*Lunch*
>  Whole wheat enriched bread, 1 slice
>  Cottage cheese, 1/2 cup
>  Fruit, unsweetened, 1/2 cup
>  Margarine, 1 tsp.
>  Tea

*Dinner*
>  Tomato juice, 1/2 cup
>  Chicken (baked), 3 oz.
>  Spinach, 1/2 cup
>  Potato, baked, 1 small
>  Margarine, 1 tsp.

*Snack*
>  Skim milk, 8 oz.
>  Banana, 1/2 small

For 1200 kcal, add 1 meat, 1 bread, and 1 fat.

*Food Procurement and Food Preparation for Special Diets.*    Skills in food procurement and preparation in which elderly, independently living persons can be instructed include the following:

1.  How to obtain transportation to the market.
2.  How to obtain local information on food stores where assistance may be obtained in carrying bagged groceries to the car.
3.  Foods to buy which have a high nutrient-to-calorie ratio (Appendix Table 5).
4.  Understanding food labeling. It is advised that if the elderly person has a visual impairment, use of a magnifying lens in the market may be helpful.
5.  How and where, and which foods to procure in order to follow a therapeutic diet, e.g. low-sodium products (Appendix Table 6).

Unless sodium restriction is severe (<1000 mg/day), it is rarely necessary to deliberately shop for special low-sodium products, but rather it is necessary to explain high-sodium foods which should be avoided, including instant, dried, and canned soups (unless bearing the label ''low-sodium''), canned, smoked, and dried fish, sea food (especially if canned), ham, bacon, hot dogs, cold cuts, meat spreads, cheeses unless of the low-sodium varieties, salted snack foods including nuts, potato chips, crackers, and canned vegetables unless packed in water. For the sodium content of foods, Table 6 in the Appendix should be consulted, and a list of high-sodium foods should be given to the elderly individual. It must be stressed that sodium restriction requires that salt not be added to foods either in cooking or at the table.

When the need is to seek low-sodium staples, then markets supplying low-sodium bread, margarine, and canned goods should be identified.

When elderly people are receiving diuretics, they should usually increase potassium intake. Instructions in food sources rich in potassium should be given, and preconceived notions about bananas or oranges being the only good sources of potassium should be dispelled. Rich food sources of potassium which are also low in sodium are given in Table 6 in the Appendix.

Guidelines on obtaining and preparing low-fat and low-cholesterol diets should be given through explanation of foods to be avoided, and through instruction on foods to be selected. Verbal instruction should be supplemented by distribution of short lists of low-fat and low-cholesterol foods as in Table 7 in the Appendix. It must be emphasized that compliance with low-fat diets requires that foods should not be fried or cooked with addition of fat other than that approved by the prescribed diet.

For guidelines on foods and cooking methods which are appropriate to elderly diabetic patients, see section on diabetes in Chapter 8.

It is often important to instruct elderly men and women on good food sources of dietary fiber. In recommending high-fiber foods, it is important to remember that elderly people will often be unable to consume bulky foods or foods that require a lot of chewing. High-fiber foods appropriate for the elderly are listed in the Appendix in Table 8.

*Kitchens and Cooking for the Disabled.*  When elderly persons are physically disabled, special instruction is necessary for modifications to be made in the kitchen and in kitchen appliances to make it possible for the person to function alone. Utensils, dishes, glassware, and silverware should be within reach of a person using a walker or wheelchair. Redesign or change in the installation or modification of kitchen cabinets, stovetops, and ovens may be necessary. When the nutritionist is inexperienced in these matters, consultation should be held with the persons or societies having expertise in the rehabilitation of elderly persons following stroke or other chronic diseases associated with long-term and/or permanent handicaps.

*Information on Meal and Food Distribution Programs.*  Elderly individuals need also to be given information on locally available meal and food distribution systems, including meal facilities under Title III, Meals-on-Wheels, or local agencies providing low cost meals. Program eligibility has to be determined on the basis of income, domicile, and age. Elderly persons who are found to be eligible to receive Food Stamps may need assistance in obtaining the Food Stamps from the Department of Social Services. It may be important for the individual to be accompanied to the market, particularly if the food layout in the market is unfamiliar, if assistance is required in food selection, or if guidance is needed on obtaining special foods necessitated by therapeutic diets. Community resources which may provide for the needs of the elderly include Home Help Service, commonly made available through the Public Health Department and homemakers working under local agencies.

*Explaining Prescribed Diets.*     The interpretation of prescribed diets must include:

1. Dietary guidance which imposes the least change in the individual's pattern or food preference.
2. Menu planning such that each daily menu includes permitted food and intake of essential nutrients.

When dietary history and/or clinical anthropometric, hematological, or biochemical assessment of nutritional status indicates that prior to implementation of the special diet, the patient's nutritional status is unsatisfactory, the physician should be consulted about the need for a nutrient supplement.

If a nutrient supplement is prescribed, its composition must be such as to conform with the restriction of the diet. For example, elderly persons who have developed chronic radiation enteritis following x-ray or other radiation treatment of the abdomen for cancer usually need to adhere to a low-lactose diet. In these persons liquid nutrient supplements must also be of the low-lactose type.

*Instructions on Prevention of Gastrointestinal Symptoms.*     Practical advice on foods which are desirable to prevent gastrointestinal complaints in the elderly usually has to be combined with gentle but firm dissipation of old wives' tales like that of the constipating effects of cheese, or the idea that orange juice and sometimes a wide variety of foods are "too acid" and therefore to be avoided by the elderly for fear of digestive disorders. It should be taught that common beverages likely to cause heartburn and upper abdominal pain or discomfort are coffee and alcohol. Coffee and alcohol can also potentiate signs of rosacea with flushing of the face and particularly of the nose, which is most marked at certain times of the day and week (i.e. when these beverages are taken in greatest amount or volume). More acute upper-right-sided abdominal pain, in a patient with a history of gall bladder disease, is usually due to intake of fatty foods. Lower abdominal pain with discomfort and gassy diarrhea can be due to lactose intolerance following radiation therapy to the abdomen, or is associated with alcohol abuse. Constipation with attendant abdominal discomfort can be due to:

1. Intake of a low fiber (lower residue) diet.
2. Failure to consume breakfast or to take a warm early morning beverage which will initiate the gastrocolic reflex.
3. Inactivity leading to weakness of the abdominal muscles so that expelling feces from the rectum is difficult.

Constipation or self-diagnosed constipation associated with intermittent diarrhea is associated with the irritable bowel syndrome but also with laxative abuse. Constipation per se is also associated with intake of therapeutic drugs which are constipating, particular examples being the narcotic analgesics used to relieve intractable pain such as that associated with metastasis and inoperable cancer which have not responded to chemotherapy or radiation therapy.

Intermittent constipation and diarrhea in the elderly may occur in diverticular disease as well as with mismanagement of the diet, e.g. sudden or irregular change from a low-fiber to a high-fiber diet (hemicellular rich foods), or intake of foods high in lignin, i.e. foods which contain seeds and pips such as strawberries and tomatoes. Diarrhea can be due to gluten-sensitive enteropathy and inflammatory bowel disease, as well as lactose intolerance and laxative abuse.

It cannot be overemphasized that in the elderly abdominal symptoms are frequently associated with underlying serious abdominal disease or intake of therapeutic drugs which are necessitated for the control of systemic disease.

Other common causes of abdominal symptoms are abuse of food substances including coffee and alcohol, or abuse of drugs such as laxatives and cathartics, as well as dietary mismanagement.

Abdominal symptoms, particularly constipation, may be due to debility and muscle weakness, particularly if the individual has been confined to bed for long periods of time or because wheelchair confinement or obesity give little opportunity or inclination for physical exercise.

The elderly may complain excessively of abdominal symptoms or may relate abdominal symptoms to the types of food consumed or to the methods of cooking (particularly institutional cooking) when in fact no such relationships exist. The nutritionist from whom advice is sought by an elderly person or by another person taking care of the elderly individual should not offer dietary advice unless the cause of the abdominal symptoms has been established by a physician, nurse, or clinician and causes other than diet have been eliminated. Dietary guidelines appropriate to elderly persons with commonly encountered abdominal symptoms are indicated in Table 10-3.

*Meals and Medication Usage.*     Elderly persons or their attendants need information which can be given by the nutritionist, but only after consultation with the patient's physician and the pharmacist on eating times which will allow optimum absorption of prescribed drugs. For lists of drugs which are better absorbed in the fasting or fed state, the nutritionist should consult Tables 9-1 and 9-2 in Chapter 9.

Modification of eating schedules to promote compliance with therapeutic drug instructions may require a change in meal times or advising the individual to take milk and iron-containing foods away from times of drug (tetracycline) intake. It may also be necessary to discuss with the patient appropriate small snacks to take with drugs to lessen gastric distress. A cracker or rusk may be

**TABLE 10-3  Dietary Guidelines for Elderly Patients with Gastrointestinal Symptoms**

All elderly persons with gastrointestinal symptoms or change in bowel function should be examined by a physician to exclude upper GI, colon, and rectal cancer. Dietary guidelines given here are for elderly persons with GI symptoms which are not due to cancer or accompanied by other gastrointestinal pathology requiring surgical or drug therapy.

*Indigestion or flatulence.* Avoid fruit and fatty food, alcohol, coffee.

*Bloating or "Gas."* Avoid large meals, boiled or baked beans, and very large volumes of citrus fruit juice.

*Constipation.* Establish cause. Increase intake of high fiber foods including foods containing cereal brans such as bran breakfast cereals, breads and muffins. Increase intake of carrots, squash, celery, and leafy green vegetables as well as fruits including apples and apple sauce. Drink one (4 oz.) glass of prune juice per day. Drink warm beverages on arising each morning at breakfast and make a regular visit to the toilet thereafter.

*Diarrhea.* Establish cause. If due to chronic radiation enteritis with nonreversible malabsorption and lactose intolerance, omit milk and substitute other high-calcium foods. Decrease fat intake. If due to gluten-sensitive enteropathy, omit breads and other foods containing gluten.

taken with antibiotics such as tetracycline without impairment of drug absorption.

*Combatting Fad Diets.* Elderly persons are attracted by fad diets because of advertisements in magazines and claims made in fad diet books which suggest that adherence to a particular diet will protect the individual from acute or chronic illness, will increase vitality or will relieve health complaints which are commonly associated with aging. Writers of fad diet books may also advocate intake of "health foods" or megadoses of nutrients including amino acids such as lysine, sugars such as fructose, vitamins, minerals, and trace elements. The nutritionist working with the elderly should be familiar with current fad diet literature and should be able to point out to their elderly clients the fallacies and dangers of the fad diet regimen which has attracted interest or is being followed. High protein-high fat diets impose special health risks in elderly persons whose hepatic, pancreatic, or renal function is impaired. Complications arising from intake of these diets include liver failure (high protein), acute pancreatitis (high fat), and renal failure (high protein). Weight-reducing diets which suggest an intake of soups and bouillon high in sodium can precipitate congestive heart failure.

Counselling on avoidance of fad diets requires that the nutritionist gain the complete confidence of the elderly client and that a rational alternative diet be provided which will ameliorate or modify health problems from which the person is seeking relief. In the event that a fad diet is being followed as an alternative measure to proper medical care, the elderly person should be assisted in obtaining primary health care from a family physician or, if appropriate, from a medical specialist.

*Need for Socialization at Mealtime.* Loneliness is a very common problem among elderly persons. Contributory causes are loss by death, institutionalization of or separation from spouse or long-term companion, breakdown of family ties, lack of participation in social organizations such as Senior Citizens or church groups, lack of transportation, eccentricity, physical disability, depression, and insensitivity of younger persons (including care givers) to the special needs of older people.

The nutritionist can help to relieve loneliness in elderly clients or patients by giving advice on congregate meal plans for independently living persons or obtaining Meals-on-Wheels with the special opportunity for conversation with the delivery persons for housebound elderly. Elderly patients in nursing homes should be encouraged to eat their meals with other patients in a communal dining room, in a group in the recreation area, or around the nursing station. When elderly persons have organic brain syndromes and are likely to disturb other patients having their meals by making noise or by unattractive eating habits, it is often possible to find patients with similar problems to eat together. Socialization at mealtimes for patients in nursing homes requires establishment of specific, stepwise goals in the patient care plan, whereby the withdrawn individual is encouraged both by the nutritionist and/or the dietitian, by the nurse, and by the social worker to gradually accept the presence of other patients during eating times, to take a pride in his or her personal appearance when at meals with others, to learn to enjoy interchange of conversation or words with other patients, and to make friends.

*Combatting Alcohol Abuse.* Alcohol abuse is a problem in the elderly as in younger age groups. Nutritionists have special opportunities to identify the problem, to counsel clients on temperance, and to initiate referral to alcoholism counselling services. Alcohol abuse is indicated by observation of liquor, beer, or wine bottles in the home, particularly in unusual places such as in arm chairs, at the back of the sofa, or at the bedside, by dietary history indicating a high level of daily intake or binge drinking, by admitted intake of single or multiple medications containing alcohol, by history of alcoholism or hospitalization for alcohol-related diseases, by erratic or unusual behavior suggesting inebriation during visits by the nutritionist or nutrition aide, by a history of blackouts, frequent falls, or by impairment of nutritional status which fails to respond to changing diet or administration of nutrient supplements.

Nutrition counselling for elderly alcoholics cannot be successful unless the patient becomes abstinent through medical supervision, alcoholism counselling, or use of an alcohol-aversive drug. Use of an alcohol-aversive drug (Disulfiram—Antabuse) may be hazardous for elderly persons with severe impairment of liver function or who are receiving interactive drugs. When abstinence is achieved, alcoholics will often crave sweet foods and may eat a diet low in essential nutrients though adequate in calories. The nutritionist counselling such a patient should develop menu plans which encourage use of foods that are high in essential nutrients. Milk may not be tolerated by newly abstinent, elderly alcoholics who are lactose intolerant. Restricted protein intake is necessary for elderly alcoholics with liver disease, and fat restriction is necessary for patients with alcoholic pancreatitis. Restriction of sodium intake is necessary for cirrhotic patients with ascites (Roe, 1979).

Nutrition counselling for the alcoholic must be preceded by consultation between the nutritionist and the patient's physician. Diets must be prescribed by a physician, and it is the nutritionist's responsibility to promote dietary compliance.

*Advice on Nutrient Supplements.*    The administration of specific vitamin and/or mineral supplements should be based on need defined by clinical and biochemical assessment of nutritional status. However, all nutritionists should be fully aware that alcohol excess produces damage to the liver, bone marrow, and brain which increases the requirements for B vitamins including riboflavin, folacin, vitamins $B_6$ and $B_{12}$, and thiamin. While diets high in these vitamins should be recommended to all elderly patients who have had a recent or long-term history of alcohol abuse, therapeutic doses of folic acid should *not* be recommended until pernicious anemia has been excluded, and thiamin needs to avoid alcoholic brain damage (Korsakoff's psychosis) must be either determined on the basis of biochemical tests (erythrocyte transketolase assay) or may be derived from standard recommendations for amount of the vitamin required. The experienced clinical nutritionist will often be the member of the health care team who can best emphasize to the physician the urgent need for high doses of parenteral thiamin for the elderly alcoholic who has been subsisting on a semistarvation diet. Pharmacologic doses of thiamin given intravenously by the physician to these patients is prophylaxis against development of the permanent brain damage associated with Korsakoff's psychosis.

*Food Budgeting.*    Intake of an inadequate diet by elderly people may be related to the high prices of foods which are thought to be most nutritious. Elderly people who are conservative in their food habits need encouragement by a nutritionist to use cheaper foods which are alternate sources of essential nutrients but are seldom used because of unfamiliarity or prejudice. Food likes and dislikes must be carefully assessed before meal planning in order to increase the chance of dietary compliance.

## COMMUNITY FEEDING PROGRAMS FOR
## THE ELDERLY IN THE UNITED STATES:
## TITLE VII AND TITLE III PROGRAMS

In 1973 the Congress of the United States first appropriated monies to establish a feeding program for the elderly on a national basis. The Nutrition Program for Older Americans (NPOA) was mandated by the 1972 Title VII Amendment to the Older Americans Act of 1965. The Commission on Aging, Director of the Administration on Aging (AoA) within the Department of Health, Education, and Welfare was empowered to administer the Title VII program through AoA in consultation with other departments of the federal government. AoA is divided into 10 regional offices, each containing 3 to 8 states. The regional offices must review and approve the annual operating plans of states and territories in their regions and carry the responsibility for providing assistance to state offices on aging for development of their Title VII plans. The State Agencies on Aging are responsible for producing operating plans to carry out the Title VII program in accordance with federal goals and guidelines. The State Agencies award funds to local projects.

From the annual appropriation, Title VII funds were made available to 50 states and also to the District of Columbia, Guam, American Samoa, the Virgin Islands, and the Trust Territories of the Pacific Islands. The funds that were made available supported up to 90 percent of the cost of development and implementation of the Title VII program.

State agencies were responsible for:

1. Identification of eligible target groups among the elderly in the state and approval of projects serving these individuals.
2. Establishing a minimum project size for effective program implementation.
3. Approval of local project plans and awarding of Title VII grants.
4. Monitoring and evaluating the program.
5. Reviewing project menus.

Community-based meals are now provided under the Title III program whereas formerly community-based meals were under Title VII. Meals are served to people over 60 years of age. Congregate meals, which constitute most of the meals served, are made available at Title III sites, which may be senior citizens centers, religious facilities, schools, public housing, restaurants, or community centers. Local nutrition projects under the County Offices of the Aging are responsible, under the State Agency or Area Agency, for delivery of services. Local community projects have some professional administrative staff and direct providers of services including dietitians, nurses, and social workers, as well as nonprofessional paid staff and volunteers. Paid staff are assisted by volunteers in the provision and delivery of congregate and home-delivered meals.

Local goals of the Title III program administrative staffs are:

1. To establish nutrition projects which serve at least one hot meal a day for the elderly in congregate meal settings and by home delivery.

2. To assure that the meal provided includes a minimum of one third of the Recommended Dietary Allowances.

3. To serve individuals 60 years of age or older who may not eat adequately, either because they cannot afford to do so, because they do not have the requisite skills to purchase and prepare nourishing meals, because they have limited mobility, or because they do not have the motivation to prepare meals. Persons having these characteristics, as well as minority individuals, are "target" groups.

4. To set up feeding sites as close to the eligible individuals as possible and to furnish transportation to the sites.

5. To encourage participation of target groups.

6. To provide special menus to meet special dietary needs which may be related to health problems, religious beliefs, or ethnic preference.

7. To provide health and welfare counselling and nutrition education.

8. To provide training to paid staff and volunteers who are purchasing, preparing, transporting, and serving meals.

9. To give staffing preferences to persons 60 years of age or older.

10. To undertake program evaluation.

There is no cost for meals, but individuals may make a voluntary contribution. There is no test of eligibility by income. Main meals that are delivered to homes are the same or similar to those served at the congregate sites.* An additional light meal consisting of a sandwich, a piece of fruit, and milk may be packed with the hot meal and delivered to provide food for supper. In most Title III programs the aim is to provide five hot meals per week. Weekend meals may be delivered to the home in some sites.

Local, state, and federal goals in program evaluation are to examine program inputs and outputs in relation to effects and benefits of the Title III program. Program inputs include food, funds, staff, equipment, program consultants, and technical equipment. Program outputs include meals, transportation, outreach, referral services, nutrition education, counselling, and escort services. Effects which may be examined include program satisfaction, improved nutrient intake of those served, increased socialization, increased availability of services, target group of elderly persons served, and the financial savings for participants. Long-term benefits which may be evaluated are the improved health and nutritional status of those served, an improvement in mental and social well-being, and maintenance of an independent life style.

Program evaluations have shown that the major positive effects are increased socialization and improved life satisfaction of participants. Partici-

---

*Meals-on-Wheels is a separate program under the auspices of local volunteer groups.

pants have also found that their food bills have been reduced. Diet, nutrition, and health benefits have varied. In several studies it has been shown that the diet of participants has a higher nutrient content than the diet of nonparticipants. Criticism of the program by participants has included dissatisfaction with Title III meals. Elderly persons expressing satisfaction with the programs have also reported the most benefits (Posner, 1979).

Nonparticipation in the Title III program by eligible persons may reflect an ability to cope with food purchase and preparation, the provision of meals by family members or others, or a disinterest in eating and health.

Several experimental programs have been undertaken by Area Agencies on Aging. These have been designed to cover unmet nutritional needs of the elderly or to assist those who have not been reached by the regular Title III program (Watkin, 1977).

A formula-type food has been provided consisting of milk powder with added nutrients which can be made up into a milk shake by adding water. The nutrient content of the drink is equivalent to the nutrient content of the Title III meal. This formula food can have special usefulness in serving the needs of persons for whom home delivery of meals is temporarily discontinued or not yet available.

Freeze-dried foods which can be reconstituted with hot water have been provided under the auspices of NASA.

Shopping aides make food purchases for elderly shut-in clients. The elderly clients give shopping lists to the aides who shop at local markets. The shopping aides are not trained to advise clients on a formal basis on foods needed to provide nutritious meals.

## DIETETIC SERVICES IN NURSING HOMES IN THE UNITED STATES

The Social Security Amendments of 1972 (P.L. 92-603) require the development of uniform dietetic standards for all skilled nursing facilities. Standards are mandated for facilities certified under Medicare and Medicaid (Federal Register, 1974). These standards pertain to 1) staffing, 2) menus and nutritional adequacy, 3) therapeutic diets, 4) preparation and service of foods, 5) hygiene of staff, and 6) sanitary conditions.

### Staffing

A full-time dietetic service supervisor must be employed. This person must either be a qualified dietitian, a graduate of a dietetic technicians program or a dietetic assistant training program approved by The American Dietetic Association, or a graduate of a state-approved course of instruction in food service management, and have had experience as a supervisor in a health care or military facility. If the dietetic service supervisor is a food service manager, then consultation must be provided by a qualified dietitian. If the supervisor of dietetic services is not a dietitian, then consultant visits are supposed to be of sufficient duration and frequency to meet the dietetic needs of the facility.

## Menus and Nutritional Adequacy

Menus need to be planned and followed following physicians' orders to meet the nutritional needs of patients. The Recommended Dietary Allowances are to be followed to the extent that it is medically possible. All menus are to be approved by the full-time or consultant dietitian.

## Therapeutic Diets

Therapeutic diets are to be prescribed by the physician. Special therapeutic menus must be planned in writing, and prepared and served as ordered with supervision by the dietitian or in consultation with the dietitian. An up-to-date diet manual, approved by the dietitian, must be available to the attending physician, nursing staff, and dietetic personnel in the facility.

## Preparation and Service of Food

At least three meals or their equivalent must be served daily, at regular hours, with not more than 14 hours between a substantial evening meal and breakfast.

To the extent that it is medically possible, bedtime nourishments are to be offered to all patients.

Foods are to be prepared by methods that conserve nutritive value, flavor, and appearance, and be attractively served at the proper temperatures and in a form to meet individual needs. If a patient refuses food served, appropriate substitutes of similar nutritive value are to be served.

## Hygiene of Staff

Dietetic service personnel are to be free of communicable disease. They must practice hygienic food-handling techniques.

In the event that food service employees are assigned duties outside the dietetic service, these duties must not interfere with the sanitation, safety, or time required for dietetic work assignments.

## Sanitary Conditions

Food must be procured from sources approved or considered satisfactory by federal, state, or local authorities. Food must also be stored, prepared, distributed, and served under sanitary conditions. Waste must be disposed of properly.

Written reports of inspections by state and local health authorities must be kept on file at the facility, with notations made of action taken by the facility to comply with any recommendations.

Conditions for participation of skilled nursing homes under Medicare and Medicaid which apply to physicians' and nurses' services also pertain to the nutritional care of patients. Each patient's total program of care must be reviewed by the attending physician and/or medical director of the facility at least once every 30 days or more often as required for the first 90 days. The total program of care includes dietary orders which must be reviewed by the physician, and decisions made as to whether the orders should be continued, changed, or discontinued according to the patient's needs. Dietary needs of each patient are to be identified with the assistance of the dietitian.

Nursing personnel are required to gain awareness of the nutritional needs of the patients. Nurses must also monitor and record the food and fluid intake of patients. They are further required to assist patients with their meals whenever such help is needed. It is expected that a close liaison will be established between physicians, nurses, and dietary service personnel in skilled nursing homes.

State guidelines for dietary services as well as medical and nursing services relating to the nutritional care of patients in skilled nursing homes are generally similar to federal guidelines. Intermediate care homes which may be designated "health-related" must comply with the 1974 federal standards in order to be certified and to participate in Medicare and Medicaid. Domiciliary care facilities, also known as personal care homes, residential care facilities for adults, and rest homes, are not covered by the federal or state standards set for Skilled Nursing and Intermediate Care Homes. Guidelines for the management of their food service operations are set by state departments of social services.

Responsibilities of the operator or administrator of skilled nursing homes relating to dietary services are as follows:

1. To organize and administer the dietetic service.
2. To integrate the dietetic service into administrative and patient care services and assure that the dietetic service is represented on all committees whose work affects dietetic service operations and provision of nutritional services.
3. To maintain records of diet orders and changes, nutritional care plans, and nutrition counselling afforded to patients.
4. To develop a monitoring system that provides for "appropriate and timely review" of the nutritional care provided to all patients.
5. To prepare patients for discharge by providing information and methods to the patient to manage his or her own nutritional care or transferring appropriate information to another agency or facility for continuity of care.
6. To furnish evidence that sufficient and appropriate foods have been purchased, prepared, and served to patients and to maintain such records for one year.
7. To ensure that the dietetic service select food and drink and prepare menus with regard to the cultural background and food habits of patients and that they write and date menus and keep records of general and therapeutic diets.
8. To provide a dining room area equipped and arranged for regular use by all patients who can get there unaided or come assisted for regularly scheduled meals.

9. To maintain a file on specifications and maintenance for all major and fixed dietetic service equipment.
10. To provide the dietary service with sufficient and suitable space and equipment to ensure efficient sanitary operation of all required functions.
11. To assure that all employees, including those in the dietary service, maintain personal cleanliness and hygiene.
12. To maintain the following records for the dietary service:
    a) a plan for organization, management, and day-to-day operations
    b) a master plan and weekly work schedules for staffing
    c) the name, qualifications, and terms of agreement with the dietitian
    d) a current diet manual.

The standards of the Joint Commission on Accreditation of Extended Care Facilities also require that pertinent information on each patient should be assembled and that short- and long-term goals should be established. Discharge plans must also be formulated.

Patient care and discharge plans should include nutritional components. It is the duty of the dietitian to assemble information from the physician, nurses, and social workers which may relate to the patient's nutrition. The dietitian and physician together should make a nutritional assessment of each patient and determine nutritional needs (Treadwell, 1974).

Patient care plans are the joint responsibility of the health team in long-term care facilities, including skilled nursing home and intermediate care home. The health team includes the medical director and/or the attending physician, the nurse directly responsible for the care of the particular patient, the social worker and, in some instances, other health professionals such as a physical therapist and an occupational therapist. At weekly meetings within the facility, at which patient care plans are developed and reviewed, the administrator of the facility is usually also present.

The nutrition component of the patient care plan is developed by the dietitian. It must be integrated into the total patient care plan. Goals must be set by each team member. These nutritional goals include:

1. Providing each patient with food of sufficient energy and nutrient content to meet his or her needs.
2. Evaluating change in the nutritional and health status of the patient in response to general or therapeutic diets.
3. Retraining the patient to feed himself or herself.
4. Increasing socialization at eating times.
5. Responding to the patient's food-related concerns.

Plans must be developed which detail procedures by which these goals can be accomplished. The procedures are then implemented insofar as this is feasible in a sequential manner. Evaluation of progress in meeting the nutritional goals is a primary responsibility of the dietitian but other members of the health team may well contribute. For example, the nurse will be able to provide records of the patient's food intake and body weight and the physician will have reports on blood counts and a biochemical profile which should include screening tests of nutritional status. If the dietitian is employed on a consultant basis, then the supervisor of the dietetic service, whether a food service manager or a dietetic technician, must evaluate progress when the dietitian is absent. Actual consumption of food and beverages by the patient should be monitored.

Modification in nutritional care plans must be undertaken to deal with the following conditions:

1. Patient refusal to eat or dislike of the diet.
2. Physical signs and laboratory test results indicating unwanted change in nutritional and/or health status.
3. Identification of special or newly present nutritional needs relating to poor appetite, disease, or medications.
4. Special behavioral problems.

When the patient is ready for discharge or is to be sent to another facility offering a higher or lower level of care, nutrition discharge plans made by the dietitian should include guidelines for the person(s) who will be undertaking the care of the patient or instructions to the patient, if the patient will be caring for him– or herself, relating to diet, food preparation, appetite, eating problems, and more recent nutritional assessment.

## Problems Relating to Nutritional Care of Patients in Skilled Nursing Homes

Dietetic services are inadequate when:

1. The dietetic service supervisor is not a dietitian.
2. Standards for nutritional adequacy of menus are not followed.
3. Presented therapeutic diets are not followed.
4. Meals are badly cooked and/or served.
5. Food-borne infection occurs because nutrition staff does not follow hygienic food-handling practices.

Nursing service is inadequate when:

1. Food and beverage intake is not monitored, or not monitored regularly.
2. Patients are not weighed.
3. Patients are not assisted in feeding themselves.

Physican service is inadequate when:

1. The physician is ignorant of the nutritional needs of patients.
2. The physician prescribes an inappropriate therapeutic diet.
3. The attending physician rarely sees the patient.
4. An assessment of nutritional status is not carried out.

Team problems include:

1. Inadequate concern for the patient.
2. The desire to meet standards only to pass federal or state inspection.

## NUTRITION EDUCATION PROGRAMS

Nutrition education programs for the elderly are quite frequently initiated by nutritionists or by nutrition students, not only for the purpose of dietary counselling but also with the aim of imparting nutrition knowledge which is unrelated or only indirectly related to diets. Such nutrition education programs may be provided at senior citizens centers, at congregate meal sites supplying Title III meals to the elderly, in churches, in domiciliary care facilities, and even in nursing homes. One or more lectures are usually given. The topics are likely to be chosen by the speaker although sometimes choice of subject matter is decided by college teachers or by social program directors in community organizations. The elderly target groups are assumed to be eager to have the latest information on advances in nutritional science and may retain this information. Whereas this assumption may be correct when the talk or talks are being given to socially and intellectually active elderly, it is naive to believe that nutritional science or even tips on good nutrition are of concern to elderly people who are either intellectually impaired or whose diet and nutrition is the responsibility of others (Templeton, 1978).

Realistic goals of nutrition education programs for the elderly are:

1. To provide reliable nutrition information to active older people on topics of current interest or dispute.
2. To provide basic nutrition education to such groups when this is requested by group members.
3. To explain recent policy changes at the federal or local level on food assistance programs to the elderly.
4. To teach interested elderly how to cook special or fun dishes of high nutrient content.
5. To provide structured and reliable instruction to groups of elderly with specific chronic diseases requiring dietary management (e.g., diabetics, cardiac patients).
6. To provide recreational activity to groups of aged people inside and outside institutions.
7. To provide nutrition education experience to students in training.

Studies of nutrition education as part of group feeding programs have been conducted, and it has been reported that both improved eating habits and a greater knowledge of nutrition for the participants has come about as a result of the educational program. Kim et al. (1981), commenting on these results of nutrition education for the elderly, noted that these changes could have been brought about from the social contact of the group meal situation and not just from the nutrition education program.

Constraints on nutrition education programs for the elderly have been identified by these authors as follows:

1. The normal aging process may cause physical changes which interfere with the learning process, such as reduced hearing capacity or an inability to follow rapid speech.
2. Impaired vision can make it impossible for elderly audiences either to see slides on a screen or to read instructional materials.
3. Elderly people whose dietary practices have been shaped by an extended lifetime are not easily persuaded by talks or lectures to change their dietary practices.

In spite of these reservations about nutrition programs for the elderly, Kim et al. (1981) decided to set up a nutrition education program in a nursing home to try to improve the eating habits of nursing home residents. At the same time they established a means to evaluate the effectiveness of their program on the dietary intakes of the residents. Nutrient intakes were measured before, during, and after presentation of the nutrition education in a small nursing home. The nutrition education presentations were given to small groups of residents during the noon meal weekly for a period of four weeks. The weekly talks were videotaped and played back to the residents in a room which was next to the dining room toward the end of the noontime meal.

Changes in nutrient intake were observed in the experimental group, that is, in the residents of the nursing home receiving the nutrition education (while the program was in progress) but these improvements in nutrient intake were not maintained after the program was over. It was pointed out by the investigators that whereas it is possible that the nutrition education program was responsible for the temporary changes in nutrient intake, it could also be that the focus of attention on the nursing home residents could have altered their intakes.

Attempts have also been made to improve the food and the actual dietary intake of nursing home residents by education of the facility staff. Holme and Kim (1981) developed nutrition education lessons for weekly presentation to nursing home staffs. These sessions were conducted in one nursing home. Sessions were voluntary and considered as in-service workshops. Each presentation was for a period of one-half hour and these sessions were conducted at weekly intervals. Pretest and posttest questionnaires were developed to assess the nutrition knowledge of the nursing home staff before the lesson and thereafter. Questionnaires also investigated the staff attitudes before the presentation and after as to the importance to the residents of a nutritionally adequate diet. Material presented included food plan (the nutritional basis of a sound diet), a videotape-illustrated lecture which showed eating patterns of the elderly, changes in these eating patterns which could occur and why they occur when these people enter the nursing home, and lastly, a lecture on interpersonal relationships between the food service staff and the residents.

As a result of this program it was found that the staff increased their nutrition knowledge. The staff rated the presentations according to quality and responded positively to a videotape entitled "Meals: Then and Now." They also responded well to the opportunity to use roleplaying in the last lesson. Another positive outcome of this program was that, at its completion, 78 percent of the staff members felt that they could now talk to residents about their feelings about meals that were served in the nursing home, and that they could further encourage the residents to make better food choices.

## STUDENT GUIDE TO NUTRITION EDUCATION PROGRAMS FOR THE ELDERLY

Nutrition education programs require a definition of overall goals as well as a specific goal. One must consider the motives of the person presenting the program, learn about the characteristics of the audience, develop the program, and decide on the means of evaluation of the program, program production, and results of the program.

### Define Your Goals

What are you trying to do?

1. To provide nutrition information in response to the requests of elderly people in the community.
2. To give dietary counselling in response to patient wishes or in response to requests by an M.D. or R.N.
3. To expand the nutrition knowledge of public health nurses or home health aides having responsibility for the care of the homebound elderly.
4. To teach food service personnel or other staffs of the geriatric facility the nutritional value of food, the nutritional requirements of the elderly, meals which will meet nutritional needs, and skills which will facilitate interpersonal relationships with the residents.
5. To give individual counselling to the elderly on special diets.
6. To help elderly people spend their food dollars wisely.
7. To explain food labeling.
8. To talk to elderly people who are captive audiences (e.g., in congregate meal sites) about nutrition topics which may be relevant to their health (e.g., the dangers of high-sodium foods, drug-nutrient interactions), but said in lay terms.

### Consider Your Motives

Why are you concerned with the development of a nutrition education program for the elderly? Motives could be:

1.  To provide nutrition information to those elderly who seek it.
2.  To give information on nutrition to those elderly you think would benefit.
3.  To change the attitudes of geriatric caregivers to nutrition.
4.  To improve the quality of the diet for geriatric patients.
5.  To change the food habits of the elderly.
6.  To entertain groups of elderly people.
7.  To fulfill a class requirement.

### Find Out About Your Audience

1.  Who are they?
2.  What are their food-related or nutrition problems?
3.  Where are they going to be when you make your presentation?
4.  What is their attention span likely to be?
5.  Are they visually impaired?
6.  How long can they stay at your presentation(s)?
7.  Will the audience really come to hear you, or are they present for other primary purposes?
8.  Are they likely to find a selected topic(s) relevant and interesting?
9.  What is their educational level?
10. Will you be speaking to the same audience each time you give a talk?
11. Is the audience hearing impaired so that you will need a microphone?
12. What means will you have for determining your audience's immediate response to your presentation and whether you have fulfilled your goal?

### Develop Your Program

Bearing in mind your goals and motives, are they justifiable and appropriate to your audience?

### Example of a Nutrition Education Program for Senior Citizens

*Stimulus.*     A request has come from a senior citizens group for a nutritionist (or nutrition student) to talk to them for one hour about their need for B vitamins and how they can get these vitamins from their food.

*Goal.*     Your goal is to respond to this request. Your motive is to fulfill a class requirement. The projected audience will consist of approximately 50 women and men between the ages of 65 and 86. None of these persons are likely to be blind, but about 50 percent are visually impaired and 50 percent have hearing problems. All have at least a high school education.

The facility provided is a large, well-lit room which has a screen and a slide projector with a carousel. There is an overhead projector and a microphone.

*Program Plan.*   Handouts should include:

1. A pamphlet describing the functions of essential B vitamins written in lay language and produced in large print.
2. Charts showing food sources rich in B vitamins, preferably multicolored bar graphs.

Pretest and posttest questionnaires should be developed:

1. Pretest. A pretest quiz should be given to the audience to find out if they know what B vitamins there are, what foods are good sources of these vitamins, and why these vitamins are needed for good health.
2. Posttest questionnaires should be developed before the program to evaluate whether the audience has learned the nutrition information and to determine their overall responses to the program.

*Lecture and Time Frame.*   A 30-minute lecture is given, illustrated with slides which show elderly people eating foods containing rich sources of B vitamins. Functions of these vitamins, their food sources, and the requirements of the elderly for the major B vitamins (thiamin, folate, riboflavin, niacin, vitamin $B_6$ and vitamin $B_{12}$) are emphasized.

The overhead projector is used to show transparencies on which there are large, clearly drawn diagrams of foods which are rich sources of these vitamins. The microphone is used throughout the presentation so that those in the audience with moderate hearing impairment can hear the presentation.

A 10-minute question period follows. Questions are requested from the audience. The speaker should repeat the question asked, using the microphone. Discussion is encouraged, and the speaker should be prepared to clear up misunderstandings.

After the lecture, a second quiz is given, to find out if the audience has taken in the message, and whether they thought the talk was interesting, clear, and useful. For each of these ratings a scale should be used. Rating should also be requested for the audiovisual materials used.

*Program Record.*   Record forms should be prepared and used by the speaker or by an assistant present at the lecture, on which the following information can be tabulated:

1. The number of people present at the program.
2. The age structure of the class.
3. The female to male ratio.
4. The number of persons leaving the presentation
5. The number of pre- and posttest quizzes completed and returned.
6. The number of persons falling asleep during the class.
7. The number of questions posed at question time and after the class.
8. The number in the audience who request the speaker to return for another nutrition program.

The program can be evaluated by considering:

1. Process—program development.
2. Product—the lesson plan, its presentation, the handout materials, and the audiovisual materials.
3. Outcome—the audience evaluation of the quality of the program and the change in the nutrition knowledge of the audience.

## QUESTIONS

1. Goals of nutrition counselling for the elderly are:
   a) to explain personal food energy and nutrient needs
   b) to interpret prescribed diets
   c) to promote best use of limited food budget
   d  to encourage intake of nutrients which prevent aging
   e) to establish optimal eating times which allow optimal absorption, utilization, and tolerance of prescribed medications.

2. The Nutrition Program for Older Americans (Title III) provides meals for the elderly in which of the following locations:
   a) skilled nursing homes
   b) congregate meal centers
   c) private homes
   d) hospitals
   e) domiciliary care facilities

3. Staff of skilled nursing homes have certain responsibilities under Medicare and Medicaid in providing for the nutrition of patients. Pair the following staff members with their responsibilities:

   a) physician                  i.   Approval of diet manual
   b) dietitian                  ii.  Food purchase
   c) food service manager       iii. Rx therapeutic diets
   d) nurses                     iv.  Organization of dietetic service
   e) operator or administrator  v.   Recording food
                                      intake of patients

4. Common problems relating to the nutritional care of patients in skilled nursing homes include which of the following:
   a) patients are not weighed
   b) therapeutic diets are not followed
   c) meals are not served regularly
   d) assessment of nutritional status is not carried out
   e) the dietetic service supervisor is not a dietitian

5. In counselling elderly people on weight reduction, certain objectives should be stressed. Select the three most important and practical goals.
   a) severe food restriction
   b) moderate increase in exercise
   c) regular intake of anorectic drug
   d) development of nutritionally adequate diet
   e) menu planning to meet prescribed food energy level

## REFERENCES

CLARKE, M., and L.M. WAKEFIELD, "Food choices of institutionalized vs. independent-living elderly," *J. Amer. Dietet. Assoc.*, 66 (1975), 600–4.

HARPER, A.E., "Recommended dietary allowances for the elderly," *Geriatrics*, 33 (1978), 73–80.

HARPER, J.M., G.R. JANSEN, C.T. SHIGETOMI, and A.L. FREY, "Menu planning in the nutrition program for the elderly," *J. Amer. Dietet. Assoc.*, 68 (1976), 529–34.

HOLME, D.S., and S. KIM, "Nutrition education programs for nursing home staff," *J. Amer. Dietet. Assoc.*, 78 (1981), 366–69.

KIM, S., J.E. SCHRIVER, and K.M. CAMPBELL, "Nutrition education for nursing home residents," *J. Amer. Dietet. Assoc.*, 78 (1981), 362–68.

LAWSON, D.E.M., A.A. PAUL, A.E. BLACK, T.J. COLE, A.R. MANDAL, and M. DAVIE, "Relative contributions of diet and sunlight to vitamin D state in the elderly," *Brit. Med. J.*, 4 (1979), 303–5.

"New federal regulations for skilled nursing homes," *Commentary, J. Amer. Dietet. Assoc.*, 64 (1974), 467–69.

PELCOVITCH, S.J., "Nutrition to meet the human needs of older Americans," *J. Amer. Dietet. Assoc.*, 62 (1972), 99.

POSNER, B.M., *Nutrition and the Elderly. Policy Development, Program Planning and Evaluation.* Lexington, MA, Toronto: Lexington Books, D.C. Heath and Co., 1979.

ROE, D.A., *Alcohol and the Diet.* Westport, CT: AVI Publ. Co., 1979.

ROE, D.A., "Nutrition and chronic drug administration—effects on the geriatric patient," *American Pharmacy* NS20, 1980, 30–35.

SMITH, C.E., "Influence of standards on the nutritional care of the elderly," *J. Amer. Dietet. Assoc.*, 73 (1978), 115–19.

Social Security Administration, "Skilled nursing facilities: standards for certification and participation in Medicare and Medicaid programs," *Federal Register*, 39. 12, (Jan., 1974), 2237.

TEMPLETON, C.L., "Nutrition counseling needs in a geriatric population," *Geriatrics*, 33 (1978), 58–66.

TREADWELL, D.D., "Planning the nutrition component of long-term care," *J. Amer. Dietet. Assoc.*, 64 (1974), 56–60.

U.S. Senate Select Committee on Nutrition and Human Needs, "Nutrition and the Elderly," June 19, 1974.

WATKIN, D.M., "The nutrition program for older Americans: A successful application of current knowledge in nutrition and gerontology," *World Rev. Nutr. Dietet.*, 26 (1977), 26–40.

WURTMAN, J.J., *Eating Your Way Through Life.* New York: Raven Press, 1979, pp. 204–7.

# Appendix

**TABLE 1   Food Exchange Lists**

*Exchange Lists for Meal Planning* by committees of the American Diabetes Association, Inc., and The American Dietetic Association in cooperation with The National Institute of Arthritis, Metabolism and Digestive Diseases and the National Heart and Lung Institute, National Institutes of Health, Public Health Service, U.S. Department of Health, Education and Welfare, 1976.

### Milk Exchanges* (Includes Non-Fat Low-Fat and Whole Milk)

The list shows the kinds and amounts of milk or milk products to use for one Milk Exchange. Those which appear in bold type are non-fat. Low-Fat and Whole Milk contain saturated fat.

| | |
|---|---|
| **Non-Fat Fortified Milk** | |
| **Skim or non-fat milk** | 1 cup |
| **Powdered (non-fat dry, before adding liquid)** | 1/3 cup |
| **Canned, evaportated-skim milk** | 1/2 cup |
| **Buttermilk made from skim milk** | 1 cup |
| **Yogurt made from skim milk (plain, unflavored)** | 1 cup |
| *Low-Fat Fortified Milk* | |
| 1% fat fortified milk | 1 cup |
| (omit 1/2 Fat Exchange) | |
| 2% fat fortified milk | 1 cup |
| (omit 1 Fat Exchange) | |
| Yogurt made from 2% fortified milk (plain, unflavored) | 1 cup |
| (omit 1 Fat Exchange) | |
| *Whole Milk (Omit 2 Fat Exchanges)* | |
| Whole milk | 1 cup |
| Canned, evaporated whole milk | 1/2 cup |
| Buttermilk made from whole milk | 1 cup |
| Yogurt made from whole milk (plain, unflavored) | 1 cup |

*One Exchange of Milk contains 12 grams of carbohydrate, 8 grams of protein, a trace of fat and 80 calories.

TABLE 1   Food Exchange Lists (continued)

## Vegetable Exchanges* (All Non-Starchy Vegetables)

This list shows the kinds of vegetables to use for one Vegetable Exchange. One Exchange is 1/2 cup.

| | |
|---|---|
| Asparagus | Greens: |
| Bean Sprouts |    Mustard |
| Beets |    Spinach |
| Broccoli |    Turnip |
| Brussels Sprouts | Mushrooms |
| Cabbage | Okra |
| Carrots | Onions |
| Cauliflower | Rhubarb |
| Celery | Rutabaga |
| Cucumbers | Sauerkraut |
| Eggplant | String Beans, green or yellow |
| Green Pepper | Summer Squash |
| Greens: | Tomatoes |
|    Beet | Tomato Juice |
|    Chards | Turnips |
|    Collards | Vegetable Juice Cocktail |
|    Dandelion | Zucchini |
|    Kale | |

The following raw vegetables may be used as desired:

| | |
|---|---|
| Chicory | Lettuce |
| Chinese Cabbage | Parsley |
| Endive | Radishes |
| Escarole | Watercress |

Starchy Vegetables are found in the Bread Exchange List.

*One Exchange of Vegetables contains about 5 grams of carbohydrate, 2 grams of protein and 25 calories.

## Fruit Exchanges* (All Fruits and Fruit Juices)

This list shows the kinds and amounts of fruits to use for one Fruit Exchange.

| | | | |
|---|---|---|---|
| Apple | 1 small | Mango | 1/2 small |
| Apple Juice | 1/3 cup | Melon | |
| Applesauce (unsweetened) | 1/2 cup |    Cantaloupe | 1/4 small |
| Apricots, fresh | 2 medium |    Honeydew | 1/2 medium |
| Apricots, dried | 4 halves |    Watermelon | 1 cup |
| Bananas | 1/2 small | Nectarine | 1 small |
| Berries | | Orange | 1 small |
|    Blackberries | 1/2 cup | Orange Juice | 1/2 cup |
|    Blueberries | 1/2 cup | Papaya | 3/4 cup |
|    Raspberries | 1/2 cup | Peach | 1 medium |
|    Strawberries | 3/4 cup | Pear | 1 small |
| Cherries | 10 large | Persimmon, native | 1 medium |
| Cider | 1/3 cup | Pineapple | 1/2 cup |
| Dates | 2 | Pineapple Juice | 1/3 cup |
| Figs, fresh | 1 | Plums | 2 medium |
| Figs, dried | 1 cup | Prunes | 2 medium |
| Grapefruit | 1/2 | Prune Juice | 1/4 cup |
| Grapefruit Juice | 1/2 cup | Raisins | 2 tablespoons |
| Grapes | 12 | Tangerine | 1 medium |
| Grape Juice | 1/4 cup | | |

Cranberries may be used if no sugar is added.

*One Exchange of Fruit contains 10 grams of carbohydrate and 40 calories.

TABLE 1    Food Exchange Lists (continued)

## Meat Exchanges* (Lean Meat)

This list shows the kinds and amounts of Lean Meat and other Protein-Rich Foods to use for one Low-Fat Meat Exchange.

| | | |
|---|---|---|
| Beef: | Baby Beef (very lean), Chipped Beef, Chuck, Flank Steak, Tenderloin, Plate Ribs, Plate Skirt Steak, Round (bottom, top), All cuts Rump, Spare Ribs, Tripe | 1 oz. |
| Lamb: | Leg, Rib, Sirloin, Loin (roast and chops), Shank, Shoulder | 1 oz. |
| Pork: | Leg (Whole Rump, Center Shank), Ham, Smoked (center slices) | 1 oz. |
| Veal: | Leg, Loin, Rib, Shank, Shoulder, Cutlets | 1 oz. |
| Poultry: | Meat without skin of Chicken, Turkey, Cornish Hen, Guinea Hen, Pheasant | 1 oz. |
| Fish: | Any fresh or frozen | 1 oz. |
| | Canned Salmon, Tuna, Mackerel, Crab and Lobster | 1/4 cup |
| | Clams, Oysters, Scallops, Shrimp | 5 or 1 oz. |
| | Sardines, drained | 3 |
| Cheese containing less than 5% butterfat | | 1 oz. |
| Cottage Cheese, Dry and 2% butterfat | | 1/4 cup |
| Dried Beans and Peas (omit 1 Bread Exchange) | | 1/2 cup |

*One Exchange of Lean Meat (1 oz.) contains 7 grams of protein, 3 grams of fat and 55 calories.

## Meat Exchanges* (Medium-Fat Meat)

This list shows the kinds and amounts of Medium-Fat Meat and other Protein-Rich Foods to use for one Medium-Fat Meat Exchange.

| | | |
|---|---|---|
| Beef: | Ground (15% fat), Corned Beef (canned), Rib Eye, Round (ground commercial) | 1 oz. |
| Pork: | Loin (all cuts Tenderloin), Shoulder Arm (picnic), Shoulder Blade, Boston Butt, Canadian Bacon, Boiled Ham | 1 oz. |
| Liver, Heart, Kidney and Sweetbreads (these are high in cholesterol) | | 1 oz. |
| Cottage Cheese, creamed | | 1/4 cup |
| Cheese: | Mozzarella, Ricotta, Farmer's cheese, Neufchatel, | 1 oz. |
| | Parmesan | 3 tbs. |
| Egg (high in cholesterol) | | 1 |
| Peanut Butter (omit 2 additional Fat Exchanges) | | 2 tbs. |

*For each Exchange of Medium-Fat Meat omit 1/2 Fat Exchange.

## Meat Exchanges* (High-Fat Meats)

This list shows the kinds and amounts of High-Fat Meat and other Protein-Rich Foods to use for one High-Fat Meat Exchange.

| | | |
|---|---|---|
| Beef: | Brisket, Corned Beef Brisket, Ground Beef (more than 20% fat), Hamburger (commercial), Chuck (ground commercial), Roasts (Rib), Steaks (Club and Rib) | 1 oz. |
| Lamb: | Breast | 1 oz. |
| Pork: | Spare Ribs, Loin (Back Ribs), Pork (ground), Country style Ham, Deviled Ham | 1 oz. |
| Veal: | Breast | 1 oz. |
| Poultry: | Capon, Duck (domestic), Goose | 1 oz. |
| Cheese: | Cheddar Types | 1 oz. |
| Cold Cuts | | 4-1/2" X 1/8 " slice |
| Frankfurter | | 1 small |

*For each Exchange of High-Fat Meat omit 1 Fat Exchange.

TABLE 1    Food Exchange Lists (continued)

## Bread Exchanges* (Includes Bread, Cereal and Starchy Vegetables)

This list shows the kinds and amounts of Breads, Cereals, Starchy Vegetables and Prepared Foods to use for one Bread Exchange. Those which appear in bold type are low-fat.

*Cereal*

| | |
|---|---|
| **Bran Flakes** | 1/2 cup |
| **Other ready-to-eat unsweetened Cereal** | 3/4 cup |
| **Puffed Cereal (unfrosted)** | 1 cup |
| **Cereal (cooked)** | 1/2 cup |
| **Grits (cooked)** | 1/2 cup |
| **Rice or Barley (cooked)** | 1/2 cup |
| **Pasta (cooked)** | 1/2 cup |
| Spaghetti, Noodles, Macaroni | |
| **Popcorn (popped, no fat added)** | 3 cups |
| **Cornmeal (dry)** | 2 Tbs. |
| **Flour** | 2-1/2 Tbs. |
| **Wheat Germ** | 1/4 cup |

*Crackers*

| | |
|---|---|
| **Arrowroot** | 3 |
| **Graham, 2-1/2"** | 2 |
| **Matzoth, 4" × 6"** | 1/2 cup |
| **Oyster** | 20 |
| **Pretzels, 3-1/8" long × 1/2" dia.** | 25 |
| **Rye Wafers, 2" × 3-1/2"** | 3 |
| **Saltines** | 6 |
| **Soda, 2-1/2" sq.** | 4 |

*Dried Beans, Peas, and Lentils*

| | |
|---|---|
| **Beans, Peas, Lentils (dried and cooked)** | 1/2 cup |
| **Baked Beans, no pork (canned)** | 1/4 cup |

*Starchy Vegetables*

| | |
|---|---|
| **Corn** | 1/3 cup |
| **Corn on Cob** | 1 small |
| **Lima Beans** | 1/2 cup |
| **Parsnips** | 2/3 cup |
| **Peas, Green (canned or frozen)** | 1/2 cup |
| **Potato, White** | 1 small |
| **Potato (mashed)** | 1/2 cup |
| **Pumpkin** | 3/4 cup |
| **Winter Squash, Acorn or Butternut** | |
| **Yam or Sweet Potato** | 1/4 cup |

*Prepared Foods*

| | |
|---|---|
| Biscuit 2" dia. | 1 |
| (omit 1 Fat Exchange) | |
| Corn Bread, 2" × 2" × 1" | 1 |
| (omit 1 Fat Exchange) | |
| Corn Muffin, 2" dia. | 1 |
| (omit 1 Fat Exchange) | |
| Crackers, round butter type | 5 |
| (omit 1 Fat Excahnge) | |
| Muffin, plain small | 1 |
| (omit 1 Fat Exchange) | |
| Potatoes, French Fried, length 2" to 3-1/2" | 8 |
| (omit 1 Fat Exchange) | |
| Potato or Corn Chips | 15 |
| (omit 2 Fat Exchanges) | |
| Pancake, 5" × 1/2" | 1 |
| (omit 1 Fat Exchange) | |
| Waffle, 5" × 1/2" | 1 |
| (omit 1 Fat Exchange) | |

*One Exchange of Bread contains 15 grams of carbohydrate, 2 grams of protein and 70 calories.

## TABLE 1    Food Exchange Lists (continued)

### Fat Exchanges* (Bread, Cereal, Pasta, Starchy Vegetables, and Prepared Foods)

This list shows the kinds and amounts of Fat-Containing Foods to use for one Fat Exchange. To Plan a diet low in Saturated Fat select only those Exchanges which appear in bold type. They are Polyunsaturated.

| | |
|---|---|
| **Margarine, soft, tub or stick**** | 1 teaspoon |
| **Avocado (4" in diameter)***** | 1/8 |
| **Oil, Corn, Cottonseed, Safflower, Soy, Sunflower** | 1 teaspoon |
| **Oil, Olive***** | 1 teaspoon |
| **Oil, Peanut***** | 1 teaspoon |
| **Olives***** | 5 small |
| **Almonds***** | 10 whole |
| **Pecans***** | 2 large whole |
| **Peanuts***** | |
| **Spanish** | 20 whole |
| **Virginia** | 10 whole |
| **Walnuts** | 6 small |
| **Nuts, other***** | 6 small |
| Margarine, regular stick | 1 teaspoon |
| Butter | 1 teaspoon |
| Bacon fat | 1 teaspoon |
| Bacon, crisp | 1 strip |
| Cream, light | 2 tablespoons |
| Cream, sour | 2 tablespoons |
| Cream, heavy | 1 tablespoon |
| Cream Cheese | 1 tablespoon |
| French dressing**** | 1 tablespoon |
| Italian dressing**** | 1 tablespoon |
| Lard | 1 teaspoon |
| Mayonnaise**** | 1 teaspoon |
| Salad dressing, mayonnaise type**** | 2 teaspoons |
| Salt pork | 3/4 inch cube |

*One Exchange of Fat contains 5 grams of fat and 45 calories.
**Made with corn, cottonseed, safflower, soy or sunflower oil only.
***Fat content is primarily monounsaturated.
****If made with corn, cottonseed, safflower, soy or sunflower oil can be used on fat modified diet.
Source: P. B. Reed, *Nutrition in Applied Science.* (St. Paul, Minn.: West Publ. Co., 1980), pp. 680-83.

## TABLE 2    Exchange Units* in Serving Sizes of Certain Southern Foods

| FOOD | PORTION SIZE | PROTEIN | FAT | EXCHANGE UNITS |
|---|---|---|---|---|
| pig ears | 90 gm. | 13.2 | 6.9 | 2 lean meat |
| pg feet | 240 gm. | 12.9 | 13.2 | 2 high-fat meat |
| hog maws | 3/4 cup | 14.4 | 7.8 | 2 lean meat |
| pig tails | 180 gm. | 12.3 | 17.4 | 2 high-fat meat |
| cracklins | 1 round tsp. | 1.1 | 3.8 | 1 fat |
| chiitterlings | 1/4 cup | 3.8 | 9.4 | 2 fat |
| brains | 1/2 cup | 7.8 | 7.8 | 1 high-fat meat |
| vegetables cooked with fat | 1 exchange | 1.0 | 3.8 | 1 vegetable, 1 fat |
| fried chicken drumsticks | 1 average | 7.6 | 3.3 | 1 lean meat |
| thighs | 1 average | 7.7 | 5.4 | 1 medium-fat meat |

*Exchange Lists for Meal Planning, 1976.

From M. P. Goldsmith and J. K. Davidson, "Southern ethnic food preferences and exchange values for the diabetic diet," *J. Amer. Dietet. Assoc.,* 70: 61-64, 1977. Copyright the American Dietetic Association. Reprinted by permission.

TABLE 3 Calculation of Food Energy Intake. Nutritive Value of Common Foods[a]

| | Amount | Cal | Protein (g) | Fat (g) | Carbohydrate (g) | Calcium (mg) | Phosphorus (mg) | Iron (mg) | Sodium (mg) | Potassium (mg) | Vitamin A (IU) | Thiamin (mg) | Riboflavin (mg) | Niacin (mg) | Ascorbic acid (mg) | USDA Handbook No. 456/ Ref. no. |
|---|---|---|---|---|---|---|---|---|---|---|---|---|---|---|---|---|
| *Milk* | | | | | | | | | | | | | | | | |
| Buttermilk | 1C | 88 | 8.8 | 0.2 | 12.5 | 296 | 233 | 0.1 | 319 | 343 | 10 | 0.10 | 0.44 | 0.2 | 2 | 509b |
| Milk, skim | 1C | 88 | 8.8 | 0.2 | 12.5 | 296 | 233 | 0.1 | 127 | 355 | 10 | 0.09 | 0.44 | 0.2 | 2 | 1322b |
| Milk, whole | 1C | 159 | 8.5 | 8.5 | 12.0 | 288 | 227 | 0.1 | 122 | 351 | 350 | 0.07 | 0.41 | 0.2 | 2 | 1320b |
| *Vegetables* | | | | | | | | | | | | | | | | |
| Asparagus[b] | 4 | | | | | | | | | | | | | | | 47b |
| Green beans, frozen, french style | ½C | 14 | 1.2 | 0.1 | 3.1 | 19 | 25 | 0.5 | 1 | 99 | 443 | 0.07 | 0.08 | 0.5 | 10 | 194c |
| Beans, lima (frozen) | ½C | 84 | 5.1 | 0.1 | 16.2 | 17 | 77 | 1.5 | 86 | 362 | 195 | 0.06 | 0.03 | 0.9 | 15 | 173c |
| Beets | ½C | 27 | 1.0 | 0.1 | 6.1 | 12 | 20 | 0.5 | 37 | 177 | 15 | 0.03 | 0.04 | 0.3 | 5 | 385b |
| Beet greens,[b] spinach, collards (cooked) | ½C | 22 | 2.5 | 0.4 | 3.5 | 111 | 34 | 1.4 | 33 | 260 | 6133 | 0.07 | 0.14 | 0.6 | 36 | 393a, 2170a, 807a |
| Brussels sprouts,[b] frozen | ½C | | | | | | | | | | | | | | | 492c |
| Cabbage, raw | 1C | 21 | 1.7 | 0.2 | 4.2 | 25 | 34 | 0.5 | 12 | 189 | 200 | 0.06 | 0.06 | 0.4 | 47 | 512c |
| Cauliflower | ½C | | | | | | | | | | | | | | | 831a |
| Corn on cob, 5" (boiled) | 1 | 70 | 2.5 | 0.8 | 16.2 | 2 | 69 | 0.5 | —[c] | 151 | 310 | 0.09 | 0.08 | 1.1 | 7 | 846a |
| Peas, green, frozen | ½C | 55 | 4.1 | 0.3 | 9.5 | 15 | 69 | 1.5 | 92 | 108 | 480 | 0.22 | 0.07 | 1.4 | 11 | 1530c |
| Potato, french fried (2" to 3½" diameter) | 10 | 137 | 2.2 | 6.6 | 18.0 | 8 | 56 | 0.7 | 3 | 427 | — | 0.07 | 0.04 | 1.6 | 11 | 1789b |
| Potato, sweet, mashed | ½C | 73 | 1.1 | 0.3 | 16.8 | 21 | 30 | 0.5 | 7 | 155 | 5038 | 0.06 | 0.04 | 0.4 | 11 | 2250c |
| Potato, white, baked (2" diameter) | ½C | 59 | 1.7 | 0.1 | 13.3 | 6 | 41 | 0.5 | 3 | 316 | — | 0.07 | 0.03 | 1.2 | 13 | 1787d |
| Pumpkin,[b] carrots, winter squash | ½C | 37 | 1.1 | 0.3 | 8.9 | 27 | 32 | 0.5 | 10 | 261 | 6757 | 0.04 | 0.08 | 0.6 | 7 | 1832d, 620a, 2201a |

The following table continues on this page. Column headings (nutrient names) are not printed on this page; the numeric columns appear in this order: amount, calories, protein (g), fat (g), carbohydrate (g), calcium (mg), phosphorus (mg), iron (mg), sodium (mg), potassium (mg), vitamin A (IU), thiamin (mg), riboflavin (mg), niacin (mg), vitamin C (mg), and reference code.

| Food | Amount | Cal | Prot | Fat | Carb | Ca | P | Fe | Na | K | Vit A | Thiam | Ribo | Niac | Vit C | Ref |
|---|---|---|---|---|---|---|---|---|---|---|---|---|---|---|---|---|
| Rutabagas, mashed | ½C | 42 | 1.1 | 0.1 | 9.9 | 71 | 37 | 0.4 | 5 | 201 | 660 | 0.07 | 0.07 | 1.0 | 31 | 1920b |
| Summer squash[b] | ½C | | | | | | | | | | | | | | | 2192a |
| Celery, stalks | 3 | | | | | | | | | | | | | | | 637c |
| Cucumbers, slices | 16 | | | | | | | | | | | | | | | 942d |
| Lettuce, shredded | 1C | 9 | 0.7 | 0.1 | 2.1 | 19 | 17 | 0.6 | 18 | 133 | 290 | 0.03 | 0.04 | 0.3 | 6 | 1256c |
| Tomatoes,[b] canned and juice | ½C | 24 | 1.2 | 0.2 | 5.2 | 8 | 23 | 0.9 | 200 | 269 | 1028 | 0.06 | 0.04 | 0.9 | 20 | 2284d, 2288d |
| Tomatoes, fresh (2 2/5" diameter) | 1 | 20 | 1.0 | 0.2 | 4.3 | 12 | 25 | 0.5 | 3 | 222 | 820 | 0.05 | 0.05 | 0.6 | 21 | 2282c |
| Turnips, mashed | ½C | 26 | 0.9 | 0.3 | 5.7 | 41 | 28 | 0.5 | 39 | 216 | — | 0.05 | 0.06 | 0.4 | 26 | 2353b |
| *Fruits* | | | | | | | | | | | | | | | | |
| Apple (2½" diameter) | 1 | 61 | 0.2 | 0.6 | 15.3 | 7 | 11 | 0.3 | 1 | 116 | 100 | 0.03 | 0.02 | 0.1 | 4 | 13d |
| Applesauce, unsweetened | ½C | 50 | 0.3 | 0.3 | 13.2 | 5 | 6 | 0.6 | 3 | 95 | 50 | 0.03 | 0.01 | 0.1 | 1 | 28c |
| Banana, medium | ½ | 51 | 0.7 | 0.1 | 13.2 | 5 | 16 | 0.4 | 1 | 220 | 115 | 0.03 | 0.04 | 0.4 | 6 | 141b |
| Berries[b] (blue, black, raspberries) | ½C | 46 | 0.8 | 0.4 | 10.9 | 19 | 15 | 0.8 | 1 | 113 | 118 | 0.02 | 0.04 | 0.4 | 10 | 424b, 418a, 1851a |
| Cantaloupe (¼ of 6" diameter) | 1C | 48 | 1.1 | 0.2 | 12.0 | 22 | 26 | 0.6 | 19 | 402 | 5440 | 0.06 | 0.05 | 1.0 | 53 | 1358c |
| Citrus fruit: | | | | | | | | | | | | | | | | |
| Orange[b]/grapefruit juice | ½C | | | | | | | | | | | | | | | 1421c, 1053b |
| Orange, small | 1 | | | | | | | | | | | | | | | 1437b, 1061a |
| Grapefruit | ½ | 49 | 0.8 | 0.1 | 11.8 | 19 | 19 | 0.3 | 1 | 189 | 158 | 0.08 | 0.3 | 0.3 | 49 | 663b |
| Cherries, large | 10 | 47 | 0.9 | 0.2 | 11.7 | 15 | 13 | 0.3 | 1 | 129 | 70 | 0.03 | 0.04 | 0.3 | 7 | 1085a |
| Grapes | 12 | 41 | 0.4 | 0.2 | 10.4 | 7 | 12 | 0.2 | 2 | 104 | 60 | 0.04 | 0.02 | 0.2 | 7 | 1504e |
| Pears, water pack | 1 | 50 | 0.4 | 0.4 | 1.8 | 8 | 10 | 0.4 | 2 | 136 | — | 0.02 | 0.04 | 0.2 | 2 | 1846c |
| Raisins (1½ T) | ½ oz. | 40 | 0.4 | — | 10.8 | 9 | 14 | 0.5 | 4 | 107 | — | 0.02 | 0.01 | 0.1 | — | 2217e |
| Strawberries | 1C | 55 | 1.0 | 0.7 | 12.5 | 31 | 31 | 1.5 | 1 | 244 | 90 | 0.04 | 0.10 | 0.9 | 88 | 2424c |
| Watermelon, diced | 1C | 42 | 0.8 | 0.3 | 10.2 | 11 | 16 | 0.8 | 2 | 160 | 940 | 0.05 | 0.05 | 0.3 | 11 | |

TABLE 3 Calculation of Food Energy Intake. Nutritive Value of Common Foods[a] (continued)

| | Amount | Cal | Protein (g) | Fat (g) | Carbohydrate (g) | Calcium (mg) | Phosphorus (mg) | Iron (mg) | Sodium (mg) | Potassium (mg) | Vitamin A (IU) | Thiamin (mg) | Riboflavin (mg) | Niacin (mg) | Ascorbic acid (mg) | USDA Handbook No. 456/ Ref. no. |
|---|---|---|---|---|---|---|---|---|---|---|---|---|---|---|---|---|
| **Bread and Crackers, Enriched** | | | | | | | | | | | | | | | | |
| Biscuit (2" diameter, 1¼" high) | 1 | 103 | 2.1 | 4.8 | 12.8 | 34 | 49 | 0.4 | 175 | 33 | — | 0.06 | 0.06 | 0.5 | — | 410a |
| Cornbread, piece (2½"×2½"×1½") | 1 | 178 | 3.8 | 5.8 | 27.5 | 133 | 209 | 0.8 | 263 | 61 | 130 | 0.10 | 0.10 | 0.8 | — | 1350d |
| Frankfurter roll (6") | 1 | 119 | 3.3 | 2.2 | 21.2 | 30 | 34 | 0.8 | 202 | 38 | — | 0.11 | 0.07 | 0.9 | — | 1902c |
| Graham crackers | 2 | 55 | 1.1 | 1.3 | 10.4 | 6 | 21 | 0.2 | 95 | 55 | — | 0.01 | 0.03 | 0.2 | — | 914b |
| Hamburger bun (3½") | 1 | 119 | 3.3 | 2.2 | 21.2 | 30 | 34 | 0.8 | 202 | 38 | — | 0.11 | 0.07 | 0.9 | — | 1902c |
| Muffin, plain (2"×1½") | 1 | 118 | 3.1 | 4.0 | 16.9 | 42 | 60 | 0.6 | 176 | 50 | 40 | 0.07 | 0.09 | 0.6 | — | 1343b |
| Saltines (2½" square) | 4 | 48 | 1.0 | 1.3 | 8.0 | 2 | 10 | 0.1 | 123 | 13 | — | — | — | 0.1 | — | 916d |
| Soda crackers (2½" square) | 5 | 65 | 1.3 | 1.8 | 10.0 | 3 | 13 | 0.2 | 156 | 16 | — | — | — | 0.1 | — | 918d |
| White or whole wheat bread | 1 | 76 | 2.4 | 0.9 | 14.1 | 24 | 27 | 0.7 | 142 | 29 | — | 0.07 | 0.06 | 0.7 | — | 461b |
| **Cereals, Enriched** | | | | | | | | | | | | | | | | |
| Bran flakes, 40% | ½C | 53 | 1.8 | 0.3 | 14.1 | 10 | 63 | 6.2 | 104 | 68 | 825 | 0.20 | 0.25 | 2.1 | 6 | 441 |
| Corn flakes | ¾C | 73 | 1.5 | 0.1 | 15.9 | — | 7 | 0.4 | 188 | 22 | 885 | 0.22 | 0.26 | 2.2 | 7 | 866a |
| Farina, cooked | ½C | 51 | 1.6 | 0.1 | 10.6 | 5 | 15 | — | 176 | 11 | — | 0.05 | 0.03 | 0.5 | — | 992 |
| Grits, corn | ½C | 62 | 1.4 | 0.1 | 13.5 | 1 | 13 | 0.4 | 251 | 14 | 75 | 0.05 | 0.04 | 0.5 | — | 863a |
| Oatmeal, cooked | ½C | 66 | 2.4 | 1.2 | 11.6 | 11 | 68 | 0.7 | 262 | 73 | — | 0.09 | 0.02 | 0.1 | — | 1391 |
| Rice, cooked | 1/3C | 74 | 1.4 | 0.1 | 16.4 | 7 | 19 | 0.6 | 256 | 19 | — | 0.08 | 0.01 | 0.7 | — | 1872a |
| Wheat, puffed | 1C | 54 | 2.3 | 0.2 | 11.8 | 4 | 48 | 0.6 | 1 | 51 | — | 0.08 | 0.03 | 1.2 | — | 2458 |
| **Pasta, Enriched** | | | | | | | | | | | | | | | | |
| Noodles,[b] macaroni, spaghetti | ½C | 91 | 3.0 | 0.6 | 18.3 | 7 | 41 | 0.7 | 1 | 43 | — | 0.11 | 0.07 | 1.2 | — | 1378c, 1299c, 2159c |
| **Meat, Poultry, Fish** | | | | | | | | | | | | | | | | |
| Beef,[b] Lamb, Veal | 1 oz | 79 | 7.4 | 5.2 | — | 3 | 32 | 0.8 | 16 | 74 | 2 | 0.03 | 0.07 | 1.6 | — | 353d, 1185e, 2370e |

| Food | Measure | | | | | | | | | | | | | | | Reference |
|---|---|---|---|---|---|---|---|---|---|---|---|---|---|---|---|---|
| Beef liver | 1 oz | 65 | 7.5 | 3.0 | 1.5 | 3 | 135 | 2.5 | 52 | 108 | 15130 | 0.07 | 1.19 | 4.7 | 7.7 | 1267a |
| Bologna (1 slice, 4½″ diameter) | 1 oz | 86 | 3.4 | 7.8 | 0.3 | 2 | 36 | 0.5 | 369 | 65 | – | 0.05 | 0.06 | 0.7 | – | 1982g |
| Chicken, light meat | 1 oz | 50 | 9.4 | 1.0 | – | 3 | 80 | 0.4 | 19 | 123 | 17 | 0.01 | 0.02 | 3.5 | – | 682d |
| Cod,b haddock, halibut (broiled) | 1 oz | 48 | 6.9 | 1.8 | 0.5 | 8 | 73 | 0.3 | 40 | 121 | 80 | 0.01 | 0.02 | 1.4 | – | 795d, 1118d, 1104d |
| Ham, cured | 1 oz | 92 | 6.3 | 7.1 | – | 3 | 52 | 0.8 | 227 | 71 | – | 0.15 | 0.06 | 1.1 | – | 1779f |
| Hot dog | 1 | 139 | 5.6 | 12.4 | 0.8 | 3 | 60 | 0.9 | 495 | 99 | – | 0.07 | 0.09 | 1.2 | – | 1994c |
| Pork, fresh | 1 oz | 103 | 6.8 | 8.1 | – | 3 | 73 | 0.9 | 17 | 78 | – | 0.26 | 0.07 | 1.6 | – | 1716c |
| Shrimp | 1 oz | 37 | 7.7 | 0.4 | 0.2 | 37 | 84 | 1.0 | – | 39 | 20 | – | 0.01 | 0.6 | – | 2045c |
| Tuna, canned in oil | 1 oz | 82 | 6.9 | 5.8 | – | 2 | 83 | 0.3 | 227 | 85 | 26 | 0.01 | 0.02 | 2.9 | – | 2323h |
| Egg, large | 1 | 82 | 6.5 | 5.8 | 0.5 | 27 | 103 | 1.2 | 61 | 65 | 590 | 0.05 | 0.15 | – | – | 968b |
| **Cheese** | | | | | | | | | | | | | | | | |
| Cheddar, domestic | 1 oz | 113 | 7.1 | 9.1 | 0.6 | 213 | 136 | 0.3 | 198 | 23 | 370 | 0.01 | 0.13 | – | – | 646p |
| Cottage cheese, small curd, creamed | ½C | 112 | 14.3 | 4.4 | 3.1 | 98 | 160 | 0.3 | 241 | 90 | 180 | 0.03 | 0.26 | 0.1 | – | 647d |
| Peanut Butter | 2T | 188 | 8.0 | 16.2 | 6.0 | 18 | 122 | 0.6 | 194 | 200 | – | 0.04 | 0.04 | 4.8 | – | 1499f |
| **Dried Beans and Peas** | | | | | | | | | | | | | | | | |
| Navy beans,b kidney beans, split peas | ½C | 114 | 7.5 | 0.4 | 20.6 | 32 | 123 | 2.2 | 8 | 342 | 15 | 0.12 | 0.07 | 0.8 | – | 115b, 161d, 1533a |
| **Fats** | | | | | | | | | | | | | | | | |
| Bacon, crisp, slices | 2 | 86 | 3.8 | 7.8 | 0.5 | 2 | 34 | 0.5 | 153 | 35 | – | 0.08 | 0.05 | 0.8 | – | 126d |
| Cream,b light, 20% or half & half | 1T | 26 | 0.5 | 2.5 | 0.7 | 16 | 13 | – | 7 | 19 | 100 | – | 0.02 | – | – | 929b, 928b |
| French or Italian dressingb | 1T | 75 | 0.1 | 7.6 | 1.9 | 2 | 2 | 0.1 | 267 | 8 | – | – | – | – | – | 1932b, 1936b |
| Margarine/butterb | 1t | 34 | – | 3.8 | – | 1 | 1 | – | 46 | 1 | 160 | – | – | – | – | 1317d, 505d |
| Mayonnaise,b salad dressing | 1T | 83 | 0.2 | 8.8 | 1.3 | 3 | 4 | 0.1 | 86 | 3 | 35 | – | – | – | – | 1938b, 1940b |
| Oils | 1T | 120 | – | 13.6 | – | – | – | – | – | – | – | – | – | – | – | 1401j |
| **Nuts** | | | | | | | | | | | | | | | | |
| Unsalted peanuts, pecans, walnuts, almonds | 2T | 103 | 2.9 | 9.6 | 2.9 | 20 | 64 | 0.5 | 19 | 102 | 5 | 0.07 | 0.05 | 1.0 | – | 1496b, 1536j, 2421e, 81 |

**TABLE 3** Calculation of Food Energy Intake. Nutritive Value of Common Foods[a] (continued)

| | Amount | Cal | Protein (g) | Fat (g) | Carbohydrate (g) | Calcium (mg) | Phosphorus (mg) | Iron (mg) | Sodium (mg) | Potassium (mg) | Vitamin A (IU) | Thiamin (mg) | Riboflavin (mg) | Niacin (mg) | Ascorbic acid (mg) | USDA Handbook No. 456/Ref. no. |
|---|---|---|---|---|---|---|---|---|---|---|---|---|---|---|---|---|
| *Desserts* | | | | | | | | | | | | | | | | |
| Brownies, with nuts (1¾"X1¾"X7/8") | 1 | 97 | 1.3 | 6.3 | 10.2 | 8 | 30 | 0.4 | 50 | 38 | 40 | 0.04 | 0.02 | 0.1 | — | 813 |
| Cake, chocolate (3"X3"X2") | 1 piece | 322 | 4.2 | 15.1 | 45.8 | 65 | 121 | 0.8 | 259 | 123 | 130 | 0.02 | 0.09 | 0.2 | — | 525c |
| Cake, plain (3"X3"X2") | 1 piece | 313 | 3.9 | 12.0 | 48.1 | 55 | 88 | 0.3 | 258 | 68 | 150 | 0.02 | 0.08 | 0.2 | — | 534c |
| Chocolate pudding | ½C | 193 | 4.1 | 6.1 | 33.4 | 125 | 128 | 0.7 | 73 | 223 | 195 | 0.03 | 0.18 | 0.2 | — | 1823 |
| Cookies, chocolate chip | 2 | 99 | 1.1 | 4.4 | 14.6 | 8 | 24 | 0.4 | 84 | 28 | 26 | 0.01 | 0.01 | 0.1 | — | 818b |
| Custard, baked | ½C | 153 | 7.2 | 7.3 | 14.7 | 149 | 155 | 0.6 | 105 | 194 | 465 | 0.06 | 0.25 | 0.2 | — | 948 |
| Gelatin dessert | ½C | 71 | 1.8 | — | 16.9 | — | — | — | 61 | — | — | — | — | — | — | 1032b |
| Ice cream, vanilla | 4 fl. oz. | 129 | 3.0 | 7.0 | 13.9 | 97 | 77 | 0.1 | 42 | 121 | 295 | 0.03 | 0.14 | 0.1 | — | 1139d |
| Pie, apple (9" diameter) | 1/8 pie | 302 | 2.6 | 13.1 | 45.0 | 9 | 26 | 0.4 | 355 | 94 | 40 | 0.02 | 0.02 | 0.5 | 1 | 1566c |
| Sherbet, orange | 4 fl oz | 130 | 0.9 | 1.2 | 29.7 | 16 | 13 | — | 10 | 21 | 60 | 0.01 | 0.03 | — | 2 | 2041b |
| Vanilla wafers | 5 | 93 | 1.1 | 3.2 | 14.9 | 8 | 13 | 0.1 | 51 | 15 | 25 | 0.01 | 0.02 | 0.1 | — | 833b |
| *Sweets* | | | | | | | | | | | | | | | | |
| Milk chocolate | 1 oz | 147 | 2.2 | 9.2 | 16.1 | 65 | 65 | 0.3 | 27 | 109 | 80 | 0.02 | 0.10 | 0.1 | — | 587 |
| Molasses,[b] jams, jelly, maple syrup | 1T | 52 | 0.1 | — | 13.4 | 16 | 3 | 0.8 | 2 | 17 | — | — | 0.01 | — | — | 2050b, 1149e, 2049d |
| Soft drinks | 6 fl oz | 72 | — | — | 18.5 | — | — | — | — | — | — | — | — | — | — | 404a |
| Sugar | 1T | 46 | — | — | 11.9 | — | — | — | — | — | — | — | — | — | — | 2230b |

[a]Approximate values. All values have been rounded to the nearest decimal point.
[b]Average value for the group of foods listed.
[c]Dash indicates a true amount of nutrient that contributes to serving size.

From U.S. Department of Agriculture, Nutritive value of American foods, in *Agriculture Handbook No. 456* (Washington, D.C.: Government Printing Office).

**TABLE 4  Moderately High Fiber Diet**

*Breakfast*
1/2 c. stewed prunes
1 c. shredded wheat cereal
1/2 c. milk
hot beverage

*Lunch*
2 oz. sliced turkey
2 sl. whole wheat bread, with lettuce, tomato, and mayonnaise
1/2 c. applesauce
beverage

*Dinner*
3 oz. chopped beef
1/2 c. mashed potatoes
1/2 c. peas
1 small banana
beverage

*Snack*
1 c. milk
fresh orange

---

**TABLE 5  Foods to Buy Which Have a High Nutrient-to-Calorie Ratio**

1. Skim milk
2. Cheese (from part-skim milk)
3. Cottage cheese
4. Lean meat, poultry, and low-fat fish
5. Fortified breakfast cereals
6. Whole wheat enriched bread
7. Orange juice and other citrus fruit juices
8. Fresh fruits, e.g. oranges, grapefruit, cantaloupe, banana
9. Green, leafy vegetables, e.g. spinach, broccoli
10. Dark yellow vegetables, e.g. carrots, squash

## TABLE 6 Average Sodium and Potassium Content of Common Foods

The following tables are reprinted from the second edition of the U.S. Dietary Goals. The Goals recommend restricting salt intake to about 5 g a day, which effectively means reducing sodium intake to about 2 g (2000 mg). No recommendation is made for the daily consumption of potassium, but people taking diuretics, instructed by their physicians to eat foods high in potassium to replace losses, may be interested to see what foods contain large amounts of this mineral.

| FOOD | WEIGHT (g) | SODIUM (mg) | POTASSIUM (mg) |
|---|---|---|---|
| *Meat, fish, or poultry, cooked without added salt* | | | |
| Average | 30 | 33 | 125 |
| Clams, soft | 100 | 36 | 239 |
| Clams, hard | 100 | 205 | 311 |
| Crab, canned | 100 | 1000 | 110 |
| Crab, steamed | 100 | 456 | 271 |
| Flounder | 100 | 237 | 587 |
| Frankfurters (2) | 100 | 1100 | 220 |
| Frozen fish (cod) | 100 | 400 | 400 |
| Haddock | 100 | 177 | 348 |
| Kidneys, beef | 100 | 253 | 324 |
| Lobster, canned | 100 | 210 | 180 |
| Lobster, fresh | 100 | 325 | 258 |
| Oysters, raw | 100 | 73 | 121 |
| Salmon, canned | 100 | 522 | 349 |
| Salmon, salt-free, canned | 100 | 48 | 391 |
| Scallops, fresh | 100 | 265 | 476 |
| Shrimp, raw | 100 | 140 | 220 |
| Shrimp, frozen or canned | 100 | 140 | 200-312 |
| Sweet breads | 100 | 116 | 433 |
| Tuna, canned | 100 | 800 | 240 |
| Tuna, salt-free, canned | 100 | 46 | 382 |
| *Cheese* | | | |
| American cheese | 30 | 341 | 25 |
| Cream cheese | 30 | 75 | 22 |
| Cottage cheese | 30 | 76 | 28 |
| Cottage cheese, unsalted | 30 | 6 | — |
| Low-sodium cheese (cheddar) | 30 | 3 | 120 |
| *Egg* | | | |
| Whole, fresh and frozen (1) | 50 | 61 | 65 |
| Whites, fresh and frozen | 50 | 73 | 70 |
| Yolks, fresh | 50 | 26 | 49 |
| *Milk* | | | |
| Buttermilk, cultured | 120 | 135 | 192 |
| Condensed sweetened milk | 120 | 135 | 377 |
| Evaporated milk, unduiluted | 120 | 142 | 364 |
| Powdered milk, skim | 30 | 160 | 544 |
| Low-sodium milk, canned | 120 | 6 | 288 |
| Whole milk | 240 | 120 | 346 |
| Yogurt (skim milk) | 100 | 51 | 143 |

| FOOD | WEIGHT (g) | SODIUM (mg) | POTASSIUM (mg) |
|---|---|---|---|
| *Potato* | | | |
| White, baked in skin | 100 | 4 | 323 |
| White, boiled | 100 | 2 | 285 |
| Instant, prepared with water, milk, fat | 100 | 256 | 290 |
| Sweet (canned soild pack) | 100 | 48 | 200 |
| | | | |
| *Breads* | | | |
| Bakery, white | 25 | 127 | 26 |
| Bakery, whole wheat | 25 | 132 | 68 |
| Bakery, rye | 25 | 139 | 36 |
| Low-sodium (local) | 25 | 4 | 25 |
| Plain muffin | 40 | 132 | 38 |
| English muffin | 57 | 215 | 57 |
| A-protein rusk (1) | 11 | 4 | 5 |
| Graham crackers (2) | 14 | 93 | 53 |
| Low-sodium crackers (2) | 9 | 10 | 11 |
| Vanilla wafers (5) | 14 | 35 | 10 |
| Yeast doughnut | 30 | 70 | 24 |
| Cake doughnut | 35 | 160 | 32 |
| *Cereal, dry* | | | |
| Kellogg's Corn Flakes | 30 | 282 | 15 |
| Puffed Rice | 15 | trace | 7 |
| Rice Krispies | 30 | 267 | 15 |
| Special K | 30 | 244 | 17 |
| Puffed Wheat | 15 | trace | 21 |
| Shredded Wheat | 20 | 1 | 52 |
| Kellogg's Sugar Frosted Flakes | 30 | 200 | 19 |
| Sugar Pops | 30 | 67 | 22 |
| Bran Flakes | 30 | 118 | 151 |
| | | | |
| *Cereal, cooked without added salt* | | | |
| Corn grits, enriched, regular | 100 | 1 | 11 |
| Farina, enriched, regular | 100 | 2 | 9 |
| Farina, instant cooking | 100 | 7 | 13 |
| Farina, quick cooking | 100 | 190 | 10 |
| Oatmeal or Rolled Oats | 100 | 2 | 61 |
| Pettijohn's Wheat | 100 | trace | 84 |
| Rice | 100 | 5 | 28 |
| Rice, instant | 100 | trace | trace |
| Wheat, rolled | 100 | trace | 84 |
| Wheatena | 100 | trace | 84 |
| | | | |
| *Fat* | | | |
| Bacon (1 strip) | 7 | 73 | 17 |
| Butter | 5 | 49 | 3 |
| Margarine | 5 | 49 | 1 |
| Mayonnaise | 15 | 90 | 5 |
| Mayonnaise, low-sodium | 15 | 17 | 1 |
| Low-sodium butter | 15 | 1 | 3 |
| Unsalted margarine (Fleishman's) | 5 | 1 | 1 |
| Vegetable oil | 15 | 0 | 0 |

**TABLE 6**  Average Sodium and Potassium Content of Common Foods (continued)

| FOOD | WEIGHT (g) | SODIUM (mg) | POTASSIUM (mg) |
|---|---|---|---|
| *Cream* | | | |
| Coffee Mate | 1* | 4 | 27 |
| Half-and-half | 30 | 14 | 39 |
| Heavy whipping cream (30 percent) | 30 | 10 | 27 |
| Poly-perx | 30 | — | — |
| Sour cream (Sealtest) | 30 | 13 | 43 |
| Table cream (18 percent) | 30 | 13 | 37 |
| Whipped topping | 30 | 4 | 6 |
| *Gravy* | | | |
| Low sodium | 30 | 10 | 25 |
| Regular | 30 | 210 | 28 |
| *Peanut butter* | | | |
| Cellu, Salt free | 15 | 1 | 100 |
| Regular, made with small amounts of added fat and salt | 15 | 91 | 100 |
| *Desserts* | | | |
| Baked custard (Delmark) | 120 | 128 | 174 |
| D'zerta | 120 | 35 | 0 |
| Gelatin | 120 | 51 | 1 |
| Ice cream (4-oz cup) | 60 | 23 | 49 |
| Sherbet | 60 | 6 | 14 |
| Water ice | 60 | trace | 2 |
| *Cakes* | | | |
| All varieties except gingerbread and fruit cakes (both mixes and recipes) | 50† | 123 | 50 |
| With low-sodium shortening and baking powder | 50† | 10-20 | 75-150 |
| *Pies* | | | |
| All varieties except raisin, mince (1/8 of 9-inch pie) | 320† | 375 | 180 |
| *Candy* | | | |
| Hard candy (1 equals 5 g) | 100 | 32 | 4 |
| Gum drops (8 small equals 10 g) | 100 | 35 | 5 |
| Jelly beans | 100 | 12 | 1 |
| *Salt* | | | |
| 1 g NaCl—1 packet salt | — | 400 | — |
| 5 g NaCl-1 tsp | — | 2000 | — |
| *Salt substitutes* | | | |
| Diamond Crystal | 500‡ | 1 | 220 |
| Co-salt | 500‡ | 0 | 185 |
| Adolph's | 500‡ | 0 | 241 |
| McCormick's | 500‡ | 0 | 234 |
| Morton | 500‡ | 0 | 250 |

| FOOD | WEIGHT (g) | SODIUM (mg) | POTASSIUM (mg) |
|---|---|---|---|
| *Sugar substitutes* | | | |
| Saccharine (1/4-gr tablet) | 1 | 1 | 0 |
| Sucaryl | 500‡ | 0 | 0 |
| Sweet-10 | 500‡ | 0 | 0 |
| Adolph's | 500‡ | 0 | 0 |
| Morton | 500‡ | 0 | 0 |
| Diamond Crystal | 500‡ | 0 | 0 |
| *Beverages* | | | |
| Beer | 100 | 7 | 25 |
| Chocolate syrup (2 tsp) | 10 | 5 | 29 |
| Coca-Cola | 100 | 4 | 1 |
| Coffee, instant (beverage) | — | 1 | 50 |
| Cranberry juice | 100 | 1 | 10 |
| Diet Seven-Up | 100 | 10 | 0 |
| Egg nog, reconstituted | 240 | 250 | 630 |
| Fresca | 100 | 18 | 0 |
| Frozen lemonade, reconstituted | 100 | trace | 16 |
| Gingerale | 100 | 6 | 2 |
| Hot chocolate (Carnation 1 pack— 6 oz water) | 100 | 104 | 190 |
| Kool-Aid, reconstituted | 240 | trace | 0 |
| Meritene, reconstituted | 240 | 250 | 740 |
| Pepsi Cola | 100 | 2 | 4 |
| Royal Crown Cola | 100 | 3 | trace |
| Seven-Up | 100 | 9 | 0 |
| Sprite | 100 | 16 | 0 |
| Tab | 100 | 5 | 0 |
| Tea, instant (beverage) | — | trace | 25 |

Fresh fruits and fruit juices are naturally very low in sodium and thus are not listed individually in this table.

*In teaspoons.

†Average serving.

‡In milligrams.

| FOOD | SODIUM (mg) |
|---|---|
| *Group I Vegetables (0-20 mg/100 g, average 7.4 mg)*** | |
| Asparagus | 7 |
| Broccoli | 12 |
| Brussels sprouts | 14 |
| Cabbage, common | 14 |
| Cauliflower | 9 |
| Chicory | 7 |
| Collards | 16 |
| Corn | 2 |
| Cow peas | 1 |
| Cucumbers | 6 |
| Eggplant | 1 |
| Endive | 14 |
| Escarole | 14 |

| FOOD | SODIUM (mg) |
|------|-------------|
| Green peppers | 13 |
| Kohlrabi | 6 |
| Leeks | 5 |
| Lentils | 3 |
| Lettuce | 9 |
| Lima beans, not frozen | 1 |
| Mushrooms, raw | 15 |
| Mustard green | 10 |
| Navy beans | 7 |
| Okra | 2 |
| Onions | 7 |
| Parsnips | 8 |
| Peas, dried, split, cooked | 13 |
| Peas, green | 1 |
| Potatoes, baked in skin | 4 |
| Potatoes, boiled, pared before cooking | 3 |
| Radishes | 18 |
| Rutabagas | 4 |
| Squash, summer or winter | 1 |
| String beans | 2 |
| Sweet potato | 10 |
| Tomatoes | 4 |
| Turnip greens | 17 |
| Wax beans | 2 |
| Yams | 4 |

*Group II Vegetables (23-60 mg/100 g, average 40 mg)*

| | |
|---|---|
| Artichoke | 30 |
| Beets | 43 |
| Black-eyed peas, frozen only | 39 |
| Carrots | 33 |
| Chinese cabbage | 23 |
| Dandelion greens | 44 |
| Kale | 43 |
| Parsley | 45 |
| Red cabbage | 26 |
| Spinach | 50 |
| Turnips | 34 |
| Watercress | 52 |

*Group III Vegetables (75-126 mg/100 g, average 81 mg)*

| | |
|---|---|
| Beet greens | 76 |
| Celery | 88 |
| Chard, Swiss | 86 |

This table assumes the use of fresh vegetables without salt added in cooking. The amount of salt added to canned and frozen vegetables can vary. *Agricultural Handbook No. 8* from the USDA estimates that canned vegetables average 235 mg sodium per 100 g edible portion. Frozen vegetables range from almost no sodium to as high as 125 mg sodium per 100 g edible portion.

**A 100-g portion for most vegetables is about a 1/2-c to 1-c serving.

Select Committee on Nutrition and Human Needs, *Dietary Goals for the United States,* 2nd ed. (Washington, D.C.: Government Printing Office, 1977), pp. 80-83. The Senate's tables are taken from information in U.S. Department of Agriculture, Agricultural Research Service, Composition of foods: Raw, processed, prepared, *Agricultural Handbook No. 8* (Washington, D.C.: Government Printing Office, 1963).

### TABLE 7 Low Fat, Low Cholesterol Foods of Animal Origin

| | SERVING SIZE | CHOLESTEROL mg | FAT g |
|---|---|---|---|
| **Milk and Milk Products** | | | |
| Milk, skim | 1 c | 7 | — |
| Milk, 2 percent | 1 c | 15 | 4.9 |
| Cottage cheese[1] | | 5 | 1.0 |
| Yogurt[2] | | 6 | 0.9 |
| Ice cream | 1/2 c | 5 | 2.5 |
| **Meat and Fish** | | | |
| Beef, lean, cooked[3] | 3 oz | 100 | 6.7 |
| Lamb, lean, cooked | 3 oz | 100 | 7.3 |
| Cod, cooked | 3 oz | 100 | 3.0 |
| Fish, cooked | 3 oz | 54 | 0.9 |

[1] uncreamed

[2] made from partially skimmed milk

[3] boiled, steamed, baked or broiled (no fat added)

Low fat diet = selection of foods listed above plus bread, cereals, breakfast rice, fruit and vegetables to give ≤ 50 g fat/day.

Low cholesterol diet = selection of foods listed above plus bread, cereals, breakfast rice, fruit and vegetables and *all* vegetable margarine to give ≤ 200 mg cholesterol/day.

Values, converted to domestic measures, are from A. A. Paul and D. A. T. Southgate, McCance and Widdowson's 4th Revised Edition of MRC Special Report No. 297, HMSO, London, 1978, and from E. M. N. Hamilton and E. N. Whitney, *Nutrition Concepts and Controversies* (St. Paul, New York, Los Angeles, San Francisco: West Publ. Co., 1979).

### TABLE 8 High Fiber Foods

| FOOD | DIETARY FIBER g/100 g |
|---|---|
| *Cereals* | |
| Wheat bran | 44.0 |
| All-bran | 8.4 |
| Shredded wheat | 12.3 |
| Special K | 5.5 |
| Whole wheat bread ("whole meal") | 8.5 |
| Crispbread rye | 11.7 |
| *Fruits* | |
| Apples, raw (flesh only) | 2.0 |
| Bananas | 3.4 |
| Prunes, stewed with sugar | 7.7 |
| *Vegetables* | |
| Broccoli, cooked | 4.1 |
| Carrots | 3.1 |
| Peas | 5.2 |
| Spinach | 6.3 |

Values are from A. A. Paul and D. A. T. Southgate, McCance and Widdowson's 4th Revised Edition of MRC Special Report No. 297, HMSO, London, 1978.

**TABLE 9  Folacin Activity of Frozen Convenience Foods**

TOTAL AND FREE FOLACIN ACTIVITY IN FROZEN DINNERS AFTER DEFROSTING AND AFTER REHEATING

| | FREE FOLACIN ACTIVITY* | | | | TOTAL FOLACIN ACTIVITY* | | | |
| | AFTER DEFROSTING | | AFTER REHEATING | | AFTER DEFROSTING | | AFTER REHEATING | |
| DINNER | RANGE | MEAN | RANGE | MEAN | RANGE | MEAN | RANGE | MEAN |
|---|---|---|---|---|---|---|---|---|
| | | | ← mcg. folic acid/100 gm. dinner → | | | | | |
| No.  1. Chinese-style | 1.7- 3.1 | 2.7 | | | 3.1- 7.8 | 5.6 | | |
| No.  2. Swiss steak | 5.9- 7.1 | 6.3 | 5.2-6.2 | 5.6 | 8.3-18.6 | 14.7 | 15.7-17.8 | 16.4 |
| No.  3. Loin of pork | 2.3- 5.6 | 4.1 | 1.8-2.2 | 2.0 | 3.4-11.6 | 6.4 | 5.5-14.2 | 8.7 |
| No.  4. Ham | 3.9- 8.6 | 5.5 | 3.6-6.3 | 4.6 | 6.0-11.7 | 8.9 | 12.0-17.3 | 15.3 |
| No.  5. Salisbury steak | 3.8- 6.7 | 5.5 | | | 6.1-15.6 | 11.1 | | |
| No.  6. Turkey | 4.1- 6.6 | 5.3 | 4.0-4.8 | 4.5 | 7.1-13.2 | 11.5 | 9.8-16.4 | 12.3 |
| No.  7. Fried chicken | 4.0- 5.2 | 4.5 | | | 6.0-10.4 | 9.0 | | |
| No.  8. Salisbury steak | 4.2- 6.2 | 5.1 | 4.5-9.1 | 7.7 | 8.5-18.4 | 14.2 | 15.1-17.3 | 16.2 |
| No.  9. Beef | 5.2- 8.8 | 6.8 | 4.6-5.7 | 5.1 | 8.3-15.5 | 11.4 | 13.5-16.7 | 15.1 |
| No. 10. Turkey | 4.0- 6.1 | 5.2 | | | 8.1-17.4 | 13.4 | | |
| No. 11. Chopped sirloin beef | 5.9-11.6 | 9.0 | 5.3-6.3 | 5.6 | 9.6-18.8 | 13.6 | 15.6-19.4 | 18.0 |
| No. 12. Beef | 4.3- 9.3 | 7.2 | 6.0-7.1 | 6.5 | 16.2-19.5 | 17.6 | 18.9-21.3 | 20.2 |
| No. 13. Fried chicken | 2.7- 8.0 | 4.8 | | | 9.2-14.5 | 12.6 | | |
| No. 14. Turkey | 2.5- 5.7 | 4.5 | 1.5-3.2 | 2.6 | 6.5-10.8 | 8.9 | 5.3- 6.6 | 6.1 |

| Dinner | | | | | | | | |
|---|---|---|---|---|---|---|---|---|
| No. 15. Chinese-style | 2.1 | 1.7-2.8 | 1.9-3.0 | 2.3 | 6.0 | 4.3-9.6 | 2.8-5.7 | 4.2 |
| No. 16. Chinese-style | 2.8 | 2.4-3.3 | 1.9-2.1 | 2.0 | 6.3 | 5.8-6.8 | 3.5-5.9 | 4.9 |
| No. 17. Chinese-style | 2.2 | 1.8-2.5 | | | 5.6 | 4.7-6.4 | | |
| No. 18. Chinese-style | 2.7 | 2.2-3.3 | | | 6.8 | 4.3-8.3 | | |
| No. 19. Shrimp and chips | 8.4 | 6.9-9.2 | | | 18.0 | 14.3-19.3 | | |
| No. 20. Fish and chips | 8.7 | 7.1-9.6 | 6.9-8.1 | 7.4 | 14.8 | 8.8-18.3 | 16.1-17.7 | 17.0 |
| No. 21. Macaroni and cheese | 2.0 | 1.3-3.0 | | | 6.0 | 2.5-12.7 | | |
| No. 22. Macaroni and beef | 3.6 | 3.2-4.1 | 1.0-2.2 | 1.5 | 7.6 | 6.3-10.3 | 3.7-4.3 | 4.1 |
| No. 23. Fried chicken | 4.7 | 3.9-5.5 | | | 15.0 | 11.8-18.2 | | |
| No. 24. Spaghetti and meatballs | 6.2 | 3.7-7.7 | | | 15.3 | 12.9-18.3 | | |
| No. 25. Meatballs | 2.9 | 2.2-3.3 | 1.8-2.4 | 2.1 | 6.4 | 3.3-9.3 | 4.9-5.7 | 5.3 |
| No. 26. Beef | 2.1 | 1.6-2.7 | | | 5.8 | 5.2-6.3 | | |
| No. 27. Chinese-style | 2.6 | 1.7-3.1 | | | 7.1 | 5.7-8.9 | | |
| No. 28. Chinese-style | 3.7 | 3.0-4.0 | | | 10.4 | 9.5-11.3 | | |
| No. 29. Chinese-style | 1.7 | 1.2-2.1 | | | 7.0 | 5.9-8.3 | | |
| No. 30. Shrimp | 12.8 | 12.0-13.8 | 6.3-8.9 | 7.6 | 25.2 | 22.7-26.7 | 12.2-15.6 | 14.5 |
| mean, all dinners . . . | 5.8*† | 1.8-13.8 | 1.0-8.9 | 4.5 | 11.5 | 3.4-26.7 | 2.8-21.3 | 11.9 |

*Results obtained on four dinners. Expressed as folic acid.
†Means with different letters are significantly different at $P < 0.05$.

TABLE 9   Folacin Activity of Frozen Convenience Food (continued)

## TOTAL AND FREE FOLACIN ACTIVITY OF COMPONENTS
## OF PREPARED FROZEN DINNERS AFTER DEFROSTING

| DINNER AND COMPONENT | FREE FOLACIN ACTIVITY* | | TOTAL FOLACIN ACTIVITY* | |
| --- | --- | --- | --- | --- |
| | PER 100 gm. | PER DINNER | PER 100 gm. | PER DINNER |
| | ← *mcg.* → | | | |
| No.  1.  Chinese-style | | | | |
| rice | 2.1 | 1.7 | 5.3 | 4.2 |
| sauce | 2.2 | 0.7 | 6.2 | 1.9 |
| breaded shrimp | 6.3 | 2.9 | 7.5 | 3.4 |
| chicken chow mein | 2.0 | 3.6 | 6.1 | 11.0 |
| whole dinner | 2.7 | 8.9 | 6.1 | 20.5 |
| No.  2.  Swiss steak | | | | |
| potato, mashed | 5.4 | 4.6 | 8.1 | 6.8 |
| vanilla pudding | 4.4 | 2.0 | 3.9 | 1.7 |
| mixed vegetables | 30.6 | 17.5 | 39.5 | 22.6 |
| steak, gravy | 3.7 | 5.2 | 7.7 | 10.8 |
| whole dinner | 9.0 | 29.3 | 12.9 | 41.9 |
| No.  3.  Loin of pork | | | | |
| French fried potatoes | 4.8 | 2.3 | 26.5 | 12.7 |
| lemon muffin | 8.1 | 2.9 | 11.7 | 4.2 |
| apple sauce | 0.1 | 0.07 | 0.8 | 0.6 |
| loin of pork, gravy | 0.3 | 0.4 | 3.3 | 4.8 |
| whole dinner | 1.9 | 5.7 | 7.3 | 22.3 |
| No.  4.  Ham | | | | |
| potatoes, mashed | 5.6 | 5.4 | 16.5 | 16.0 |
| corn muffin | 5.1 | 1.8 | 7.3 | 2.6 |
| peas and carrots | 15.5 | 8.4 | 45.0 | 24.4 |
| ham, gravy | 0.1 | 0.1 | 2.8 | 3.7 |
| whole dinner | 5.0 | 15.7 | 14.9 | 46.7 |
| No.  5.  Salisbury steak | | | | |
| vanilla pudding | 5.1 | 4.6 | 7.4 | 6.7 |
| peas | 12.5 | 5.6 | 89.5 | 40.3 |
| potatoes, mashed | 3.5 | 3.0 | 8.1 | 6.9 |
| steak, gravy | 2.1 | 3.4 | 4.9 | 8.0 |
| chicken noodle sourp | 0.2 | 0.2 | 1.0 | 1.1 |
| whole dinner | 3.4 | 16.8 | 12.7 | 63.0 |
| No.  6.  Turkey | | | | |
| apple crisp | 1.9 | 1.9 | 4.1 | 4.1 |
| peas | 19.6 | 9.5 | 35.5 | 17.2 |
| potatoes, mashed | 5.7 | 4.5 | 7.1 | 5.6 |
| turkey, gravy | 2.8 | 4.5 | 6.1 | 9.9 |
| cream of tomato soup | 2.7 | 3.1 | 7.3 | 8.4 |
| whole dinner | 4.7 | 23.7 | 9.0 | 45.2 |
| No.  7.  Fried chicken | | | | |
| potatoes, whipped | 5.5 | 5.8 | 9.2 | 9.8 |
| chicken | 6.0 | 5.9 | 14.8 | 14.6 |
| whole dinner | 5.7 | 11.7 | 11.9 | 24.4 |
| No.  8.  Salisbury steak | | | | |
| French fried potatoes | 9.8 | 10.4 | 18.0 | 19.1 |
| steak | 3.7 | 2.9 | 9.7 | 7.7 |
| whole dinner | 7.2 | 13.3 | 14.5 | 26.8 |

TABLE 9  Folacin Activity of Frozen Convenience Food (continued)

## TOTAL AND FREE FOLACIN ACTIVITY OF COMPONENTS
## OF PREPARED FROZEN DINNERS AFTER DEFROSTING

| DINNER AND COMPONENT | FREE FOLACIN ACTIVITY* | | TOTAL FOLACIN ACTIVITY* | |
|---|---|---|---|---|
| | PER 100 gm. | PER DINNER | PER 100 gm. | PER DINNER |
| | ← mcg. → | | | |
| No. 9. Beef | | | | |
| apple cake cobbler | 3.5 | 2.6 | 5.6 | 4.2 |
| corn | 22.3 | 11.5 | 39.7 | 20.4 |
| potatoes, hashed | 3.1 | 2.0 | 17.8 | 11.3 |
| beef, gravy | 1.4 | 2.2 | 4.6 | 7.1 |
| tomato soup | 3.4 | 3.7 | 8.3 | 9.1 |
| whole dinner | 4.8 | 22.0 | 11.5 | 52.1 |
| No. 10. Turkey | | | | |
| potatoes, mashed | 3.8 | 3.4 | 11.8 | 10.6 |
| cranberry sauce | 0.3 | 0.1 | 1.6 | 0.5 |
| peas | 20.1 | 10.3 | 40.2 | 20.7 |
| turkey, gravy | 4.1 | 7.0 | 9.0 | 15.3 |
| whole dinner | 6.0 | 20.8 | 13.6 | 47.1 |
| No. 11. Chopped sirloin beef | | | | |
| French fried potatoes | 10.0 | 4.4 | 22.4 | 9.9 |
| blueberry muffin | 7.8 | 2.7 | 9.6 | 3.3 |
| peas | 22.5 | 12.8 | 50.6 | 28.8 |
| beef, gravy | 1.4 | 2.3 | 5.8 | 9.4 |
| whole dinner | 7.5 | 22.2 | 17.3 | 51.4 |
| No. 12. Beef | | | | |
| corn | 16.9 | 9.4 | 56.5 | 31.5 |
| hashed brown potatoes | 2.8 | 1.5 | 17.0 | 8.9 |
| peas | 22.6 | 12.2 | 55.6 | 30.0 |
| beef, gravy | 2.2 | 3.6 | 5.4 | 8.9 |
| whole dinner | 8.2 | 26.7 | 24.2 | 79.3 |
| No. 13. Fried chicken | | | | |
| potatoes | 6.4 | 5.4 | 16.2 | 13.7 |
| diced apples | 0.4 | 0.2 | 2.6 | 1.0 |
| mixed vegetables | 12.4 | 7.2 | 48.4 | 28.0 |
| fried chicken | 3.8 | 5.1 | 11.4 | 15.4 |
| whole dinner | 5.7 | 17.9 | 18.4 | 58.1 |
| No. 14. Turkey | | | | |
| potatotes, whipped | 4.6 | 4.4 | 12.3 | 11.9 |
| turkey, gravy | 3.5 | 5.9 | 9.7 | 16.3 |
| whole dinner | 3.9 | 10.3 | 10.7 | 28.2 |
| No. 15. Chinese-style | | | | |
| spareribs | 0.7 | 0.6 | 3.3 | 2.6 |
| almond chicken | 2.6 | 2.5 | 5.2 | 4.9 |
| chicken fried rice | 1.3 | 2.7 | 3.3 | 7.0 |
| whole dinner | 1.5 | 5.8 | 3.8 | 11.5 |
| No. 16. Chinese-style | | | | |
| pineapple chicken | 1.7 | 1.7 | 2.9 | 2.8 |
| egg rolls | 4.1 | 1.0 | 5.5 | 1.3 |
| chicken fried rice | 1.1 | 0.9 | 3.2 | 2.6 |
| chicken chow mein | 2.5 | 5.2 | 4.8 | 10.0 |
| whole dinner | 2.1 | 8.8 | 4.0 | 16.7 |

TABLE 9   Folacin Activity of Frozen Convenience Food (continued)

## TOTAL AND FREE FOLACIN ACTIVITY OF COMPONENTS OF PREPARED FROZEN DINNERS AFTER DEFROSTING

| DINNER AND COMPONENT | FREE FOLACIN ACTIVITY* | | TOTAL FOLACIN ACTIVITY* | |
|---|---|---|---|---|
| | PER 100 gm. | PER DINNER | PER 100 gm. | PER DINNER |
| | ← mcg. → | | | |
| No. 17.  Chinese-style | | | | |
| pineapple chicken | 1.5 | 1.4 | 2.9 | 2.7 |
| chicken fried rice | 1.3 | 1.3 | 1.9 | 2.0 |
| chicken chow mein | 1.9 | 4.0 | 4.8 | 10.1 |
| whole dinner | 1.6 | 6.7 | 3.6 | 14.8 |
| No. 18.  Chinese-style | | | | |
| fried rice | 1.8 | 2.8 | 2.9 | 4.6 |
| chicken with vegetable | 2.2 | 2.5 | 5.3 | 6.1 |
| spareribs | 0.1 | 0.1 | 1.9 | 1.5 |
| whole dinner | 1.6 | 5.4 | 3.5 | 12.2 |
| No. 19.  Shrimp and chips | | | | |
| shrimp | 7.4 | 7.4 | 9.6 | 9.6 |
| French fried potatoes | 9.5 | 13.7 | 19.2 | 27.7 |
| sweet and sour sauce | 0.9 | 0.2 | 2.5 | 0.5 |
| whole dinner | 8.1 | 21.3 | 11.3 | 37.8 |
| No. 20.  Fish and chips | | | | |
| haddock | 2.8 | 3.4 | 7.2 | 8.7 |
| French fried potatoes | 8.7 | 13.2 | 26.7 | 40.5 |
| whole dinner | 6.1 | 16.6 | 18.0 | 49.2 |
| No. 23.  Fried chicken | | | | |
| apple brown betty | 1.8 | 1.8 | 4.8 | 4.8 |
| corn | 16.9 | 8.5 | 46.1 | 23.2 |
| potatoes, mashed | 3.7 | 3.3 | 8.8 | 8.0 |
| chicken | 3.7 | 4.5 | 11.2 | 13.7 |
| vegetable soup | 1.6 | 1.8 | 4.3 | 4.8 |
| whole dinner | 4.2 | 19.9 | 11.5 | 54.5 |
| No. 24.  Spaghetti and meatballs | | | | |
| apple sauce | 0.4 | 0.3 | 2.3 | 1.9 |
| peas | 19.6 | 10.6 | 70.0 | 37.8 |
| spaghetti and meatballs | 4.6 | 10.0 | 10.4 | 22.6 |
| whole dinner | 5.9 | 20.9 | 17.6 | 62.3 |
| No. 25.  Meatballs | | | | |
| potatoes, whipped | 4.4 | 4.9 | 8.3 | 9.2 |
| meatballs, gravy | 2.3 | 4.0 | 7.0 | 12.1 |
| whole dinner | 3.1 | 8.9 | 7.5 | 21.3 |
| No. 26.  Beef | | | | |
| potatoes, whipped | 3.6 | 3.6 | 5.6 | 5.6 |
| beef, gravy | 1.5 | 2.3 | 4.9 | 7.5 |
| whole dinner | 2.3 | 5.9 | 5.2 | 13.1 |
| No. 27.  Chinese-style | | | | |
| chicken | 4.8 | 4.8 | 8.8 | 8.8 |
| breaded chicken and pineapple | 1.5 | 1.3 | 3.0 | 2.6 |
| chicken fried rice | 2.4 | 4.8 | 7.4 | 14.9 |
| whole dinner | 2.8 | 10.9 | 6.7 | 26.3 |

**TABLE 9** Folacin Activity of Frozen Convenience Food (continued)

### TOTAL AND FREE FOLACIN ACTIVITY OF COMPONENTS OF PREPARED FROZEN DINNERS AFTER DEFROSTING

| DINNER AND COMPONENT | FREE FOLACIN ACTIVITY* PER 100 gm. | FREE FOLACIN ACTIVITY* PER DINNER | TOTAL FOLACIN ACTIVITY* PER 100 gm. | TOTAL FOLACIN ACTIVITY* PER DINNER |
|---|---|---|---|---|
| | ← *mcg.* → | | | |
| No. 28. Chinese-style | | | | |
| breaded sweet and sour shrimp | 5.7 | 5.4 | 9.0 | 8.5 |
| shrimp fried rice | 3.4 | 2.5 | 10.7 | 8.0 |
| shrimp chow mein | 4.0 | 8.8 | 15.7 | 34.4 |
| whole dinner | 4.3 | 16.7 | 13.1 | 50.9 |
| No. 29. Chinese-style | | | | |
| chicken fried rice | 2.7 | 2.0 | 7.3 | 5.5 |
| breaded sweet and sour spareribs | 1.6 | 1.8 | 3.8 | 4.2 |
| chicken chow mein | 3.7 | 8.2 | 8.0 | 17.7 |
| whole dinner | 2.9 | 12.0 | 6.7 | 27.4 |

*Results obtained from pooled components of four dinners. Expressed as folic acid.

### TOTAL FOLACIN ACTIVITY OF THREE GROUPS OF FROZEN CONVENIENCE DINNERS

| GROUP | TOTAL FOLACIN ACTIVITY* RANGE | TOTAL FOLACIN ACTIVITY* MEAN |
|---|---|---|
| | *mcg./100 gm.* | |
| 1 | 9.0-24.2 | 15.4 |
| 2 | 3.5-13.1 | 5.9 |
| 3 | 5.2-14.5 | 10.3 |

*Expressed as folic acid.

Taken from K. Hoppner, B. Lampi and D. E. Perrin, "Folacin activity of frozen convenience foods," *J. Amer. Dietet. Assoc.* 63: 536-39, 1973.

**TABLE 10  Folacin Content of Foods in Terms of 100 gm. Edible Portion and of Specified Units***

| ITEM NUMBER | FOOD AND DESCRIPTION | PER 100 gm. EDIBLE PORTION | | APPROXIMATE MEASURE | PER SPECIFIED UNIT | | |
|---|---|---|---|---|---|---|---|
| | | FREE FOLACIN | TOTAL FOLACIN | | WEIGHT | FREE FOLACIN | TOTAL FOLACIN |
| | | ← mcg. → | | | gm. | ← mcg. → | |
| *Cereal grains and their products* | | | | | | | |
| 1 | barley, pot | 9 | 20 | 1 c. | 200 | 18 | 40 |
| 2 | corn, whole grain | 15 | 19 | | | | |
| 3 | cornmeal, degermed | 9 | 24 | 1 c. | 122 | 11 | 29 |
| 4 | macaroni, dry form | 4 | 12 | 8-oz. pkg. | 227 | 9 | 27 |
| | rice | | | | | | |
| 5 | brown | 12 | 16 | 1 c. | 185 | 22 | 30 |
| 6 | white | −† | 10 | 1 c. | 185 | — | 18 |
| 7 | parboiled | 9 | 11 | 1 c. | 185 | 17 | 20 |
| 8 | rice bran | — | 39 | | | | |
| 9 | rice germ | — | 64 | | | | |
| 10 | rye flour, sifted | 31 | 78 | 1 c. | 88 | 27 | 69 |
| 11 | sorghum, grain | 18 | 27 | | | | |
| 12 | spaghetti, dry form | 4 | 12 | 8-oz. pkg. | 227 | 9 | 27 |
| 13 | wheat, whole grain | 39 | 52 | | | | |
| | wheat flour | | | | | | |
| 14 | whole | 40 | 54 | 1 c. | 120 | 48 | 65 |
| 15 | clear | 29 | 32 | | | | |
| | patent | | | | | | |
| 16 | bread, sifted | 19 | 25 | 1 c. | 115 | 22 | 29 |
| 17 | all-purpose, sifted | 18 | 21 | 1 c. | 115 | 21 | 24 |
| 18 | wheat bran | 134 | 258 | | | | |
| 19 | wheat germ | 257 | 328 | | | | |
| | breakfast cereals, dry | | | | | | |
| 20 | farina | — | 24 | 1 c. | 180 | — | 43 |
| 21 | farina, wheat germ added | 17 | 34 | 1 c. | 180 | 31 | 61 |
| 22 | oatmeal | 16 | 52 | 1 c. | 80 | 13 | 42 |
| | breakfast cereals, ready-to-eat; not fortified with folacin | | | | | | |

| # | Food | | | Measure | Weight (g) | | |
|---|---|---|---|---|---|---|---|
| 23 | cornflakes | 9 | 12 | 1 oz. | 28 | 3 | 3 |
| 24 | oats, with added wheat glutten | 8 | 22 | 1 oz. | 28 | 2 | 6 |
| 25 | rice, puffed | 8 | 23 | 1 oz. | 28 | 2 | 6 |
| 26 | rice, with added protein concentrate and wheat glutten | 14 | 31 | 1 oz. | 28 | 4 | 9 |
| 27 | wheat germ, toasted | 125 | 420 | 1 oz. | 28 | 35 | 118 |
| 28 | wheat and malted barley granules | 15 | 54 | 1 oz. | 28 | 4 | 15 |
| 29 | wheat, shredded | 10 | 50 | 1 oz. | 28 | 3 | 14 |
| | bakery products | | | | | | |
| | bread | | | | | | |
| 30 | rye | 6 | 23 | 1 slice | 25 | 2 | 6 |
| 31 | white | 13 | 39 | 1 slice | 25 | 3 | 10 |
| 32 | whole wheat | 27 | 58 | 1 slice | 28 | 8 | 16 |
| | cakes | | | | | | |
| 33 | chocolate with icing | 4 | 6 | 1 slice (3" high; 2 3/8" arc) | 99 | 4 | 6 |
| 34 | sponge | 3 | 7 | 1 slice (3" high; 2 1/4" arc) | 44 | 1 | 3 |
| | cookies | | | | | | |
| 35 | chocolate chip | 4 | 9 | 1 cookie | 10 | <0.5 | 1 |
| 36 | shortbread | 4 | 9 | 1 cookie | 8 | <0.5 | 1 |
| | doughnuts | | | | | | |
| 37 | cake type | 5 | 8 | 1 doughnut | 32 | 2 | 3 |
| 38 | yeast leavened | 5 | 22 | 1 doughnut | 35 | 2 | 8 |
| 39 | pie, apple | 2 | 4 | 1/6 of pie | 158 | 3 | 6 |

*Leguminous seeds and their products*

| # | Food | | | Measure | Weight (g) | | |
|---|---|---|---|---|---|---|---|
| | beans, common, mature seeds | | | | | | |
| | white | | | | | | |
| 40 | raw, dry | 25 | 129 | 1 c. | 205 | 51 | 264 |
| 41 | canned, baked with tomato sauce | 8 | 24 | 1 c. | 255 | 20 | 61 |
| | red | | | | | | |
| 42 | raw, dry | 24 | 133 | 1 c. | 185 | 44 | 246 |
| 43 | cooked | — | 37 | 1 c. | 185 | — | 68 |

**TABLE 10  Folacin Content of Foods in Terms of 100 gm. Edible Portion and of Specified Units* (continued)**

| ITEM NUMBER | FOOD AND DESCRIPTION | PER 100 gm. EDIBLE PORTION | | PER SPECIFIED UNIT | | | |
|---|---|---|---|---|---|---|---|
| | | FREE FOLACIN | TOTAL FOLACIN | APPROXIMATE MEASURE | WEIGHT | FREE FOLACIN | TOTAL FOLACIN |
| | | ← mcg. → | | | gm. | ← mcg. → | |
| | *Leguminous seeds and their products, continued* | | | | | | |
| | pinto, mature seeds, dry | | | | | | |
| 44 | raw, dry | 57 | 216 | 1 c. | 190 | 108 | 410 |
| 45 | cooked | — | 59 | 1 c. | 190 | — | 112 |
| 46 | canned, drained | — | 51 | 1 c. | 190 | — | 97 |
| | beans, Lima, mature seeds | | | | | | |
| 47 | raw, dry | 25 | 113 | 1 c. | 190 | 48 | 215 |
| 48 | cooked | — | 43 | 1 c. | 190 | — | 82 |
| 49 | beans, mung, mature seeds, dry | 26 | 133 | 1 c. | 210 | 55 | 279 |
| 50 | beans, mungo, mature seeds, dry | 28 | 108 | | | | |
| | chickpeas or garbanzos, mature seeds | | | | | | |
| 51 | raw, dry | 32 | 199 | 1 c. | 200 | 64 | 398 |
| 52 | roasted | 22 | 139 | | | | |
| 53 | canned, drained | — | 102 | | | | |
| | cowpeas, mature seeds | | | | | | |
| 54 | raw, dry | 69 | 133 | 1 c. | 170 | 117 | 226 |
| 55 | canned, drained | — | 80 | 1 c. | 165 | — | 132 |
| 56 | lentils, mature seeds, dry | 19 | 36 | 1 c. | 190 | 36 | 68 |
| 57 | peanuts, roasted | 24 | 106 | 1 c. | 144 | 35 | 153 |
| 58 | peanut butter | 20 | 79 | 1 Tbsp. | 16 | 3 | 13 |
| 59 | pigeon peas, mature seeds, dry | 20 | 110 | | | | |
| 60 | soybeans, mature seeds, dry | 75 | 171 | 1 c. | 210 | 158 | 359 |
| | soybean products, fermented | | | | | | |
| 61 | natto | 95 | 126 | | | | |
| 62 | tempeh | 12 | 156 | | | | |
| 63 | soy sauce | 8 | 28 | 1 Tbsp. | 18 | 1 | 5 |

*Nuts and seeds (other than leguminous seeds)*

| No. | Item | | | | | | |
|---|---|---|---|---|---|---|---|
| 64 | almonds | 33 | 96 | 1 c. | 142 | 47 | 136 |
| 65 | Brazil nuts, shelled | 1 | 4 | 1 c. | 140 | 1 | 6 |
| 66 | cashew nuts, roasted | 8 | 68 | 1 c. | 140 | 11 | 95 |
| 67 | coconut, shredded | 10 | 24 | 1 c. | 130 | 13 | 31 |
| 68 | filberts (hazelnuts), shelled | 23 | 72 | 1 c. | 135 | 31 | 97 |
| 69 | pecans, shelled | 13 | 24 | 1 c. | 108 | 14 | 26 |
| 70 | pistachio nuts | 10 | 58 | | | | |
| 71 | sesame seeds | 49 | 96 | | | | |
| 71a | sesame seeds | | | 1 Tbsp. | 8 | 4 | 8 |
| 71b | sesame seeds | | | 1 c. | 150 | 74 | 144 |
| 72 | walnuts, English, shelled | 52 | 66 | 1 c. | 100 | 52 | 66 |

*Vegetables*

| No. | Item | | | | | | |
|---|---|---|---|---|---|---|---|
| 73 | asparagus, raw | 58 | 64 | 1 c. | 135 | 78 | 86 |
| 74 | bean sprouts, canned | 7 | 10 | 1 c. | 125 | 9 | 12 |
| | beans, snap | | | | | | |
| | green | | | | | | |
| 75 | raw | 33 | 44 | 1 c. | 110 | 36 | 48 |
| 76 | cooked, drained | – | 40 | 1 c. | 125 | – | 50 |
| 77 | frozen | 8 | 33 | 1 c. | 125 | 10 | 41 |
| | yellow or wax | | | | | | |
| 78 | raw | 32 | 40 | 1 c. | 110 | 35 | 44 |
| 79 | frozen | 8 | 34 | 1 c. | 125 | 10 | 42 |
| 80 | beans, Lima, frozen | 9 | 31 | 1 c. | 160 | 14 | 50 |
| 81 | beets, common, red raw | 69 | 93 | 1 c. | 135 | 93 | 126 |
| 82 | cooked | 38 | 78 | 1 c. | 170 | 65 | 133 |
| | broccoli | | | | | | |
| | spears | | | | | | |
| 83 | raw | 51 | 69 | 3 medium | 354 | 181 | 244 |
| 84 | cooked | 27 | 56 | 1 medium | 180 | 49 | 101 |
| 85 | flower, raw | 102 | 105 | | | | |
| 86 | stem, raw | 35 | 59 | | | | |
| | Brussels sprouts | | | | | | |

**TABLE 10  Folacin Content of Foods in Terms of 100 gm. Edible Portion and of Specified Units* (continued)**

| ITEM NUMBER | FOOD AND DESCRIPTION | PER 100 gm. EDIBLE PORTION | | PER SPECIFIED UNIT | | | |
|---|---|---|---|---|---|---|---|
| | | FREE FOLACIN | TOTAL FOLACIN | APPROXIMATE MEASURE | WEIGHT | FREE FOLACIN | TOTAL FOLACIN |
| | | ← mcg. → | | | gm. | ← mcg. → | |
| *Vegetables, continued* | | | | | | | |
| 87 | raw | 55 | 78 | 6 medium | 114 | 63 | 89 |
| 88 | cooked | 6 | 36 | 1 c. (7-8 sprouts) | 155 | 9 | 56 |
| | cabbage, common varieties | | | | | | |
| 89 | raw | 33 | 66 | 1 c. | 90 | 30 | 59 |
| 90 | cooked | 2 | 18 | 1 c. | 145 | 3 | 26 |
| 91 | red, raw | 23 | 34 | 1 c. | 90 | 21 | 31 |
| | cabbage, Chinese (also called celery cabbage or petsai) | | | | | | |
| 92 | raw | 42 | 83 | 1 c. | 75 | 32 | 62 |
| 93 | cooked | 5 | 19 | | | | |
| | carrots | | | | | | |
| 94 | raw | 14 | 32 | 1 medium | 59 | 8 | 19 |
| 95 | cooked | 2 | 24 | 1 c. | 155 | 3 | 37 |
| | cauliflower | | | | | | |
| 96 | raw | 31 | 55 | 1 c. | 100 | 31 | 55 |
| 97 | cooked | 2 | 34 | 1 c. | 125 | 2 | 42 |
| 98 | celery, raw | 6 | 12 | 1 c. | 100 | 6 | 12 |
| 99 | chicory greens, raw | 33 | 52 | | | | |
| 100 | collards, raw | — | 102 | 1 c. | 55 | — | 56 |
| | corn, sweet | | | | | | |
| 101 | raw, whole kernel | 27 | 33 | 1 c. | 165 | 45 | 54 |
| 102 | frozen | 2 | 21 | 1 c. | 162 | 3 | 35 |
| 103 | cucumber, raw, pared | 12 | 15 | 1 small | 128 | 15 | 19 |

| No. | Food | | | Measure | | | |
|---|---|---|---|---|---|---|---|
| | eggplant | | | | | | |
| 104 | raw | 9 | 31 | 1 c. | 200 | 4 | 32 |
| 105 | cooked | 2 | 16 | 1 c. | 50 | — | 24 |
| 106 | endive, raw | — | 49 | 1 c. | 110 | 48 | 66 |
| 107 | kale, raw | 44 | 60 | | | | |
| | lettuce, raw | | | | | | |
| 108 | leaf or head | 34 | 37 | 1 c. | 55 | 19 | 20 |
| 109 | romaine | 60 | 179 | 1 c. | 55 | 33 | 98 |
| 110 | mushrooms, raw | 20 | 23 | 1 c. | 68 | 14 | 16 |
| 111 | okra, raw | 10 | 24 | 1 c. | 100 | 10 | 24 |
| 112 | onion, mature, dry | 10 | 25 | | | | |
| 112a | onion, mature, chopped | | | 1 c. | 170 | 17 | 42 |
| 112b | onion, mature, chopped | | | 1 Tbsp. | 10 | 1 | 2 |
| | onion, young green, raw | | | | | | |
| 113 | bulbs and white portion of top | 40 | 36 | | | | |
| 113a | bulbs and white portion of top | | | 1 c. | 100 | 40 | 36 |
| 113b | bulbs and white portion of top | | | 1 Tbsp. | 6 | 2 | 2 |
| 114 | tops only (green portion) | 52 | 80 | | | | |
| 114a | tops only (green portion), chopped | | | 1 c. | 100 | 52 | 80 |
| 114b | tops only (green portion), chopped | | | 1 Tbsp. | 6 | 3 | 5 |
| | onion, Welsh, raw | | | | | | |
| 115 | bulbs and white portion of top | 16 | 66 | | | | |
| 116 | tops only (green portion) | 49 | 105 | | | | |
| 117 | parsnips, raw | 57 | 67 | 1 c. | 130 | 74 | 87 |
| 118 | parsley, raw | 41 | 116 | 1 Tbsp. | 4 | 2 | 5 |
| 119 | peas, green, frozen | 17 | 53 | 1 c. | 145 | 25 | 77 |
| 120 | peppers, hot, mature, red, raw | 23 | 52 | 1 medium | 164 | 13 | 31 |
| 121 | peppers, sweet, immature, green, raw | 8 | 19 | 1 medium | 122 | 13 | 23 |
| | potatoes | | | | | | |
| 122 | raw | 11 | 19 | | | | |
| | cooked | | | | | | |
| 123 | French fried | 8 | 22 | 10 pieces | 50 | 4 | 11 |
| 124 | hashed brown | 3 | 17 | 1 c. | 155 | 5 | 26 |
| 125 | mashed | 5 | 10 | 1 c. | 210 | 10 | 21 |

**TABLE 10  Folacin Content of Foods in Terms of 100 gm. Edible Portion and of Specified Units\* (continued)**

| ITEM NUMBER | FOOD AND DESCRIPTION | PER 100 gm. EDIBLE PORTION | | PER SPECIFIED UNIT | | | |
|---|---|---|---|---|---|---|---|
| | | FREE FOLACIN | TOTAL FOLACIN | APPROXIMATE MEASURE | WEIGHT | FREE FOLACIN | TOTAL FOLACIN |
| | | ← mcg. → | | | gm. | ← mcg. → | |
| *Vegetables, continued* | | | | | | | |
| | pumpkin | | | | | | |
| 126 | raw | 5 | 36 | | | | |
| 127 | cooked | 2 | 19 | 1 c. | 245 | 5 | 47 |
| 128 | radishes, common, raw | 18 | 24 | 4 small | 36 | 6 | 9 |
| | rutabagas | | | | | | |
| 129 | raw | 23 | 27 | | | | |
| 130 | cooked | 9 | 21 | 1 c. | 140 | 32 | 38 |
| 130a | cooked, cubed | | | 1 c. | 170 | 15 | 36 |
| 130b | cooked, mashed | | | 1 c. | 240 | 22 | 50 |
| | spinach | | | | | | |
| 131 | raw | 119 | 193 | 1 c. | 55 | 65 | 106 |
| 132 | cooked | 60 | 91 | 1 c. | 180 | 108 | 164 |
| | squash, summer | | | | | | |
| 133 | raw | 23 | 31 | 1 c. | 130 | 30 | 40 |
| 134 | frozen, cooked | 2 | 10 | 1 c. | 210 | 4 | 21 |
| | sweet potatoes | | | | | | |
| 135 | raw | 33 | 50 | 1 medium | 146 | 48 | 73 |
| 136 | cooked | 7 | 18 | 1 medium | 146 | 10 | 26 |
| 137 | tomatoes, raw | 21 | 39 | 1 medium | 135 | 28 | 53 |
| 138 | tomato juice, canned | 10 | 26 | 1 c. | 243 | 24 | 63 |
| 138a | tomato juice, canned | | | 6-oz. glass | 182 | 18 | 47 |
| 138b | tomato juice, canned | | | 1 c. | 130 | 22 | 26 |
| 139 | turnips, raw | 17 | 20 | | | | |
| 140 | turnip greens, raw | – | 95 | 1 c. | 55 | – | 52 |

*Fruits*

| No. | | | | | Weight | | |
|---|---|---|---|---|---|---|---|
| 141 | apples, raw | 3 | 8 | 1 medium | 166 | 5 | 13 |
| 142 | applesauce, sweetened | 1 | 1 | 1 c. | 255 | 3 | 3 |
| 143 | apricots, dried | 10 | 14 | 10 halves | 35 | 4 | 5 |
| 143a | apricots, dried | | | 1 c. | 130 | 13 | 18 |
| 143b | apricots, dried | | | | | | |
| 144 | avocados, raw | 31 | 51 | ½ medium | 115 | 36 | 59 |
| 145 | bananas, raw | 22 | 28 | 1 medium | 119 | 26 | 33 |
| 146 | blueberries, raw | 2 | 6 | 1 c. | 145 | 3 | 9 |
| | cantaloupe, see muskmelon | | | | | | |
| 147 | cherries, raw | 6 | 8 | 1 c. | 117 | 7 | 9 |
| 147a | cherries, raw | | | 10 cherries | 68 | 4 | 5 |
| 177b | cherries, raw | 1 | 2 | 1 c. | 91 | 1 | 2 |
| 148 | cranberries, raw | | | | | | |
| 149 | currants, dried | | | | | | |
| 150 | dates, dried | 4 | 11 | 1 c. | 178 | 25 | 37 |
| 150a | dates, dried | | | 10 dates | 80 | 11 | 17 |
| 150b | dates, dried | | | | | | |
| 151 | figs, dried | 14 | 21 | 1 large | 21 | 1 | 2 |
| 152 | grapefruit, raw | 3 | 9 | ½ medium | 98 | 8 | 11 |
| 153 | grapefruit juice, fresh or frozen reconstituted | 8 | 11 | 1 c. | 247 | 20 | 52 |
| 153a | grapefruit juice, fresh or frozen reconstituted | | | 6-oz. glass | 185 | 15 | 39 |
| 153b | grapefruit juice, fresh or frozen reconstituted | 8 | 21 | 1 c. | 152 | 6 | 11 |
| 154 | grapes, red or white, raw | 4 | 7 | 1 c. | 253 | 5 | 5 |
| 155 | grape juice, canned or frozen reconstituted | | | | | | |
| 156 | lemon, raw | 2 | 2 | 1 medium | 74 | 9 | 9 |
| 157 | lemonade | 12 | 12 | 1 c. | 248 | 5 | 12 |
| 157a | lemonade | 2 | 5 | 6-oz. glass | 185 | 4 | 9 |
| 157b | lemonade | | | | | | |
| 158 | limes, raw | 6 | 4 | 1 lime | 67 | 4 | 3 |

**TABLE 10** Folacin Content of Foods in Terms of 100 gm. Edible Portion and of Specified Units* (continued)

| ITEM NUMBER | FOOD AND DESCRIPTION | PER 100 gm. EDIBLE PORTION | | PER SPECIFIED UNIT | | | |
|---|---|---|---|---|---|---|---|
| | | FREE FOLACIN | TOTAL FOLACIN | APPROXIMATE MEASURE | WEIGHT | FREE FOLACIN | TOTAL FOLACIN |
| | | ← mcg. → | | | gm. | ← mcg. → | |
| *Fruits, continued* | | | | | | | |
| 159 | muskmelon or cantaloupe | 30 | 30 | ½ medium | 272 | 82 | 82 |
| 160 | nectarines, raw | 7 | 5 | 1 medium | 138 | 10 | 7 |
| 161 | oranges, raw | 32 | 46 | 1 medium | 141 | 45 | 65 |
| 162 | orange juice, fresh or frozen reconstituted | 34 | 55 | | | | |
| 162a | orange juice, fresh or frozen reconstituted | | | 1 c. | 248 | 84 | 136 |
| 162b | orange juice, fresh or frozen reconstituted | | | 6-oz. glass | 185 | 63 | 102 |
| 163 | peaches, raw | 2 | 8 | 1 medium | 100 | 2 | 8 |
| 164 | pears, raw | 5 | 14 | 1 medium | 164 | 8 | 23 |
| 165 | pineapple, raw | 9 | 11 | 1 c. | 155 | 14 | 17 |
| 166 | plantain (baking banana), raw | 2 | 16 | 1 medium | 263 | 5 | 42 |
| 167 | plums, raw | 4 | 6 | 1 medium | 55 | 2 | 3 |
| 168 | prunes, dried, softenized, raw | 1 | 4 | 1 medium | 26 | <0.5 | 1 |
| 169 | raisins, natural (unbleached), raw | 3 | 4 | 1 c. | 145 | 4 | 6 |
| 170 | rhubarb, raw | 9 | 7 | 1 c. | 122 | 11 | 9 |
| 171 | strawberries, raw | 15 | 16 | 1 c. | 149 | 22 | 24 |
| 172 | tangerines, raw | 19 | 21 | 1 medium | 86 | 16 | 18 |
| 173 | watermelon, raw | 2 | 8 | 1 wedge, 4" × 8" | 426 | 9 | 34 |
| *Meat* | | | | | | | |
| | beef, separable lean | | | | | | |
| 174 | raw | 4 | 7 | | | | |
| 175 | cooked | – | 4 | 3 oz. | 85 | – | 3 |
| | beef, ground | | | | | | |

| No. | Food | | | Measure | (g) | | |
|---|---|---|---|---|---|---|---|
| 176 | raw | 3 | 7 | 3 oz. | 85 | — | 3 |
| 177 | cooked | — | 4 | | | | |
| | kidney | | | | | | |
| 178 | beef, raw | 63 | 80 | 3 oz. | 85 | — | 27 |
| | lamb | | | | | | |
| 179 | raw | 24 | 42 | 3 oz. | 85 | — | 3 |
| 180 | cooked | — | 32 | | | | |
| | lamb | | | | | | |
| 181 | raw | 1 | 4 | | | | |
| 182 | cooked | — | 3 | | | | |
| | liver | | | | | | |
| | beef, lamb, or pork | | | | | | |
| 183 | raw | 80 | 219 | 3 oz. | 85 | — | 123 |
| 184 | cooked | — | 145 | | | | |
| | pork | | | | | | |
| | separable lean | | | | | | |
| 185 | raw | 3 | 8 | 3 oz. | 85 | — | 4 |
| 186 | cooked | — | 5 | 3 oz. | 85 | — | 9 |
| 187 | ham, smoked | — | 11 | | | | |
| | veal | | | | | | |
| 188 | raw | 4 | 5 | 3 oz. | 85 | — | 3 |
| 189 | cooked | — | 3 | | | | |
| | sausages, cold cuts, and luncheon meats | | | | | | |
| 190 | beerwurst | 1 | 3 | 1 slice (1 oz.) | 28 | <0.5 | 1 |
| 191 | bologna | 2 | 5 | 1 slice (1 oz.) | 28 | 1 | 1 |
| 192 | frankfurters, unheated | 2 | 4 | 1 (5" long, ¾" diam.) | 45 | 1 | 2 |
| 193 | head cheese | 1 | 2 | 1 slice (1 oz.) | 28 | <0.5 | 1 |
| 194 | liverwurst | 20 | 30 | 1 slice (1 oz.) | 28 | 6 | 8 |
| | luncheon meats | | | | | | |

**TABLE 10  Folacin Content of Foods in Terms of 100 gm. Edible Portion and of Specified Units\* (continued)**

| ITEM NUMBER | FOOD AND DESCRIPTION | PER 100 gm. EDIBLE PORTION | | APPROXIMATE MEASURE | PER SPECIFIED UNIT | | |
| --- | --- | --- | --- | --- | --- | --- | --- |
| | | FREE FOLACIN | TOTAL FOLACIN | | WEIGHT | FREE FOLACIN | TOTAL FOLACIN |
| | | ← mcg. → | | | gm. | ← mcg. → | |
| *Meats, continued* | | | | | | | |
| 195 | boiled ham | 1 | 4 | 1 slice (1 oz.) | 28 | <0.5 | 1 |
| 196 | pork, spiced | 1 | 3 | 1 slice (1 oz.) | 28 | <0.5 | 1 |
| 197 | sausage, pork, raw | – | 14 | 3 oz. | 85 | – | 12 |
| *Poultry* | chicken, without skin | | | | | | |
| | dark meat | | | | | | |
| 198 | raw | 5 | 11 | | | | |
| 199 | cooked | – | 7 | 3 oz. | 85 | – | 6 |
| | light meat | | | | | | |
| 200 | raw | 3 | 6 | | | | |
| 201 | cooked | – | 4 | 3 oz. | 85 | – | 3 |
| | liver, chicken | | | | | | |
| 202 | raw | – | 364 | | | | |
| 203 | cooked | – | 240 | 3 oz. | 85 | – | 204 |
| | turkey, without skin | | | | | | |
| | dark meat | | | | | | |
| 204 | raw | 8 | 11 | | | | |
| 205 | cooked | – | 7 | 3 oz. | 85 | – | 6 |
| | light meat | | | | | | |
| 206 | raw | 4 | 9 | | | | |
| 207 | cooked | – | 5 | 3 oz. | 85 | – | 4 |
| *Fish and shellfish* | | | | | | | |
| 208 | cod, frozen | 6 | 18 | 3 oz. | 85 | 5 | 15 |
| 209 | crab, frozen | 2 | 20 | 3 oz. | 85 | 2 | 17 |

| No. | Food | | | Measure | | | |
|---|---|---|---|---|---|---|---|
| 210 | haddock, frozen | 4 | 10 | 3 oz. | 85 | 3 | 8 |
| 211 | halibut, frozen | 4 | 12 | 3 oz. | 85 | 3 | 10 |
| 212 | lobster, canned | 8 | 17 | 3 oz. | 85 | 7 | 14 |
| 213 | ocean perch, frozen | 5 | 9 | 3 oz. | 85 | 4 | 8 |
| | salmon | | | | | | |
| 214 | canned | 10 | 20 | 3 oz. | 85 | 8 | 17 |
| 215 | frozen | 4 | 26 | 3 oz. | 85 | 3 | 22 |
| 216 | sardines, canned | 13 | 16 | 1 fish | 12 | 2 | 2 |
| 217 | scallops, frozen | 18 | 16 | 3 oz. | 85 | 15 | 14 |
| | shrimp | | | | | | |
| 218 | canned | 8 | 15 | 3 oz. | 85 | 7 | 13 |
| 219 | frozen | 8 | 11 | 3 oz. | 85 | 7 | 9 |
| 220 | smelt, frozen | 6 | 16 | 3 oz. | 85 | 5 | 14 |
| 221 | sole, frozen | 5 | 11 | 3 oz. | 85 | 4 | 9 |
| 222 | tuna, canned | 8 | 15 | 3 oz. | 85 | 7 | 13 |

*Eggs and egg products*

| No. | Food | | | Measure | | | |
|---|---|---|---|---|---|---|---|
| | eggs | | | | | | |
| | whole | | | | | | |
| 223 | raw | 46 | 65 | 1 medium | 44 | 20 | 29 |
| 224 | hard-cooked | – | 49 | 1 medium | 44 | – | 22 |
| 225 | white, raw | 3 | 16 | 1 medium | 29 | 1 | 5 |
| 226 | yolk, raw | 121 | 152 | 1 medium | 15 | 18 | 23 |
| 227 | eggnog | <0.5 | 1 | ½ c. | 128 | – | 1 |

*Dairy products*

| No. | Food | | | Measure | | | |
|---|---|---|---|---|---|---|---|
| 228 | butter | 1 | 3 | 1 Tbsp. | 14 | <0.5 | <0.5 |
| 228a | butter | | | 1 c. | 227 | 2 | 7 |
| 228b | butter | | | | | | |
| | cheeses, natural | | | | | | |
| 229 | Cheddar | 1 | 18 | 1 c. shredded | 113 | 1 | 20 |
| 229a | Cheddar | | | 1 oz. | 28 | <0.5 | 5 |
| 229b | Cheddar | | | | | | |

TABLE 10  Folacin Content of Foods in Terms of 100 gm. Edible Portion and of Specified Units* (continued)

| ITEM NUMBER | FOOD AND DESCRIPTION | PER 100 gm. EDIBLE PORTION | | PER SPECIFIED UNIT | | | |
|---|---|---|---|---|---|---|---|
| | | FREE FOLACIN ← mcg. → | TOTAL FOLACIN | APPROXIMATE MEASURE | WEIGHT gm. | FREE FOLACIN ← mcg. → | TOTAL FOLACIN |
| *Dairy products, continued* | | | | | | | |
| 230 | cottage | — | 12 | 1 c., packed | 245 | — | 29 |
| 231 | cream | — | 13 | | | | |
| 231a | cream | | | 8-oz. pkg. | 227 | — | 30 |
| 231b | cream | | | 3-oz. pkg. | 85 | — | 11 |
| 231c | cream | | | 1 cu. in. | 16 | — | 2 |
| 232 | cheese spread, pasteurized process | 3 | 7 | 1 oz. | 28 | 1 | 2 |
| | cream, fluid | | | | | | |
| 233 | half and half | 2 | 2 | | | | |
| 233a | half and half | | | 1 c. | 242 | 5 | 5 |
| 233b | half and half | | | 1 Tbsp. | 15 | <0.5 | <0.5 |
| 234 | light coffee or table | 1 | 2 | | | | |
| 234a | light coffee or table | | | 1 c. | 240 | 2 | 5 |
| 234b | light coffee or table | | | 1 Tbsp. | 15 | <0.5 | <0.5 |
| 235 | sour, cultured | — | 11 | | | | |
| 235a | sour, cultured | | | 1 c. | 230 | — | 25 |
| 235b | sour, cultured | | | 1 Tbsp. | 12 | — | 1 |
| 236 | whipping, light | 2 | 4 | | | | |
| 236a | whipping, light | | | 1 c. | 239 | 5 | 10 |
| 236b | whipping, light | | | 1 Tbsp. | 15 | <0.5 | 1 |
| 237 | ice cream, vanilla | 2 | 2 | 1 c. | 133 | 3 | 3 |
| | milk, cow, fluid | | | | | | |
| 238 | whole, pasteurized | 5 | 5 | 1 c. | 244 | 12 | 12 |
| 239 | skim, raw | 3 | — | 1 c. | 245 | 7 | — |
| 240 | evaporated | 4 | 8 | 1 c. | 252 | 10 | 20 |
| 241 | milk, goat | 1 | 1 | 1 c. | 244 | 2 | 2 |
| 242 | milk, human | 3 | 5 | 1 fl. oz. | 31 | 1 | 2 |
| 243 | yogurt | <0.5 | 11 | 1 c. | 245 | — | 27 |

## Mixed dishes, frozen

| No. | Food | | | Measure | | | |
|---|---|---|---|---|---|---|---|
| 244 | beef with one vegetable | 2 | 5 | 1 pkg. | 254 | 5 | 13 |
| 245 | beef with two vegetables, soup, dessert | 5 | 12 | 1 pkg. | 456 | 23 | 55 |
| 246 | beef with three vegetables | 8 | 24 | 1 pkg. | 327 | 26 | 78 |
| 247 | chicken, fried, with one vegetable | 6 | 12 | 1 pkg. | 205 | 12 | 25 |
| 248 | chicken, fried, with two vegetables, dessert | 6 | 18 | 1 pkg. | 315 | 19 | 57 |
| 249 | haddock with one vegetable | 6 | 18 | 1 pkg. | 273 | 16 | 49 |
| 250 | ham with two vegetables, dessert | 5 | 15 | 1 pkg. | 314 | 16 | 47 |
| 251 | lasagna | — | 22 | 10 oz. portion | 280 | — | 62 |
| 252 | pizza cheese | — | 37 | 1/8 pie, 13¾" diam. | 65 | — | 24 |
| 253 | pepperoni | — | 38 | 1/8 pie, 13¾" diam. | 67 | — | 25 |
| 254 | sausage | — | 35 | 1/8 pie, 13¾" diam. | 67 | — | 23 |
| 255 | pork with one vegetable, one fruit, dessert | 2 | 7 | 1 pkg. | 303 | 6 | 21 |
| 256 | poultry, Oriental style with rice, vegetables | 2 | 4 | 1 pkg. | 415 | 8 | 17 |
| 257 | shrimp, Oriental style with rice, vegetables | 4 | 13 | 1 pkg. | 388 | 16 | 50 |
| 258 | shrimp with one vegetable | 8 | 14 | 1 pkg. | 264 | 21 | 37 |
| 259 | shrimp with two vegetables | 9 | 22 | 1 pkg. | 234 | 21 | 51 |
| 260 | spaghetti with meatballs, one vegetable, dessert | 6 | 18 | 1 pkg. | 354 | 21 | 64 |
| 261 | turkey with one vegetable | 4 | 11 | 1 pkg. | 264 | 11 | 29 |
| 262 | turkey with two vegetables, dessert | 6 | 14 | 1 pkg. | 346 | 21 | 48 |

**TABLE 10** Folacin Content of Foods in Terms of 100 gm. Edible Portion and of Specified Units* (continued)

| ITEM NUMBER | FOOD AND DESCRIPTION | PER 100 gm. EDIBLE PORTION | | PER SPECIFIED UNIT | | | |
|---|---|---|---|---|---|---|---|
| | | FREE FOLACIN | TOTAL FOLACIN | APPROXIMATE MEASURE | WEIGHT | FREE FOLACIN | TOTAL FOLACIN |
| | | ← mcg. → | | | gm. | ← mcg. → | |
| | *Baby foods—strained, canned* | | | | | | |
| 263 | applesauce | <0.5 | 1 | | | | |
| 263a | applesauce | | | 1 jar | 134 | — | 1 |
| 263b | applesauce | | | 1 oz. | 28 | — | <0.5 |
| 264 | apricots | <0.5 | 1 | | | | |
| 264a | apricots | | | 1 jar | 134 | — | 1 |
| 264b | apricots | | | 1 oz. | 28 | — | <0.5 |
| 265 | bananas | 1 | 2 | | | | |
| 265a | bananas | | | 1 jar | 134 | 1 | 3 |
| 265b | bananas | | | 1 oz. | 28 | <0.5 | 1 |
| 266 | beans, green or wax | 1 | 6 | | | | |
| 266a | beans, green or wax | | | 1 jar | 128 | 1 | 8 |
| 266b | beans, green or wax | | | 1 oz. | 28 | <0.5 | 2 |
| 267 | beef with broth | 1 | 6 | | | | |
| 267a | beef with broth | | | 1 jar | 99 | 1 | 6 |
| 267b | beef with broth | | | 1 oz. | 28 | <0.5 | 2 |
| 268 | beets | 2 | 10 | | | | |
| 268a | beets | | | 1 jar | 128 | 3 | 13 |
| 268b | beets | | | 1 oz. | 28 | 1 | 3 |
| 269 | carrots | 1 | 2 | | | | |
| 269a | carrots | | | 1 jar | 128 | 1 | 3 |
| 269b | carrots | | | 1 oz. | 28 | <0.5 | 1 |
| 270 | chicken with broth | 1 | 2 | | | | |
| 270a | chicken with broth | | | 1 jar | 99 | 1 | 2 |
| 270b | chicken with broth | | | 1 oz. | 28 | <0.5 | 1 |
| 271 | corn, creamed | 1 | 3 | | | | |

| No. | Food | | | Measure | Weight | | |
|---|---|---|---|---|---|---|---|
| 271a | corn, creamed | | | 1 jar | 128 | 1 | 4 |
| 271b | corn, creamed | | | 1 oz. | 28 | <0.5 | 1 |
| 272 | egg yolk | 8 | 20 | | | | |
| 272a | egg yolk | | | 1 jar | 94 | 8 | 19 |
| 272b | egg yolk | | | 1 oz. | 28 | 2 | 6 |
| 273 | fruit, mixed | 1 | 1 | | | | |
| 273a | fruit, mixed | | | 1 jar | 134 | 1 | 1 |
| 273b | fruit, mixed | | | 1 oz. | 28 | <0.5 | <0.5 |
| 274 | ham with broth | <0.5 | 6 | | | | |
| 274a | ham with broth | | | 1 jar | 99 | <0.5 | 6 |
| 274b | ham with broth | | | 1 oz. | 28 | <0.5 | 2 |
| 275 | lamb with vegetables | 1 | 8 | | | | |
| 275a | lamb with vegetables | | | 1 jar | 99 | 1 | 8 |
| 275b | lamb with vegetables | | | 1 oz. | 28 | <0.5 | 2 |
| 276 | oatmeal | — | 4 | | | | |
| 276a | oatmeal | | | 1 jar | 135 | — | 5 |
| 276b | oatmeal | | | 1 oz. | 28 | — | 1 |
| 277 | peas | 1 | 7 | | | | |
| 277a | peas | | | 1 jar | 128 | 1 | 9 |
| 277b | peas | | | 1 oz. | 28 | <0.5 | 2 |
| 278 | spinach, creamed | 2 | 4 | | | | |
| 278a | spinach, creamed | | | 1 jar | 128 | 3 | 5 |
| 278b | spinach, creamed | | | 1 oz. | 28 | 1 | 1 |

*Measure and weight apply to edible part of food only.
†Dash denotes value not available.

Taken from B. P. Perloff and R. R. Butrum, "Folacin in selected foods," *J. Amer. Dietet. Assoc.* 70: 161-69, 197.

**TABLE 11** Fiber in Breakfast Cereals

*Fiber content of breakfast cereals*

| CEREAL NAME | COMPANY | NO. SAMPLES TESTED | MOISTURE AVG (%) | NDF ("AS EATEN") AVG (%) | NDF (DRY BASIS) AVG (%) |
|---|---|---|---|---|---|
| | | DETERMINED BY THE NEUTRAL DETERGENT FIBER (NDF) METHOD | | | |
| All Bran | Kellogg | 9 | 3.3 | 28.0 | 29.0 ± 0.26 |
| Alpha Bits | General Foods | 9 | 4.6 | 1.1 | 1.2 ± 0.03 |
| Apple Jacks | Kellogg | 3 | 2.7 | 0.7 | 0.7 ± 0.05 |
| Body Buddies- Brown Sugar & Honey | General Mills | 3 | 3.6 | 0.9 | 0.9 ± 0.08 |
| 100% Bran | Nabisco | 3 | 4.4 | 28.2 | 29.5 ± 0.51 |
| | | 9 | 2.7 | 30.0 | 30.8 ± 0.31 |
| Bran Buds | Kellogg | 3 | 3.7 | 26.5 | 27.5 ± 0.89 |
| Bran Chex | Ralston Purina | 3 | 2.7 | 15.4 | 16.7 ± 0.55 |
| 40% Bran Flakes | General Foods | 9 | 7.1 | 13.7 | 14.8 ± 0.18 |
| Buc Wheats | General Mills | 3 | 5.6 | 4.6 | 4.9 ± 0.03 |
| Cap'N Crunch | Quaker | 3 | 3.7 | 1.2 | 1.2 ± 0.05 |
| Cap'N Crunch Peanut Butter | Quaker | 3 | 3.1 | 1.2 | 1.2 ± 0.04 |
| Cheerios | General Mills | 3 | 6.5 | 3.8 | 4.1 ± 0.13 |
| Cocoa Krispies | Kellogg | 3 | 2.8 | 0.3 | 0.3 ± 0.05 |
| Cocoa Pebbles | General Foods | 9 | 3.8 | 0.3 | 0.3 ± 0.03 |
| Cocoa Puffs | General Mills | 3 | 4.6 | 0.4 | 0.4 ± 0.09 |
| Cookie Crisp-Choc. Chip | Ralston Purina | 3 | 3.1 | 0.4 | 0.4 ± 0.05 |
| Cookie Crisp-Oatmeal | Ralston Purina | 3 | 2.7 | 0.6 | 0.6 ± 0.09 |
| Cookie Crisp-Vanilla | Ralston Purina | 3 | 2.4 | 0.4 | 0.4 ± 0.09 |
| Corn Bran | Quaker | 4 | 2.5 | 18.1 | 18.6 ± 0.24 |
| Corn Chex | Ralston Purina | 3 | 3.5 | 1.0 | 1.0 ± 0.21 |
| Corn Flakes | Kellogg | 3 | 4.8 | 0.5 | 0.5 ± 0.11 |
| | | 12 | 5.4 | 1.1 | 1.2 ± 0.05 |
| Corny Snaps | Kellogg | 3 | 3.4 | 0.9 | 0.9 ± 0.13 |
| Count Chocula | General Mills | 3 | 3.3 | 1.7 | 1.8 ± 0.10 |
| Country Crisp | General Foods | 9 | 5.0 | 1.0 | 1.1 ± 0.09 |

| Product | Company | n | | | |
|---|---|---|---|---|---|
| Country Morning Raisins & Dates | Kellogg | 3 | 6.9 | 2.6 | 2.8 ± 0.07 |
| Cracklin Bran | Kellogg | 3 | 3.6 | 12.2 | 12.7 ± 0.62 |
| Crazy Cow-Chocolate | General Mills | 3 | 3.5 | 0.7 | 0.7 ± 0.08 |
| Crazy Cow-Strawberry | General Mills | 3 | 4.2 | 0.7 | 0.7 ± 0.09 |
| Crunch Berries | Quaker | 3 | 3.3 | 1.1 | 1.1 ± 0.03 |
| C. W. Post | General Foods | 9 | 5.0 | 2.4 | 2.5 ± 0.05 |
| C. W. Post- Raisins | General Foods | 9 | 5.6 | 1.8 | 1.9 ± 0.19 |
| Familia (Swiss Import) | Somalon Ag | 3 | 10.7 | 6.2 | 7.0 ± 0.13 |
| Fortified Oat Flakes | General Foods | 9 | 5.8 | 2.6 | 2.8 ± 0.03 |
| Frankenberry | General Mills | 3 | 3.1 | 1.6 | 1.7 ± 0.07 |
| Frosted Flakes | Kellogg | 3 | 3.5 | 0.6 | 0.6 ± 0.09 |
| Frosted Mini-Wheats | Kellogg | 3 | 5.4 | 6.3 | 6.7 ± 0.16 |
| Frosted Mini-Wheats Brown Sugar & Cinnamon | Kellogg | 3 | 6.4 | 6.4 | 6.8 ± 0.41 |
| Frosted Rice | Kellogg | 3 | 3.5 | 0 | 0 |
| Frosted Rice Krinkles | General Foods | 9 | 4.0 | 0.1 | 0.1 ± 0.02 |
| Fruit Loops | Kellogg | 3 | 3.2 | 0.6 | 0.6 ± 0.04 |
| Fruity Pebbles | General Foods | 9 | 4.1 | 0 | 0 |
| Golden Grahams | General Mills | 3 | 4.4 | 1.7 | 1.8 ± 0.07 |
| Grape Nuts | General Foods | 9 | 6.5 | 4.8 | 5.1 ± 0.01 |
| Grape Nuts Flakes | General Foods | 9 | 6.6 | 6.4 | 6.9 ± 0.05 |
| Heartland Natural Cereal Coconut | Pet | 3 | 3.7 | 4.8 | 5.0 ± 0.23 |
| Heartland Natural Cereal Raisins | Pet | 3 | 4.5 | 4.6 | 4.8 ± 0.12 |
| Honey Combs | General Foods | 9 | 4.7 | 1.2 | 1.3 ± 0.01 |
| Kix | General Mills | 3 | 5.2 | 1.4 | 1.5 ± 0.10 |
| Life-Cinnamon | Quaker | 3 | 5.0 | 3.5 | 3.7 ± 0.12 |
| Life-Plain | Quaker | 12 | 5.5 | 3.0 | 3.2 ± 0.06 |
| Lucky Charms | General Mills | 3 | 3.6 | 2.0 | 2.1 ± 0.11 |
| Most | Kellogg | 4 | 3.8 | 11.2 | 11.7 ± 0.09 |
| 100% Natural | Quaker | 3 | 3.4 | 3.7 | 3.8 ± 0.09 |

**TABLE 11  Fiber in Breakfast Cereals (continued)**

*Fiber content of breakfast cereals*

| | | DETERMINED BY THE NEUTRAL DETERGENT FIBER (NDF) METHOD | | | |
|---|---|---|---|---|---|
| CEREAL NAME | COMPANY | NO. SAMPLES TESTED | MOISTURE AVG (%) | NDF ("AS EATEN") AVG (%) | NDF (DRY BASIS) AVG (%) |
| 100% Natural Apples & Cinnamon | Quaker | 3 | 3.2 | 4.5 | 4.7 ± 0.26 |
| 100% Natural Raisins & Dates | Quaker | 3 | 5.5 | 3.8 | 4.0 ± 1.00 |
| Natural Cereal-Plain | Giant Food | 3 | 3.3 | 4.2 | 4.4 ± 0.01 |
| Natural Cereal-Raisins | Giant Food | 3 | 5.5 | 4.4 | 4.7 ± 0.21 |
| Nature Valley Granola Cinnamon & Raisins | General Mills | 3 | 6.0 | 3.7 | 3.9 ± 0.32 |
| Nature Valley Granola Fruit & Nut | General Mills | 3 | 6.5 | 3.4 | 3.6 ± 0.03 |
| Post Toasties | General Foods | 9 | 7.1 | 1.8 | 1.9 ± 0.06 |
| Product 19 | Kellogg | 3 | 5.2 | 0.8 | 0.9 ± 0.09 |
| Protein Concentrate 40% High Quality | Kellogg | 3 | 4.2 | 1.3 | 1.4 ± 0.18 |
| Puffed Rice | Quaker | 3 | 7.1 | 0 | 0 |
| Puffed Wheat | Quaker | 3 | 6.4 | 3.4 | 3.6 ± 0.02 |
| Quisp | Quaker | 3 | 3.6 | 1.2 | 1.3 ± 0.05 |
| Raisin Bran | General Foods | 9 | 8.3 | 10.5 | 11.5 ± 0.14 |
| Raisin Bran | Kellogg | 3 | 9.2 | 8.4 | 9.3 ± 0.03 |
| Rice Chex | Ralston Purina | 3 | 3.4 | 0 | 0 |
| Rice Krispies | Kellogg | 3 | 4.0 | 0 | 0 |
| Shredded Wheat | Nabisco | 3 | 6.5 | 8.6 | 9.2 ± 0.15 |
| | | 12 | 6.7 | 9.4 | 10.0 ± 0.12 |
| Special K | Kellogg | 3 | 4.4 | 0.5 | 0.5 ± 0.01 |
| | | 12 | 5.8 | 0.8 | 0.9 ± 0.04 |

| | | | | | |
|---|---|---|---|---|---|
| Sugar Corn Pops | Kellogg | 3 | 3.2 | 0.4 | 0.4 ± 0.12 |
| Sugar Smacks | Kellogg | 3 | 4.4 | 1.0 | 1.1 ± 0.04 |
| Super Sugar Crisp | General Foods | 9 | 5.0 | 1.4 | 1.5 ± 0.05 |
| Team | Nabisco | 3 | 4.7 | 1.0 | 1.0 ± 0.05 |
| Total | General Mills | 12 | 4.9 | 6.8 | 7.2 ± 0.19 |
| | | | 5.2 | 7.0 | 7.4 ± 0.08 |
| Trix | General Mills | 3 | 4.9 | 0.5 | 0.5 ± 0.03 |
| Vita Crunch-Regular | Organic Milling Co. | 3 | 6.3 | 3.6 | 3.9 ± 0.06 |
| Vita Crunch-Almonds | Organic Milling Co. | 3 | 6.3 | 3.6 | 3.9 ± 0.06 |
| Vita Crunch-Raisins | Organic Milling Co. | 3 | 6.6 | 3.3 | 3.5 ± 0.08 |
| Wheat Chex | Ralston Purina | 3 | 3.4 | 6.8 | 7.1 ± 0.11 |
| Wheaties | General Mills | 3 | 5.6 | 6.3 | 6.7 ± 0.04 |

*Distribution of NDF Value for 81 Cereal Brands*

| NDF RANGE (DRY BASIS %) | NO. OF BRANDS | PERCENT OF TOTAL |
|---|---|---|
| 0-0.9 | 24 | 29.6 |
| 1-4.9 | 37 | 45.7 |
| 5-9.9 | 10 | 12.3 |
| 10-14.9 | 5 | 6.2 |
| 15-19.9 | 2 | 2.5 |
| 20-24.9 | 0 | 0 |
| 25-32 | 3 | 3.7 |

*Nested Analysis of Variance*

| VARIANCE SOURCE | PERCENT |
|---|---|
| Total | 100.0 |
| Brand name | 99.70 |
| Lot | 0.20 |
| Box | 0.05 |
| Analytical error | 0.05 |

Tables taken from D. Baker and J. M. Holden, "Fiber in breakfast cereals," *J. Food Sci.* 46: 396-98, 1981.

**TABLE 12** Vitamin $B_6$ Contents of Edible Portions of Food Items "as Served"*

| FOOD ITEM | RECIPE REFERENCE | NUMBER OF SAMPLES | VITAMIN $B_6$ | |
|---|---|---|---|---|
| | | | MEAN | RANGE |
| | | | mg/100gm | |
| *Cereal-based item* | | | | |
| biscuits, baking powder | D-1 (2) | 2 | 0.029 | 0.028-0.030 |
| bread | | | | |
| cornbread, southern style | D-14 | 2 | 0.081 | 0.064-0.098 |
| French, garlic toasted | D-7 | 3 | 0.027 | 0.000-0.060 |
| French toast | D-7 (2) | 4 | 0.036 | 0.023-0.058 |
| white | D-8 (2) | 3 | 0.035 | 0.018-0.054 |
| cake | | | | |
| applesauce | G-2 | 4 | 0.050 | 0.017-0.109 |
| gingerbread | G-17 (1) | 2 | 0.012 | 0.000-0.023 |
| peanut butter | G-20 | 2 | 0.165 | 0.160-0.170 |
| pound | G-21 (2) | 2 | 0.022 | 0.017-0.028 |
| cookies—butterscotch brownies | H-3 (2) | 2 | 0.230 | 0.155-0.305 |
| macaroni and cheese, baked | F-1 (2) | 5 | 0.023 | 0.012-0.034 |
| muffins, plain | D-30 | 2 | 0.019 | 0.000-0.038 |
| noodles | | | | |
| chow mein, canned | | 2 | 0.069 | 0.066-0.073 |
| egg, enriched | | 3 | 0.007 | 0.000-0.021 |
| pancakes | D-25 (2) | 2 | 0.020 | 0.014-0.026 |
| pie | | | | |
| blueberry | I-53-1 | 3 | 0.037 | 0.028-0.045 |
| chocolate cream | I-28 | 2 | 0.027 | 0.025-0.029 |
| pumpkin | I-45 | 3 | 0.057 | 0.030-0.075 |
| pizza, cheese and Italian sausage | D-31 (1)-6 | 2 | 0.108 | 0.102-0.114 |
| rice, fried, with pork and eggs (oven method) | E-7 (1) | 4 | 0.127 | 0.060-0.233 |
| spaghetti with meatball sauce | E-4 | 4 | 0.185 | 0.115-0.296 |
| waffles, baked (same as for pancakes above) | D-25 (2) | 2 | 0.038 | 0.037-0.040 |

| | | | | |
|---|---|---|---|---|
| *Eggs and dairy* | | | | |
| eggs, chicken—fried (griddle) | F-10 (2) | 2 | 0.082 | 0.075-0.090 |
| milk | | | | |
| cow, chocolate, 2% fat (vitamin A and D, and protein fortified) | | 2 | 0.034 | 0.030-0.037 |
| cow, whole (vitamin D fortified) | | 2 | 0.028 | 0.023-0.032 |
| *Fruits* | | | | |
| cantaloupe(s), raw | | 2 | 0.055 | 0.055-0.055 |
| cranberries, sauce | | 2 | 0.014 | 0.014-0.015 |
| grape(s), raw | | 2 | 0.126 | 0.122-0.131 |
| salads | | | | |
| cottage cheese and peach | M-13 (2) | 2 | 0.022 | 0.018-0.027 |
| jellied carrots and pineapples "Golden Glow" | M-20 | 2 | 0.011 | 0.008-0.014 |
| jellied fruit cocktail | M-26 (2) | 2 | 0.000 | 0.000-0.000 |
| *Meats, poultry, and fish* | | | | |
| beef (entrée) | | | | |
| chili con carne without beans | L-59 | 2 | 0.129 | 0.108-0.150 |
| corned, medium fat, simmered | L-44 | 2 | 0.148 | 0.138-0.157 |
| corned, hash | L-42 | 2 | 0.242 | 0.231-0.252 |
| ground, creamed | L-30 | 3 | 0.098 | 0.081-0.130 |
| liver, braised (analyzed without onions) | L-54 | 2 | 0.312 | 0.172-0.452 |
| meatballs, Swedish | L-41 (1) | 5 | 0.185 | 0.040-0.316 |
| rib roast, 70% lean | L-4 | 3 | 0.143 | 0.071-0.237 |
| round, Swiss steak with tomato sauce | L-16 (1) | 2 | 0.153 | 0.130-0.175 |
| sloppy Joe (barbecued beef sandwich, without bun) | N-27 | 2 | 0.170 | 0.115-0.224 |
| stuffed green peppers | L-40 (1) | 3 | 0.218 | 0.016-0.336 |
| chicken pot pie | L-132 (1) | 2 | 0.086 | 0.067-0.105 |

**TABLE 12** Vitamin B$_6$ Contents of Edible Portions of Food Items "as Served"* (continued)

| FOOD ITEM | RECIPE REFERENCE† | NUMBER OF SAMPLES | VITAMIN B$_6$ MEAN mg/100gm | RANGE |
|---|---|---|---|---|
| *Meats, poultry and fish, continued* | | | | |
| pork | | | | |
| chop suey | L-80 (1) | 2 | 0.207 | 0.104-0.310 |
| ham, fresh, 72% lean, roast | L-72 | 3 | 0.259 | 0.147-0.367 |
| ham steaks, fried | L-65 (2)-2 | 2 | 0.268 | 0.266-0.270 |
| loin, barbecued | L-79 (1) | 3 | 0.281 | 0.223-0.340 |
| loin slices (pork chops) | L-83 | 2 | 0.673 | 0.504-0.841 |
| sweet and sour | L-82 (1) | 2 | 0.129 | 0.097-0.161 |
| sausage | | | | |
| Knockwurst, simmered | L-63-2 | 2 | 0.147 | 0.057-0.236 |
| pork, grilled (frozen, precooked) | L-91 | 2 | 0.378 | 0.050-0.707 |
| sandwiches | | | | |
| cheeseburger with bun | N-29 | 2 | 0.095 | 0.061-0.129 |
| roast beef | N-4 | 5 | 0.263 | 0.145-0.385 |
| submarine | N-19 | 2 | 0.059 | 0.053-0.064 |
| turkey à la King | L-129 (1) | 2 | 0.253 | 0.159-0.347 |
| veal steaks, breaded | L-99 | 2 | 0.181 | 0.125-0.237 |
| fish filets, fried | L-109 | 5 | 0.153 | 0.037-0.379 |
| *Soups* | | | | |
| beef barley | P-1-1 | 2 | 0.014 | 0.011-0.016 |
| clam chowder, Manhattan style | P-12-1 | 2 | 0.054 | 0.046-0.063 |
| *Vegetables* | | | | |
| asparagus, buttered (frozen; buttered after boiled and drained) | Q-G-3 | 3 | 0.020 | 0.012-0.025 |
| beans | | | | |
| yellow wax, buttered (frozen, buttered after boiled and drained) | Q-G-3 | 3 | 0.029 | 0.016-0.041 |
| white, baked | Q-2 | 3 | 0.134 | 0.105-0.170 |

| | | | | |
|---|---|---|---|---|
| Brussels sprouts, buttered (frozen; boiled and drained) | Q-G-3 | 3 | 0.301 | 0.206-0.435 |
| cauliflower, French fried | Q-20 | 2 | 0.057 | 0.044-0.070 |
| corn, on-the-cob, buttered (frozen; buttered after boiled and drained) | Q-G-3 | 3 | 0.224 | 0.062-0.475 |
| peas, buttered (green, frozen; buttered after boiled and drained) | Q-G-3 | 2 | 0.109 | 0.073-0.145 |
| potatoes | | | | |
| baked in skin (analyzed without skin) | Q-44 | 2 | 0.138 | 0.104-0.172 |
| hashed brown | Q-46 | 2 | 0.272 | 0.206-0.338 |
| oven browned | Q-50 | 3 | 0.304 | 0.225-0.352 |
| salads | | | | |
| chef's, with lunch meat and cheese | M-7 (1) | 4 | 0.088 | 0.047-0.130 |
| coleslaw with creamy dressing | M-9 | 6 | 0.126 | 0.054-0.309 |
| kidney bean | M-31 | 7 | 0.036 | 0.020-0.100 |
| potato | M-40 (1) | 2 | 0.141 | 0.059-0.223 |
| tossed green | M-47 | 7 | 0.050 | 0.034-0.060 |
| spinach, buttered (frozen: buttered after boiled and drained) | Q-G-3 | 5 | 0.140 | 0.050-0.268 |
| squash, buttered (fresh, summer; buttered after boiled and drained) | Q-G-2 | 3 | 0.036 | 0.019-0.061 |
| succotash, buttered | Q-65 | 2 | 0.116 | 0.099-0.133 |
| sweet potatoes, with marshmallows | Q-69 | 2 | 0.059 | 0.049-0.069 |
| tomato(es) | | | | |
| juice | | 2 | 0.132 | 0.109-0.154 |
| seasoned (ripe, canned; seasoned after boiled and drained) | Q-G-1 | 2 | 0.138 | 0.099-0.176 |
| scalloped | Q-72 | 2 | 0.066 | 0.050-0.081 |
| vegetables, mixed, buttered (frozen: buttered after boiled and drained) | Q-G-3 | 2 | 0.075 | 0.061-0.088 |

*Time lapse between foods prepared and foods served ranged from 30 min. to 1½ hr.

**TABLE 13  Magnesium Content of Foodstuffs**

| FOOD | mg Mg per 100g |
|------|---------------|
| Apricot nectar juice, canned | 6.2 |
| Barbecue sauce, commercially prepared | 5.5 |
| Beef, chipped, dry | 37.6 |
| Beef stew, homemade with vegetables | 17.2 |
| Beverages, carbonated: | |
|   Club soda | 0.6 |
|   Cola: | |
|     (Coca Cola) | 1.7 |
|     (Pepsi) | 0.5 |
|   Grape | 0.7 |
|   Lemon: | |
|     (Seven Up) | 0.7 |
|     (Sprite) | 1.3 |
|   Orange | 1.7 |
|   Root beer | 1.5 |
| Bouillon cubes: | |
|   Beef | 31.0 |
|   Chicken | 8.9 |
| Bun: | |
|   Hamburger, enriched | 20.5 |
|   Hot dog, enriched | 19.8 |
| Butterscotch sauce, commercially prepared | 6.7 |
| Cabbage, Chinese, raw | 14.0 |
| Cabbage, red, raw | 13.8 |
| Cabbage, white: | |
|   Raw | 13.5 |
|   Cooked, drained | 6.3 |
| Cake, commercially prepared: | |
|   Sponge with cream filling | 7.5 |
|   Chocolate with fudge icing and cream filling | 42.2 |
|   Roll of chocolate and cream filling coated | |
|     with fudge icing | 39.5 |
| Candy: | |
|   Nougat, caramel, and peanut bar coated with | |
|     chocolate (Snickers) | 52.8 |
|   Chocolate bar with rice puffs | 51.9 |
|   Chocolate caramel roll (Tootsie Roll) | 31.8 |
|   Licorice-flavored sticks: | |
|     Red | 21.8 |
|     Black | 78.0 |
|   Peanut & nougat bar coated with chocolate (Baby Ruth) | 89.9 |
|   Malted milk balls | 55.3 |
|   Peanut butter & chocolate cup | 84.6 |
|   Nougat & caramel bar coated with chocolate: | |
|     (Milky Way) | 31.9 |
|     (Milk Shake) | 31.2 |
| Carrots, cooked, drained | 12.5 |

TABLE 13   Magnesium Content of Foodstuffs (continued)

| FOOD | mg Mg per 100g |
|---|---|
| Cereal, ready-to-eat breakfast: | |
|   Presweetened: | |
|     Corn, fruit-flavored, nutrients added (Trix) | 24.9 |
|     Corn, nutrients added (Quisp) | 40.8 |
|     Corn & graham flour, nutrients added (Golden Grahams) | 40.8 |
|     Corn & oat: | |
|       Nutrients added: | |
|       (Captain Crunch) | 37.2 |
|       (Honey Comb) | 33.7 |
|       Vitamin and mineral supplement (King Vitamin) | 34.3 |
|     Corn, wheat, & oat, nutrients added: | |
|       Apple flavored (Apple Jacks) | 23.1 |
|       Fruit flavored (Fruit Loops) | 26.8 |
|     Oat & corn, nutrients added (Alphabits) | 57.7 |
|     Oat & corn, blueberry flavored, nutrients added (Boo Berry) | 56.5 |
|     Oat, soy protein concentrate, sodium caseinate, nutrients added (Life) | 32.4 |
|     Rice puffs, cocoa-flavored, nutrients added (Cocoa Pebbles) | 31.5 |
|   Unsweetened: | |
|     Corn, nutrients added (Corn Chex) | 10.6 |
|     Corn, oat, wheat, & Rice flakes, vitamin and iron supplement (Product 19) | 31.4 |
|     Rice, nutrients added (Rice Chex) | 24.6 |
|     Wheat flakes, nutrients added (Wheaties) | 102.2 |
|     Wheat & malted barley granules, nutrients added (Grape Nuts) | 67.0 |
| Cheese: | |
|   Cream | 6.8 |
|   Mozzarella | 21.9 |
|   Spread, pasteurized, canned | 25.2 |
| Chicken, canned, deboned | 12.3 |
| Chicken pot pie, commercially prepared, frozen | 11.1 |
| Chocolate chips, semisweet | 119.2 |
| Cocoa beverages powder mix, without milk powder | 70.1 |
| Cone, ice cream, regular | 26.0 |
| Cookies: | |
|   Brownies, commercially prepared | 39.3 |
|   Caramel-peanut log coated with chocolate, commercially prepared | 63.6 |
|   Chocolate coveraged graham crackers | 41.2 |
|   Chocolate sandwich with vanilla filling, commercially prepared | 50.8 |
|   Ginger, commercially prepared | 53.2 |
|   Oatmeal, commercially prepared | 50.8 |
|   Peanut butter, homemade | 38.5 |
|   Sugar, soft, commercially prepared | 13.1 |
|   Sugar wafer | 8.9 |
| Corn bread, homemade | 32.8 |
| Corn chips | 77.4 |
| Corn & cheese snack curls | 32.0 |
| Crackers: | |
|   Cheese | 26.1 |
|   Melba toast | 62.7 |
|   Wheat, rye, malted barley (Ritz) | 22.1 |

## TABLE 13 Magnesium Content of Foodstuffs (continued)

| FOOD | mg Mg per 100g |
|---|---|
| Cream substitute, dried | 4.1 |
| Croutons, commercially prepared | 33.2 |
| Doughnut, cake-type | 22.5 |
| Egg: | |
| Hard cooked | 12.2 |
| Scrambled | 10.9 |
| Fish sticks, frozen, raw | 24.0 |
| Frozen desserts: | |
| Vanilla ice cream bar with chocolate coating | 18.4 |
| Fudge bar | 24.7 |
| Fruit punch: | |
| Orange, canned, vitamin C fortified | 3.3 |
| Tropical mixture, canned, vitamin C fortified | 4.1 |
| Tropical mixture, powder | 1.7 |
| Gelatin dessert with peaches | 2.7 |
| Gravy mix: | |
| Beef, dried | 56.2 |
| Chicken, dried | 37.8 |
| Gum, peppermint | 17.9 |
| Fish: | |
| Haddock, fillet, frozen, raw | 24.0 |
| Herring, fake fillet | 24.0 |
| Ice cream, chocolate | 22.8 |
| Jelly, apple | 3.9 |
| Macaroni & Cheese, homemade | 20.2 |
| Macaroni salad, homemade | 22.4 |
| Macaroni shells, dried, enriched | 40.8 |
| Marshmallows | 3.8 |
| Milk: | |
| 25% Fat, dry milk solids added | 11.6 |
| Nonfat dry milk solids & vegetable oil, canned (Milnot) | 25.7 |
| Muffin, English | 18.0 |
| Noodles, enriched, dry | 126.0 |
| Onion, green, raw | 20.6 |
| Orange juice, dehydrated crystals | 2.2 |
| Pastry, commercially prepared: | |
| Apple, thawed and baked | 4.6 |
| Blueberry jam, toaster-sized | 18.2 |
| Cherry, individual | 9.3 |
| Chocolate, toaster-sized | 41.3 |
| Peas, green, cooked, drained | 17.6 |
| Popcorn: | |
| Whole kernel | 156.2 |
| Caramel covered, commercially prepared | 83.8 |
| Potato: | |
| Baked | 18.2 |
| Chips made from minced potatoes | 54.6 |
| Mashed, homemade | 14.1 |
| Scalloped, homemade | 6.8 |

**TABLE 13   Magnesium Content of Foodstuffs (continued)**

| FOOD | mg Mg per 100g |
|---|---|
| Pretzels | 24.3 |
| Pudding, commercially prepared, canned: | |
|    Butterscotch | 9.5 |
|    Chocolate | 18.6 |
|    Vanilla | 8.0 |
| Rennet tablets | 10.4 |
| Roll, cinnamon Danish | 19.8 |
| Salad dressing, thousand island | 5.6 |
| Sausage: | |
|    Beef, hard | 14.9 |
|    Bologna, all meat | 13.6 |
|    Frankfurter, raw | 13.2 |
|    "Old-fashioned" loaf, with olives and pimentos | 21.3 |
|    Polish | 16.6 |
|    Pork, chopped, spiced, canned | 15.2 |
|    Pork, raw, patties | 9.8 |
|    Salami | 10.9 |
| Seaweed, canned with sugar & soy sauce | 116.0 |
| Sherbet, orange | 4.7 |
| Soup: | |
|    Chicken noodle, canned, condensed | 10.4 |
|    Cream of celery, canned, condensed | 6.2 |
|    Cream of mushroom, canned, condensed | 4.6 |
|    Vegetable, homemade | 10.8 |
| Syrup: | |
|    Maple | 23.5 |
|    Table, cane & maple | 3.4 |
| Taco shell | 103.9 |
| Topioca, dry | 3.8 |
| Tartar sauce, commercially prepared | 3.2 |
| Topping mixture, whipped cream substitute, dried | 14.2 |
| Turnips, cooked, drained | 6.7 |
| Wheat starch | 1.5 |
| Worcestershire sauce | 14.7 |

Taken from J. L. Greber, S. Marhefka, and A. H. Geissler, "A Research Note. Magnesium Content of Selected Foods," *J. Food Sci.* 43(5): 1610-12, 1978.

TABLE 14  Distribution of Magnesium in Foods Classified into Food Groups

| FOOD GROUP | NO. OF SAMPLES | MAGNESIUM CONCENTRATION | | | |
|---|---|---|---|---|---|
| | | mg/100g WET WT | | $\mu$g/KILOCALORIES | |
| | | MEAN ± S.E.M. | RANGE | MEAN ± S.E.M. | RANGE |
| Milk products (cheese, ice cream, milks, puddings) | 9 | 16.7 ± 2.6 | 6.8-25.7 | 108 ± 21 | 18-198 |
| Meat & meat alternates (chicken, dried beef, eggs, fish, sausages) | 15 | 16.9 ± 1.9 | 9.8-37.6 | 93 ± 24 | 20-353 |
| Vegetables (cabbages, carrot, onion, potato, turnip) | 7 | 14.2 ± 2.2 | 6.7-20.6 | 495 ± 107 | 196-1000 |
| Breads and Cereals (buns, cereals, cornbread, crackers, croutons, English muffin, pasta, taco shells) | 28 | 42.2 ± 5.4 | 10.6-126.0 | 112 ± 14 | 27-325 |
| Baked desserts (cakes, cookies, doughnuts, pastries, sweet rolls) | 16 | 28.9 ± 4.6 | 4.6-53.2 | 86 ± 18 | 18-307 |
| Candies (chocolates, licorice) | 11 | 52.9 ± 7.7 | 21.8-89.9 | 117 ± 16 | 63-225 |

# Answer Key

## Chapter One

1. a–g inclusive are right
2. 75 percent

3. < 5%

4. b and c
5. i—a, f
   ii—b, e
   iii—c, d

## Chapter Two

1. a, c, d
2. a, c, d
3. a, b, d

4. b, c, d
5. b, c, d
6. d, e

## Chapter Three

1. a, b, c, e
2. a, b, c
3. b, c, e

4. Institutionalized: a, d, e
   Hospitalized or
   Institutionalized: b, c, f
5. True: d, e

## Chapter Four

1. e
2. b, e
3. e

4. b
5. a, b, c, d

## Chapter Five

1. True: a, c, e
2. True: a, b, c
3. a–d do; e do not
4. a—iv; b—ii; d—i; e—iii
5. b, c e

## Chapter Six

1. a—iv; b—iii; c—iii;d—v; e—i
2. Symptoms: a, b, e, g, i
   Signs: c, d, f, h, j
3. a) skinfold thickness
   b) hemoglobin
   c) blood count—automated
   d) riboflavin status
   e) cellular immune function
4. b, d, e
5. a

## Chapter Seven

1. c, d, e
2. a
3. a—iii; b—i; c—ii
4. Acute: a, c, e, g, h
   Chronic: b, d, f, i, j
5. a) thiamin
   b) vitamin C
   c) vitamin D
   d) niacin
   e) vitamin $B_{12}$

## Chapter Eight

1. a, b, d, e
2. a, c, d, e
3. a, c, d, e
4. a, c, d
5. c

## Chapter Nine

1. b, c, d, e
2. c, d, e
3. a, c
4. a, b, c, d, e
5. c, d

## Chapter Ten

1. a, b, c, e
2. b, c
3. a—iii; b—i; c—ii; d—v; e—iv
4. a, b, d, e
5. b, d, e

# Class Projects

1. Students visit an elderly individual in the community or in an institution to find out about this person's life and about the circumstances which have determined his or her present situation. The individual is questioned about food purchases, preparation, and diet. Following the informed consent of this individual, a conversation is taped between the individual and the student or between the individual, the caregiver and the student which can be played back in class and used for instructional purposes. The elderly client or patient can be selected by the instructor or by the student with approval from the instructor.

   Practical experience has shown that these tapes have their greatest teaching value when the instructor plans discussion of:

   a. History taking.
   b. Difficulties the elderly may have in obtaining food.
   c. Problems of dietary assessment in the elderly.
   d. Determinants of independent living.

   Students should give a short preamble before playing their tape to explain whom they were interviewing, their relationship, if any, to this individual, where and when interview took place, and the constraints on the interviewing process.

2. A senior citizen comes to the class and participates in a discussion group. Best use of this is when the senior is particularly interested in the subject to be discussed and wants information on a nutrition or diet-related problem.

3.  Students take supervised field trips to

    a. A skilled nursing home.
    b. An intermediate care home.
    c. A domiciliary care unit.

    Visits are planned to include attendance at staff meetings where patient care plans are discussed (including dietary), observations of patients or residents at meal times, inspection of kitchen facilities, menus and recipe manual, and meeting with staff members including dietary staff, nurses, physical therapist, occupational therapist, social worker, and physician.

4.  Students prepare and give an in-service instruction on a nutrition-related topic to:

    a. Home health aides (working with geriatric patients).
    b. Meals-on-Wheels driver/volunteer.

5.  Students conduct a discussion group at the Senior Citizens Center on a nutrition topic chosen by the audience.

6.  Students give brief nutrition talks at a congregate meal center.

    Appropriate topics are:

    a. How to avoid high sodium intake.
    b. What foods are rich sources of potassium and why you need them.
    c. Good buys at the supermarket.
    d. How to understand food labels (with a magnifying glass).
    e. Why's and wherefore's of dietary fiber.

7.  Students prepare a diet instruction for an elderly patient who is:

    a. A diabetic.
    b. Constipated.
    c. A cardiac patient recently discharged from the hospital with congestive heart failure.

8.  Students deliver Meals-on-Wheels.

9.  Students spend a day with the public health nurse visiting elderly patients.

10. Students visit the Office for the Aging to find out about local services, state and federal services for the elderly, and the characteristics of the population over 65 years of age in their community.

# Essay Questions

Questions are based on an assigned text or case history.

Students are expected to solve one or more than one essay-type problem(s) following classroom instruction based on specific chapters of the book. Problem-solving abilities that should be acquired through these exercises include:

1. Knowing how to assess the coping skills of elderly clients and patients.
2. Being able to explain the difference between the aging process and diseases commonly occurring in the elderly.
3. Showing why geriatric diseases can increase the susceptibility of the elderly to nutritional disorders.
4. Understanding nutritional survey methods.
5. Finding the means to assess the nutritional needs of geriatric patients.
6. Deciding why the older patients change their eating habits.
7. Knowing how to measure food intake in the elderly.
8. Understanding how to select reliable methods for geriatric nutritional assessment.
9. Knowing the signs of nutritional deficiencies.
10. Being able to plan practical diets for the elderly including those who need to lose weight, those who are constipated, and those who are likely to develop congestive heart failure.
11. Having the competency to examine orders for medications and decide whether one or more of the drugs prescribed could be causing an eating disorder or a nutritional deficiency.
12. Being able to offer advice to elderly patients on food distribution programs or other nutrition support services in your area.

## Questions

1. A 68-year-old man complained of increasing fatigue, and numbness of the extremities. Neurological examination showed absence of deep-tendon reflexes and diminished vibratory and proprioceptive sensation in all extremities. The hemoglobin level was 5.4 g/dl, leukocyte count was $2.2 \times 10^9 1$, and platelet count was $150 \times 10^9 1$. The blood smear showed hypersegmented granulocytes. Aspirated marrow demonstrated marked megaloblastosis. The MCV was 125 fl. The serum cobalamin level was 42 pg/ml and the serum folate level was 14.4 ng/ml. Schilling's test results were compatible with absence of instrinsic factor.

   What is the diagnosis? Discuss the relationship between this patient's nutritional deficiency and the aging process. Describe the Schilling test.

2. A 74-year-old man was admitted to hospital because of peripheral edema, diarrhea, anorexia, polydipsia, and a loss of 5 kg in weight. The urine gave a 4+ test for protein. The serum creatinine was 1.4 mg/100 ml. Serum albumin was 1.8 g/100 ml on angiographic examination, and a large vascular mass was found in the lower pole of the right kidney.

   Explain what further nutritional assessment you would like to carry out and justify your choice of tests. What are the possible causes of malnutrition in this patient?

   On the basis of the findings given in the case history, what is the nutritional diagnosis? What could cause polydipsia?

3. Discuss the major constraints on the provision of Recommended Dietary Allowances for men and women who are $\geq 75$ years of age.

4. You are asked to make recommendations on where a 76-year-old man should go after his discharge from an acute care hospital where he has been treated for congestive heart failure. His physician has prescribed a strict low-sodium diet.

   Discuss the factors that would influence you in deciding whether he should be discharged to his own home or sent to a geriatric care facility.

5. Following the death of her husband, Mrs. Brown, who is 72, goes to live with her son and daughter-in-law. In the next three months she loses 25 pounds in weight. The daughter-in-law becomes concerned because of the weight loss and because she notices that Mrs. Brown is "not eating her meals" and seems to have "no appetite."

   How would you investigate the causes of weight loss and anorexia in this woman?

6. In a grant application, a physician states that he intends to study the caloric and nutrient intakes of a group of homebound elderly women using a 7-day dietary record. You are asked to comment on his proposed methodology and to offer an alternate method for dietary assessment of this sample population.

   Write a critique of his proposal, indicating why you have reservations about this method, and why you are suggesting another way of obtaining the necessary dietary information.

7. In an intermediate care facility, where patients eat their meals in a communal dining room, 10 of the 50 patients are found to be anemic at a time when routine blood counts are performed. Further investigation shows that 6 other patients in the facility have been found to be anemic during the past 6 months. None of these patients have had acute or chronic bleed-

ing. Iron supplements have been given, but the anemia failed to respond. In the first 6 patients found to be anemic, the blood count returned to normal after a course of B vitamins.

You are asked to find the cause of the anemia and also to find out whether the anemia could be related to the patient's diet. Explain your plan of approach to the problem and the diagnostic methods you would employ to characterize the anemia.

8. Abnormal lab reports are often overlooked in nursing homes. Since physicians may not be able to visit geriatric facilities daily, a system has been proposed by which a physician's assistant would be trained to visit each area facility daily to check lab reports for grossly abnormal values which require prompt attention. The assistant would then notify the doctor of serious hypokalemia. (Isiadinso, O.O.A. Physician's Assistant in Geriatric Medicine. *NYS J. Med.* 78: 1069−1071, 1979.)

Discuss causes of these metabolic abnormalities commonly occurring in the nursing home population.

9. *The New York Times,* May 13, 1981:

While there is no guarantee that changing your life for the sake of your health will keep you hale and hearty for the biblical three-score and ten or longer, you can certainly increase the odds of living a long and healthy life by reducing the life-style risks most strongly associated with premature death and disability. And the changes involved need not diminish the pleasures of living, though they sometimes mean exchanging one source of pleasure for another.

Give a concise account of the "life-style risks" related to nutrition and the diet which you believe are most strongly associated with premature death and disability.

10. Mr. Jones has been given a low fat, low cholesterol diet after his second myocardial infarct. Two months later he develops severe athlete's foot, for which griseofulvin is prescribed by a dermatologist. When Mr. Jones returns to the dermatologist for follow-up, he complains that his athlete's foot has not improved. Assuming that Mr. Jones has been careful to take the griseofulvin after his breakfast and dinner, explain why you think his condition has not gotten any better.

11. You have been asked to give four fifteen-minute talks on nutrition at the nearby Title III Congregate Meal Center. Choose four topics which you would like to discuss with this audience and explain the goal and plan of each talk.

12. A number of different support services are available which allow homebound elderly to live more or less independently. Discuss alternate means whereby food purchase and preparation may be provided for handicapped people.

# Resource Materials

Reference texts, manuals and supplementary teaching aids

### Gerontology

MASCRO, E.J., ed., *CRC Handbook of Physiology in Aging*. Boca Raton, Florida: CRC Press, Inc., in press.

SLESINGER, D.P., M. McDIVITT, and F.M. O'DONNELL, "Food Patterns in an urban population: age and sociodemographic correlates," *J. Gerontol.*, 35 (1980), 432–41.

WILLIAMSON, J.B., H. MUNLEY, and L. EVANS, *Aging and Society*. Chicago: Holt, Rinehart and Winston, 1980.

### Drugs

KAYNE, R.C., ed., *Drugs and the Elderly*. Univ. Calif. Press, 1978.

*Physician's Desk Reference for Non-Prescription Drugs*. Oradell, N.J. 07649: Medical Economics Corp., 1980.

RAFFAEL, P.R., J.K. COOPER, and D.W. LOVE, "Drug misuse in older people," *The Gerontologist*, 21 (1981), 146–50.

### Nursing Homes

KAHN, K.A., W. HINES, A.S. WOODSON, and G.B. ARMSTRONG, "A multidisciplinary approach to assessing the quality of care in long term care facilities," *The Gerontologist*, 17 (1977), 61–66.

### Health Status

AKHTAR, A.J.. and G.A. BROE, "Disability and dependence in the elderly at home," *Age and Aging*, 2 (1973), 102.

LAWRENCE, P.S., "Patterns of health and illness in older people," *Bull. N.Y. Acad. Sci.*, 49 (1973), 1100.

SHANAS, E., "Health status of older people. Cross-national implications," *Amer. J. Public Health*, 64 (1974), 261–64.

## Functional Assessment

HABER, L.D., "Identifying the disabled: concepts and methods in the measurement of disability," *Soc. Sci. Bull.*, 30 (1967), 17–34.
LAWTON, M.P., "Functional assessment of elderly people," *J. Amer. Geriat. Soc.*, 19 (1971), 465–81.

## Nutrition

### Nutrient Requirements

MUNRO, H.N., "Nutrition and Aging," *Brit. Med. Bull.*, 37 (1981), 83–88.

### Bibliography

METRESS, S.P., and C.S. KART, *Nutrition and Aging: A Bibliographical Survey.* Vance Bibliographers, Box 229, Monticello, IL 61856.

### Programs

HARPER, J.M., G.R. JANSEN, C.T. SHIGETAMI, and A.L. FREY, "Menu planning in nutrition programs for the elderly," *J. Amer. Dietet. Assoc.*, 68 (1976), 529–34.
KOHRS, M.B., "Recommendations for nutrition programs for the elderly," *J. Amer. Dietet. Assoc.*, 75 (1979), 543–46.

## Medical Ethics

BUTLER, R.N., "Protection of elderly research subjects," *Clin. Res.*, 28 (1980), 3–5.

## Food and Special Diets

COALE, M., Meal Planning and Exchange Lists. 80 slides. Audiocassette, 22 min. script. $60. Dept. of Family Practice, Med. Univ. South Carolina, 171 Asley Ave., Charleston, S.C. 29403.
Diabetes Education Center, Convenience Food Lists, 1979. 4959 Excelsior Blvd., Minneapolis, MN 55416.
General Mills. Meal Planning for the Golden Years. Rev. 1979. Box 1113, Minneapolis, MN 55416.
Illinois Nutrition Educators. Expanded Guide to Meal Planning, 1979. Box 1386, Evanston, IL 60204.
National Academy of Sciences. Sodium-Restricted Diets and the Use of Diuretics, 1979. 2101 Constitution Ave., N.W., Washington, D.C.

# Glossary of Medical Terms

**Alzheimer's disease**  Presenile dementia
**ariboflavinosis**  Riboflavin deficiency
**ataxia muscular incoordination**  Loss of ability to walk straight
**cachexia**  Wasting
**candidiasis**  Yeast infection
**cheilitis**  Inflammation of the lips
**cheilosis**  Redness and fissuring of lips associated with B vitamin deficiency
**cirrhosis**  Replacement of liver cells with fibrous tissue—commonly, alcohol-related liver disease
**cor pulmonale**  Heart condition secondary to chronic disease of the lungs
**decubitus ulcer**  Bed sore
**dermatitis**  Inflammation of the skin
**dermatosis**  Skin disease
**diverticulitis**  Inflammation of one or more colonic or diverticula
**diverticulosis**  Condition of the colon associated with single or multiple diverticula pouches
**dyspnea**  Breathlessness
**emphysema**  Condition in which the air sacs in the lungs become distended or ruptured
**glossitis**  Inflammation or loss of normal surface of the tongue
**gluten-sensitive enteropathy** (*syn.* **celiac-sprue syndrome**)  Malabsorption syndrome due to gluten intolerance
**hemiplegia**  Paralysis of one side of the body
**hemolysis**  Destruction of red blood cells
**icterus**  Jaundice
**intertrigo**  Superficial dermatitis of folds of skin

**koilonychia**   Spoon-shaped nails associated with iron deficiency

**metastasis**   Deposit of cancer in a secondary location

**myxedema**   Condition associated with failure of thyroid function

**neoplastic disease**   Cancer

**Parkinson's disease**   Chronic disease of the central nervous system associated with tremor

**paraplegia**   Paralysis of lower portion of the body

**pellagra**   Niacin deficiency

**pemphigoid**   Blistering disease with epidermal cell cohesion intact

**pemphigus**   Blistering disease with loss of cohesion of epidermal cells

**Plummer-Vinson syndrome**   Chronic iron deficiency plus premalignant changes in the throat or esophagus

**psychosis**   Any mental disease with or without deterioration of intellectual functioning in which individual lacks insight into his or her own condition

**purpura**   Bleeding into the skin

**scurvy**   Vitamin C deficiency

**seborrhoeic dermatitis**   Scaly, red condition of the skin of the face, scalp, chest, or skinfolds

**stomatitis**   Inflammation or loss of normal lining of the mouth

**systemic sclerosis** (*syn.* **scleroderma**)   Generalized connective tissue disease

**thyrotoxicosis**   Overactive thyroid with increased metabolic rate

**uremia**   Toxic condition associated with failure of kidney to function

**Wernicke-Korsakoff psychosis**   Thiamin-dependent syndrome associated with acute and chronic psychosis, usually in alcoholics

# Index

# E